Case-Based Nuclear Medicine
Second Edition

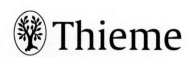

Case-Based Nuclear Medicine
Second Edition

Kevin J. Donohoe, MD

Assistant Professor of Radiology
Harvard Medical School
Attending Physician, Nuclear Medicine
Beth Israel Deaconess Medical Center
Boston, Massachusetts

Annick D. Van den Abbeele, MD

Chief, Department of Imaging
Founding Director, Center for Biomedical Imaging in Oncology
Dana-Farber Cancer Institute
Associate Professor of Radiology
Harvard Medical School
Co-director, Tumor Imaging Metrics Core
Dana-Farber/Harvard Cancer Center
Site Director, Imaging Consortium
Clinical Translational Science Award
Harvard Medical School
Boston, Massachusetts

Thieme
New York · Stuttgart

Thieme Medical Publishers, Inc.
333 Seventh Ave.
New York, NY 10001

Executive Editor: Timothy Hiscock
Managing Editor: Dominik Pucek
Editorial Director: Michael Wachinger
Production Editor: Kenneth L. Chumbley, Publication Services
International Production Director: Andreas Schabert
Vice President, International Marketing and Sales: Cornelia Schulze
Chief Financial Officer: James W. Mitos
President: Brian D. Scanlan
Compositor: Manila Typesetting Company
Printer: Gopsons Papers Limited

Library of Congress Cataloging-in-Publication Data

Case-based nuclear medicine / [edited by] Kevin J. Donohoe, Annick D. Van den Abbeele.
    p. ; cm.
    Rev ed. of: Teaching atlas of nuclear medicine / edited by Kevin J. Donohoe and Annick D. Van den Abbeele.
    2000.
    ISBN 978-1-58890-652-6 (alk. paper)
    1. Radioisotope scanning—Case studies.   2. Nuclear medicine—Case studies.   I. Donohoe, Kevin J.
        II. Van den Abbeele, Annick, 1953- III. Teaching atlas of nuclear medicine.
    [DNLM: 1. Radionuclide Imaging—Atlases.   2. Radionuclide Imaging—Case Reports. WN 17]
    RC78.7.R4T43 2011
    616.07'575—dc22
                                                                                    2010025868

Printed in India
5 4 3 2 1

ISBN 978-1-58890-652-6

To my mentors, Dennis Patton and Jim Woolfenden, who have shown me how to teach and explore. And to Mary and Lori, who pull me away from the computer now and then.

Kevin J. Donohoe, MD

To my parents, Nelly and Karel Gerard Van den Abbeele; my sister, Karyn; my brothers, Eric and Michel, and their families—for giving me the roots and the wings, for inspiring the best, and for their endless encouragement, love, and support.

Annick D. Van den Abbeele, MD

CONTENTS

SECTION III
Pulmonary Scintigraphy **131**

J. Anthony Parker

SECTION IV
Endocrine Scintigraphy..**169**

M. Elizabeth Oates and Rachel A. Powsner

SECTION V
Scintigraphy of Neoplastic Disease **207**

PART A   PET/CT

*Steven C. Burrell, Niall P. Sheehy, Victor H. Gerbaudo, Francine L. Jacobson,
and Annick D. Van den Abbeele*

PART B   Neuroendocrine Imaging **287**

Steven C. Burrell

SECTION VI
Radioisotope Therapy **317**

Steven C. Burrell and Annick D. Van den Abbeele

SECTION VII
Inflammation/Infection Imaging.. **345**

M. Elizabeth Oates

SECTION XIII
Vascular Scintigraphy 505

Steven C. Burrell and Annick D. Van den Abbeele

SECTION XIV
Pediatric Scintigraphy 539

Laura A. Drubach, Leonard P. Connolly, and S. Ted Treves

FOREWORD

This new collection of 166 cases continues to make a contribution to education in nuclear medicine. Like its predecessor, it challenges the reader to test him- or herself while acquiring new knowledge. Novice and master clinician alike should approach each case as follows:

- Read the *Clinical Presentation* and *Technique* sections.
- Examine the images and interpret them.
- State the clinical question as the referring physician should have stated it.
- Compare your image interpretation and differential diagnosis with those of the authors.
- Study the *Discussion* and *Pearls and Pitfalls* sections.
- Call up the articles in the *Suggested Reading* section to determine your interest.

This exercise will provide the reader with a systematic review of current nuclear medicine interpretation.

A casebook, unlike a textbook, is meant to be worked with, not referred to. Working with this one should be looked on as both a challenge and a joy.

Go to it!

S. James Adelstein, MD, PhD
Joint Program in Nuclear Medicine
Harvard Medical School
Boston, Massachusetts

PREFACE

This book has been written with residents in radiology and nuclear medicine in mind, but it may also be helpful to anyone interested in reviewing a spectrum of physiologic imaging studies to understand the role of nuclear medicine in the diagnosis of disease and the management of patients. Each case includes tips describing some of the more important aspects to consider in the interpretation of nuclear medicine images, as well as basic information describing how the individual procedures are done. Rather than attempting to include all possible image presentations for all possible diseases, this book focuses on the common presentations of diseases and describes the findings in a manner that will allow the reader to understand how images are affected by normal physiology and disease. The reader should then be able to apply that knowledge when encountering the innumerable variations in scan findings seen in the daily practice of medical imaging.

Individual cases are presented as they would be in clinical practice or during a board examination. A brief, clinical presentation is provided, followed by the images. Readers should try to approach the studies as they normally would during their daily practice. When they interpret the studies, all the reasons why the scans appear as they do should be considered—from the technical aspects of the imaging procedure to the disease processes involved.

The pertinent technical aspects of each study are presented after the images to further elucidate the type of study obtained, if not initially obvious. This information is followed by a differential diagnosis and then the final diagnosis. A brief discussion section outlines why the images appear as they do and discusses the specific image findings that should have helped make the final diagnosis.

In some cases, the diagnosis may be difficult. If the reader does not arrive at the same diagnosis as the author, he or she should not be discouraged, but rather should understand what the important normal and abnormal findings are and the physiology behind those findings. An understanding of the physiology is essential to the successful practice of nuclear medicine.

A list of the pearls and pitfalls encountered with each imaging procedure is also provided. The reader should consider their relevance to the specific case, including how the pearls may assist image interpretation and how the pitfalls may make an accurate diagnosis more difficult.

We have attempted to make this book challenging and fun. We hope the skills acquired in studying the cases will provide you not only with the tools necessary to pass a board examination or to recognize a specific disease process, but with an understanding of physiologic imaging that can be applied even as imaging technology evolves.

Kevin J. Donohoe, MD
Annick D. Van den Abbeele, MD

CONTRIBUTORS

Mouaz H. Al-Mallah, MD, MSc, FACC, FAHA, FESC
Associate Professor of Medicine
Wayne State University
Detroit, Michigan
Consultant Cardiologist and Division Head
Department of Cardiac Imaging
King Abdul-Aziz Cardiac Center
King Abdul-Aziz Medical City (Riyadh)
National Guard Health Affairs
Riyadh, Kingdom of Saudi Arabia

Scott H. Britz-Cunningham, MD, PhD
Instructor in Radiology
Staff Radiologist
Department of Radiology
Harvard Medical School
Brigham and Women's Hospital
Boston, Massachusetts

Steven C. Burrell, MD, FRCP
Associate Professor
Research Director
Department of Diagnostic Imaging
QEII Health Sciences Centre
Dalhousie University
Halifax, Canada

Leonard P. Connolly, MD
Assistant Professor
Harvard Medical School
Associate Radiologist
Massachusetts General Hospital Imaging
Boston, Massachusetts

Marcelo F. DiCarli, MD
Chief of Nuclear Medicine and Molecular Imaging
Director of Cardiovascular Imaging Program
Brigham and Women's Hospital
Associate Professor of Radiology and Medicine
Harvard Medical School
Boston, Massachusetts

Kevin J. Donohoe, MD
Assistant Professor of Radiology
Harvard Medical School
Attending Physician, Nuclear Medicine
Beth Israel Deaconess Medical Center
Boston, Massachusetts

Laura A. Drubach, MD
Assistant Professor
Department of Radiology
Children's Hospital
Boston, Massachusetts

Victor H. Gerbaudo, PhD
Director, Nuclear Medicine and Molecular
Imaging Program
Senior Administrative Director, Noninvasive
Cardiovascular Imaging
Department of Radiology
Brigham and Women's Hospital
Boston, Massachusetts

Francine L. Jacobson, MD, MPH
Assistant Professor of Radiology
Harvard Medical School
Staff Radiologist
Brigham and Women's Hospital
Boston, Massachusetts

M. Elizabeth Oates, MD
Professor and Chair
Department of Radiology
University of Kentucky
Director
Integrated Medical Imaging
University of Kentucky HealthCare Enterprise
Lexington, Kentucky

Umesh D. Oza, MD
Program Director
Department of Diagnostic Radiology
Baylor University Medical Center–Dallas
Dallas, Texas

J. Anthony Parker, MD, PhD
Associate Professor of Radiology
Department of Radiology
Beth Israel Deaconess Medical Center
Harvard Medical School
Boston, Massachusetts

Rachel A. Powsner, MD, MPH
Associate Professor of Radiology
Boston University Medical School
Director, Nuclear Medicine Section
Department of Radiology
Boston Veterans Administration Healthcare
    System
Boston, Massachusetts

Niall P. Sheehy, MD
Consultant Radiologist
St James's Hospital
Dublin, Ireland

S. Ted Treves, MD
Chief
Division of Nuclear Medicine and Molecular
Imaging
Children's Hospital
Professor of Radiology
Director of the Joint Program in Nuclear Medicine
Harvard Medical School
Boston, Massachusetts

Annick D. Van den Abbeele, MD
Chief, Department of Imaging
Founding Director, Center for Biomedical Imaging
    in Oncology
Dana-Farber Cancer Institute
Associate Professor of Radiology
Harvard Medical School
Co-director, Tumor Imaging Metrics Core
Dana-Farber/Harvard Cancer Center
Site Director, Imaging Consortium
Clinical Translational Science Award
Harvard Medical School
Boston, Massachusetts

Harvey A. Ziessman, MD
Professor of Radiology
Division of Nuclear Medicine
Department of Radiology
Johns Hopkins University
Baltimore, Maryland

Section I

Skeletal Scintigraphy

Kevin J. Donohoe and Umesh D. Oza

CASE 1

Clinical Presentation

A 37-year-old woman presents with the acute onset of low back pain (**Fig. 1.1**).

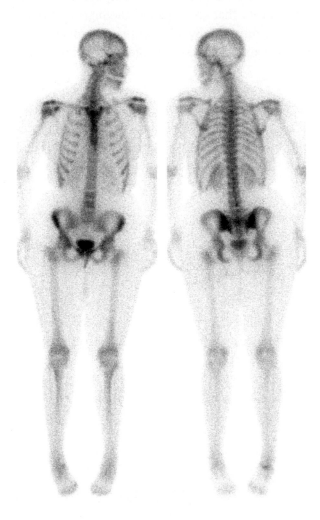

Fig. 1.1

Technique

- A 20 mCi dose of ^{99m}Tc-MDP is administered intravenously.
- Whole-body images of the skeleton are obtained 3 hours after tracer administration.
- A 1024 × 256 matrix is used for whole-body images.
- Emphasize the importance of oral hydration to improve soft tissue and bladder clearance.

Image Interpretation

Whole-body views demonstrate normal distribution of tracer throughout the bony skeleton. No focal abnormalities are noted.

Diagnosis and Clinical Follow-Up

- Bone scan was normal. No follow-up was necessary.

Discussion

Bone scans are one of the most frequently ordered studies in nuclear medicine. The superb sensitivity of the bone scan for detecting osteoblastic activity associated with bone repair makes it an excellent primary screening test for detecting malignancies that metastasize to bone and bony trauma that is not apparent on plain radiographic studies. The low specificity that accompanies the high sensitivity means that additional studies, such as plain films, computed tomography (CT), magnetic resonance imaging (MRI), and possibly biopsy, are often warranted when abnormalities are noted on the bone scan, particularly when metastatic disease is a concern.

In benign disease, the bone scan is more often done as a complementary study when the results of other imaging studies are negative and bony disease remains strongly suspected. As with malignant disease, benign abnormalities noted on the bone scan are not specific. Correlation with other information, such as the history, physical examination findings, and previously acquired anatomic imaging studies, is often necessary to determine the cause and significance of any abnormal bony uptake of tracer.

PEARLS AND PITFALLS

- Studies should be reviewed before the patient leaves the department. Additional views, such as oblique and single-photon emission computed tomography (SPECT) or SPECT/CT views, should be obtained if any question of abnormality exists.
- A short interview with the patient will often provide valuable information to assist in the interpretation of the images. Previous trauma, therapy, or symptoms are often not well documented on the study requisition yet often may cause findings on the bone scan.
- Patients should be encouraged to drink plenty of fluids and void frequently following injection of tracer. The hydration will improve soft tissue clearance and lessen the radiation dose.

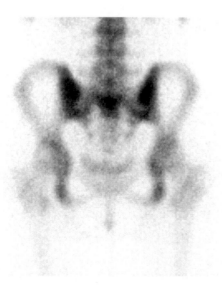

Fig. 1.2

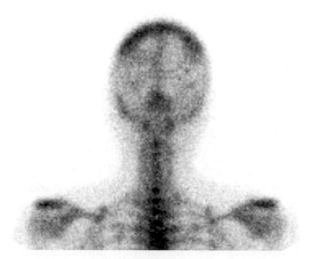

Fig. 1.3

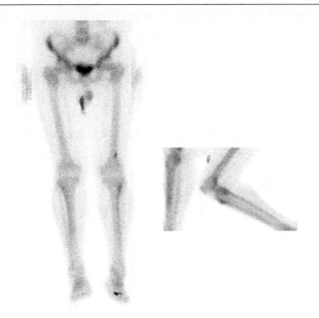

Fig. 1.4

- Delayed images at 24 hours can be obtained to allow additional soft tissue clearance or clearance from the bladder.
- A normal focus of activity caused by the sacral prominence may be mistaken for sacral metastasis (**Fig. 1.2**).
- The occipital protuberance is a normal finding that may be mistaken for skull metastasis (**Fig. 1.3**).
- Urinary contamination may be superimposed over a bone, suggesting a focal bony abnormality (**Fig. 1.4**).

Suggested Reading

Datz FL. Gamuts in Nuclear Medicine. 3rd ed. Chapter 3, 97–182. St. Louis, MO: Mosby; 1995

Mettler FA, Guiberteau MJ, eds. Essentials of Nuclear Medicine Imaging. 5th ed. The skeletal system, 243–292. New York, NY: Elsevier; 2006

CASE 2

Clinical Presentation

A middle-aged diabetic man presents with pain and swelling of the left foot (**Figs. 2.1, 2.2,** and **2.3**).

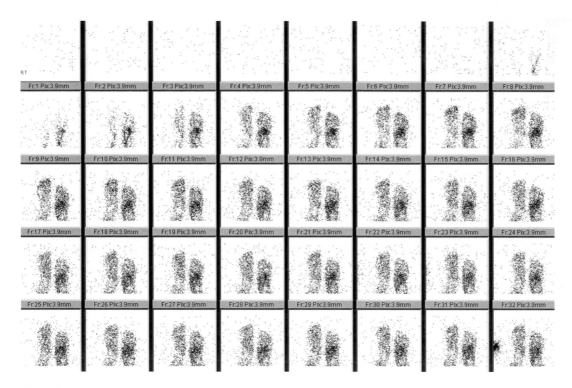

Fig. 2.1

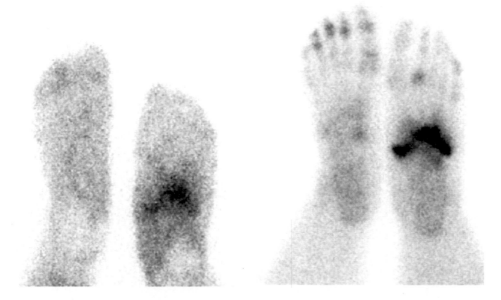

Fig. 2.2   **Fig. 2.3**

Technique

- A 20.7 mCi dose of ^{99m}Tc-HDP is administered.
- Three-phase bone scintigraphy is performed. Blood flow images of 1 second per frame are followed by blood pool images of 3 minutes duration.
- Anteroposterior (AP), lateral, and plantar views of the feet are obtained 3 hours after the administration of tracer.
- Emphasize the importance of oral hydration to improve soft tissue and bladder clearance.

Image Interpretation

Blood flow images (**Fig. 2.1**) show evidence of hyperemia in the region of the left midfoot. On the soft tissue phase (**Fig. 2.2**), there is increased tracer localization within the left midfoot. Delayed images (**Fig. 2.3**) show persistent tracer localization within the left midfoot, likely within the tarsal bones extending into the base of the metatarsals. Less intense uptake is shown within the left second metatarsophalangeal joint and interphalangeal joints of the right foot. These findings suggest arthritic/degenerative-type uptake.

Differential Diagnosis

- Charcot arthropathy
- Osteomyelitis
- Acute fractures
- Septic arthritis (**Fig. 2.4**)

Diagnosis and Clinical Follow-Up

The patient underwent AP and weight-bearing lateral radiographic evaluation (**Fig. 2.4**) of the left foot, which showed destructive changes of the navicular, cuboid, and cuneiform bones and the base of the metatarsals. There was evidence of sclerosis of the involved bones with ipsilateral dislocation of the second through fifth tarsometatarsal joints (Lisfranc fracture/dislocation) and acquired pes planus deformity. The combined radiographic and scintigraphic findings were most compatible with Charcot joint. ^{111}In-WBC scintigraphy with concomitant bone marrow scintigraphy showed no convincing evidence of osteomyelitis.

Discussion

Jean-Martin Charcot, a French neurologist, first described an arthropathy related to a neurodegenerative process resulting from syphilis. The disease process is now commonly related to diabetic neuropathy and is referred to as *Charcot arthropathy*. Other, less common causes to be considered are meningomyelocele, spinal cord injury, and syringomyelia. The classic radiographic findings include destruction of the joint space, increased sclerosis of the subchondral bone, fragmentation of bone, and deformity of the foot related to dislocation. In the foot, Charcot arthropathy results in a Lisfranc fracture/dislocation, lateral dislocation of the tarsometatarsal joint, and pes planus, as illustrated in this case. Skeletal scintigraphy is often used in combination with ^{111}In-WBC scintigraphy/marrow scintigraphy to exclude superimposed osteomyelitis. Three-phase skeletal scintigraphy is often positive

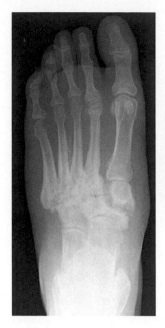
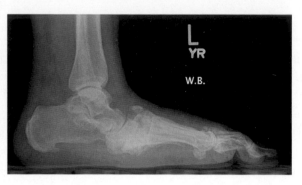

Fig. 2.4

in both Charcot arthropathy and osteomyelitis; however, cellulitis versus osseous involvement can be distinguished.

PEARLS AND PITFALLS

- Charcot arthropathy is indistinguishable from osteomyelitis on three-phase skeletal scintigraphy.
- Imaging in the plantar projection offers the best anatomic view of the osseous structures of the feet. Lateral and AP views may be better suited for ankle or hindfoot evaluation.
- Combined leukocyte/marrow scintigraphy is more specific for establishing a diagnosis of osteomyelitis in a diabetic foot.

Suggested Reading

Aliabadi P, Nikpoor N, Alparslan L. Imaging of neuropathic arthropathy. Semin Musculoskelet Radiol 2003;7(3):217–225

Palestro CJ, Mehta HH, Patel M, et al. Marrow versus infection in the Charcot joint: [111]In leukocyte and ^{99m}Tc sulfur colloid scintigraphy. J Nucl Med 1998;39(2):346–350

CASE 3

Clinical Presentation

A 49-year-old woman with a history of severe asthma presents with left shoulder pain. She also reports a remote history of right lower extremity fracture (**Figs. 3.1, 3.2, 3.3,** and **3.4**).

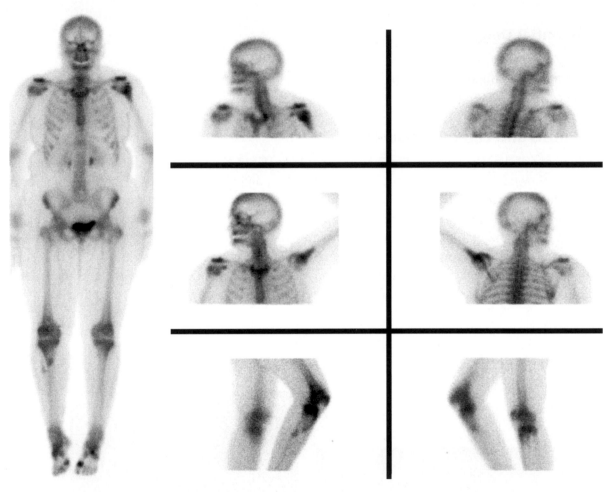

Fig. 3.1   Fig. 3.2

Technique

- A 20 mCi dose of ^{99m}Tc-MDP is administered intravenously.
- Whole-body images of the skeleton are obtained 3 hours after tracer administration.
- A 1024 × 256 matrix is used for whole-body images.
- Emphasize the importance of oral hydration to improve soft tissue and bladder clearance.

Image Interpretation

On the anterior whole-body image, there is a focal area of increased tracer localization within the left proximal humerus (**Fig. 3.1**). An additional area of increased tracer localization is shown in the right lower extremity just below the knee. Spot views (**Fig. 3.2**) confirm uptake within the osseous structures. The leg lesions are within the right proximal tibia and fibula. Uptake is also shown bilaterally in the acromioclavicular joints, knees, ankles, midfeet, and first metatarsophalangeal joints. All of the findings outside the left humerus suggest an arthritic/degenerative/post-traumatic type of uptake.

Differential Diagnosis

- Multifocal trauma
- Primary bone tumors (benign and malignant)
- Metastatic disease

Diagnosis and Clinical Follow-Up

Radiographs of the left shoulder (**Fig. 3.3**) and right knee (**Fig. 3.4**) were obtained. The left shoulder radiograph showed an aggressive cartilaginous lesion with a differential diagnosis of large enchondroma versus chondrosarcoma. The left subclavian central venous catheter shown on the radiograph was being used for immunoglobulin therapy for severe asthma. The radiographs of the right knee showed a healed fracture of the proximal right fibula and a nonaggressive chondroid lesion of the proximal tibia. CT of the right shoulder with coronal reformatted images (**Fig. 3.5**) showed a 7.8-cm lesion with endosteal scalloping. There was no cortical disruption or soft tissue mass. The patient underwent operative curettage of the left proximal humerus lesion. Pathology reported a grade 1 (low-grade) chondrosarcoma.

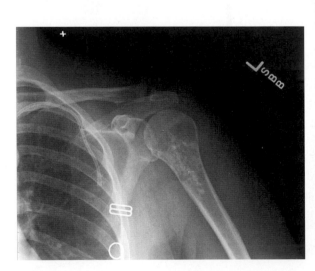

Fig. 3.3

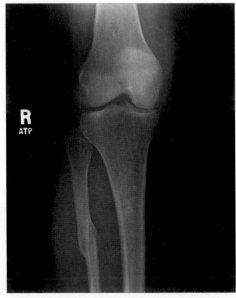

Fig. 3.4

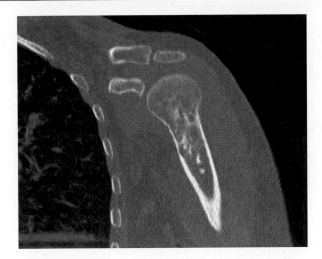

Fig. 3.5

Discussion

This case illustrates the nonspecific nature of many skeletal scintigraphic findings. Excluding the arthritic/degenerative uptake shown, the patient essentially had three focal lesions that were addressed by the clinical history and further imaging studies. The lesion in the left humerus was of greatest concern, given its size, the patient's symptoms, and the subsequent radiologic findings.

Distinguishing between chondrosarcoma and benign enchondroma is difficult by imaging alone. The role of skeletal scintigraphy is often to establish whether there is a multifocal or a unifocal process. Patients who present with pain in the region of a cartilaginous lesion are often imaged with CT or MRI to evaluate for aggressive features. Ultimately, it is the pathologist who will differentiate the two entities.

PEARLS AND PITFALLS

- Uptake of tracer in the extremities should be evaluated with additional views to better localize the lesion.
- A detailed clinical history should be obtained, with specific questions concerning sites of pain and prior trauma.
- Correlation with plain films is often useful in lesions of the extremities.
- Uptake of tracer within fractures can be seen for several years after radiographic evidence of healing.
- Maffucci syndrome is a nonhereditary disorder characterized by multiple enchondromas and hemangiomas.
- Ollier disease is a nonhereditary disorder characterized by multiple enchondromas without hemangiomas.

Suggested Reading
Wang K, Allen L, Fung E, Chan CC, Chan JC, Griffith JF. Bone scintigraphy in common tumors with osteolytic components. Clin Nucl Med 2005;30(10):655–671

CASE 4

Clinical Presentation

A young man presents with a painful, palpable mass in his right arm (**Figs. 4.1** and **4.2**).

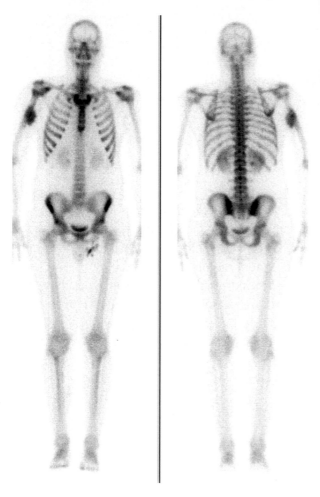

Fig. 4.1

Technique

- A 20 mCi dose of ^{99m}Tc-MDP is administered intravenously.
- Whole-body images of the skeleton are obtained 3 hours after tracer administration.
- A 1024 × 256 matrix is used for whole-body images.
- Emphasize the importance of oral hydration to improve soft tissue and bladder clearance.

Image Interpretation

On whole-body images in the anterior and posterior projections (**Fig. 4.1**), there is focally increased tracer localization within the right humeral diaphysis. The uptake involves the bone and soft tissues

Uptake along the lower pelvis was confirmed to be urine contamination on further imaging. No additional findings are shown.

Differential Diagnosis

- Osteosarcoma
- Ewing sarcoma
- Metastatic lesion
- Myositis ossificans

Diagnosis and Clinical Follow-Up

Radiographs of the right humerus (**Fig. 4.2**) showed cortical erosion, a large soft tissue mass, and an aggressive periosteal reaction with a "hair-on-end" appearance. Post-gadolinium fat saturation coronal MRI (**Fig. 4.3**) showed a large soft tissue component underestimated by both skeletal scintigraphy and radiography. The patient underwent surgical excision for Ewing sarcoma. No additional follow-up is available.

Discussion

The role of skeletal scintigraphy in primary malignant bone tumors is to assess for metastatic disease and skip lesions. Nonosseous metastasis will often show tracer uptake, although the absence of uptake does not exclude the presence of metastasis. CT is frequently used to assess for metastasis, especially in the lungs. Patients may present with pain, fever, and an elevated white blood cell count (WBC), which can mimic osteomyelitis; therefore, three-phase skeletal scintigraphy is limited in distinguishing the two entities in such clinical scenarios.

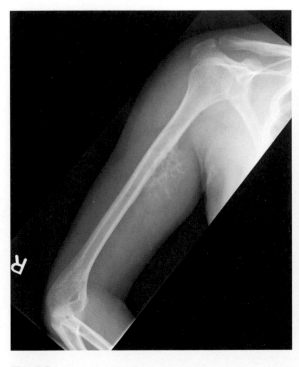

Fig. 4.2

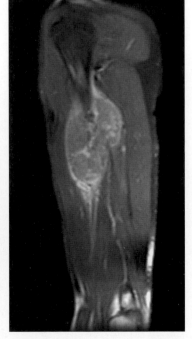

Fig. 4.3

Ewing sarcoma is typically a monostotic lesion that involves the long bones and flat bones of the pelvis. Radiographic findings that show aggressive features, as in this case, warrant further evaluation. MRI remains the best modality to evaluate the soft tissue component and tumor extent.

PEARLS AND PITFALLS

- Extremity lesions should be correlated with radiographs as initial workup.
- In patients with known primary malignant bone tumors, nonosseous structures should be carefully interrogated to evaluate for metastatic disease.
- Intraosseous (regional metastasis) and transarticular surfaces should be assessed for involvement.
- Skeletal scintigraphy underestimates the soft tissue component of sarcomas and sometimes overestimates the osseous extent of lesions secondary to adjacent osseous hyperemia or reactive changes.
- Patients with Ewing sarcoma may present with fever, pain, and an elevated WBC, mimicking osteomyelitis.

Suggested Reading

Davies AM, Makwana NK, Grimer RJ, Carter SR. Skip metastases in Ewing's sarcoma: a report of three cases. Skeletal Radiol 1997;26(6):379–384

McLean RG, Murray IP. Scintigraphic patterns in certain primary malignant bone tumours. Clin Radiol 1984;35(5):379–383

CASE 5

Clinical Presentation

A 57-year-old woman presents with bone pain (**Figs. 5.1** and **5.2**).

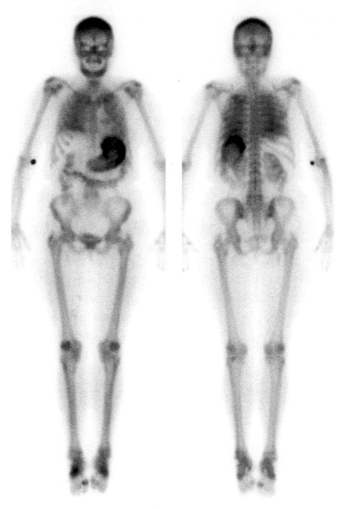

Fig. 5.1   Fig. 5.2

Technique

- A 20 mCi dose of ^{99m}Tc-MDP is administered intravenously.
- Whole-body images of the skeleton are obtained 3 hours after tracer administration.
- A 1024 × 256 matrix is used for whole-body images.
- Emphasize the importance of oral hydration to improve soft tissue and bladder clearance.

Image Interpretation

An anterior projection whole-body image (**Fig. 5.1**) shows diffuse increased uptake throughout the osseous structures, with visualization of the urinary bladder. There is extraosseous uptake of tracer within the lungs, stomach, and colon. A posterior projection whole-body image (**Fig. 5.2**) shows tracer localization within the cortex of the kidneys. Increased tracer localization within the midfeet bilaterally and the right first metatarsophalangeal joint is likely degenerative/post-traumatic in nature. The injection was into the right antecubital fossa.

Differential Diagnosis

- Metastatic calcification
- Primary hyperparathyroidism
- End-stage renal disease and secondary hyperparathyroidism
- Widespread osseous metastatic disease
- Prior administration of tracer

Diagnosis and Clinical Follow-Up

Metastatic calcification due to primary hyperparathyroidism was diagnosed. The patient had initially presented to her physician with leg pain and fatigue. Her serum calcium level was 15.5 mg/dL (normal range, 8.4–10.2 mg/dL), and her parathyroid hormone level was higher than 1200 pg/mL (normal range, 10–65 pg/mL). The patient underwent a parathyroidectomy, with normalization of the calcium and parathyroid hormone levels.

Discussion

In metastatic calcification, the calcium is usually deposited within tissues that have an alkaline environment, such that uptake in the lungs, stomach, and kidneys bilaterally is typical on skeletal scintigraphy. Some reports have suggested skeletal muscle, spleen, cardiac, and thyroid calcium deposition as well. The tracer localization within the colon is not a typical finding. The patient had undergone parathyroid scintigraphy with ^{99m}Tc-sestamibi (**Fig. 5.3**) the prior day. Most of the clearance of sestamibi is through the hepatobiliary system, with one-third excreted into the feces, thus explaining the visualization of the colon on skeletal scintigraphy.

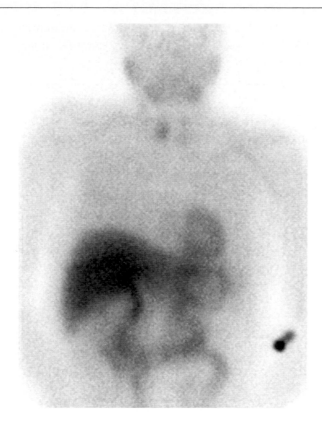

Fig. 5.3

PEARLS AND PITFALLS_____

- Free pertechnetate appears as abnormal tracer localization within the stomach, salivary glands, and thyroid gland.
- Metastatic calcification of hyperparathyroidism typically appears as uptake of tracer within the stomach, kidneys, and lungs.
- Always review the history for prior radiopharmaceutical administration.

Suggested Reading

Amico S, Lucas P, Diebold MD, Liehn JC, Petit J, Valeyre J. Metastatic calcification in the thyroid gland demonstrated on bone scan in a patient with primary hyperparathyroidism. J Nucl Med 1986;27(3):373–376

Hwang GJ, Lee JD, Park CY, Lim SK. Reversible extraskeletal uptake of bone scanning in primary hyperparathyroidism. J Nucl Med 1996;37(3):469–471

Rosenthal DI, Chandler HL, Azizi F, Schneider PB. Uptake of bone imaging agents by diffuse pulmonary metastatic calcification. AJR Am J Roentgenol 1977;129(5):871–874

CASE 6

Clinical Presentation

An 84-year-old man presents with lower back pain (**Figs. 6.1, 6.2,** and **6.3**).

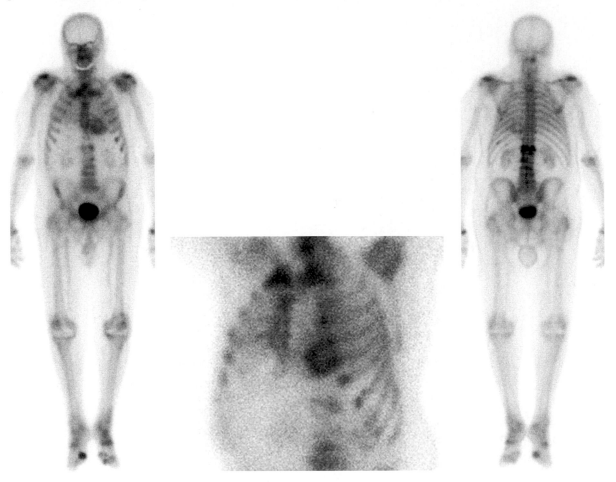

Fig. 6.1   Fig. 6.2   Fig. 6.3

Technique

- A 20 mCi dose of ⁹⁹ᵐTc-MDP is administered intravenously.
- Whole-body images of the skeleton are obtained 3 hours after tracer administration.
- A 1024 × 256 matrix is used for whole-body images.
- Emphasize the importance of oral hydration to improve soft tissue and bladder clearance.

Image Interpretation

Extraosseous uptake of tracer is shown over the left side of the chest on the anterior whole-body image (**Fig. 6.1**). Left anterior oblique projection confirms the intrathoracic location (**Fig. 6.2**). A focal area of abnormal tracer localization within the T12 vertebral body is best shown on the posterior whole-body image (**Fig. 6.3**). The relative absence of tracer localization within the knee joints bilaterally and mild uptake of tracer peripherally are compatible with bilateral knee prostheses. Focal uptake of tracer in the right first metatarsophalangeal joint is post-traumatic per patient interview. Uptake of tracer in the cervical spine, multiple levels of the lumbar spine, both acromioclavicular joints, both sternoclavicular junctions, the sternomanubrial junction, and both wrists, midfeet, and ankles suggests multifocal arthritic/degenerative uptake. Uptake of tracer in the medial thighs correlates with vascular atherosclerotic calcification.

Differential Diagnosis

- Amyloidosis
- Myocarditis/pericarditis
- Recent myocardial infarct
- Pericardial calcification
- Recent cardiac nuclear scintigraphy

Diagnosis and Clinical Follow-Up

Cardiac Amyloidosis

The patient underwent an MRI of the lumbar spine (**Fig. 6.4**), which showed an acute compression fracture of T12 with compression of the neural canal caused by retropulsion of fragments. The patient has a history of monoclonal gammopathy, which was thought to be the underlying cause of the compression fracture and amyloidosis.

Discussion

The accumulation of skeletal scintigraphy agents within the myocardium has been reported in cases of amyloidosis. Diffuse hepatic uptake and symmetric focal periarticular uptake of skeletal scintigraphy agents have also been reported. The patient's history of monoclonal gammopathy suggests that the amyloidosis is likely related to this systemic disease.

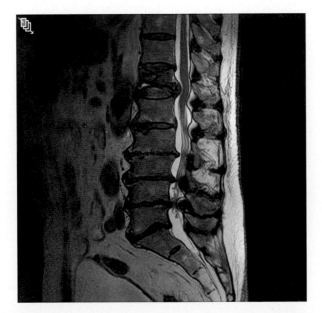

Fig. 6.4

- Myocardial uptake of skeletal scintigraphy agents is uncommon, but when it occurs, it is often caused by unsuspected disease that should not be overlooked.
- Myocardial tracer uptake may be mistaken for overlying chondral calcification. Lateral, oblique views or SPECT or SPECT/CT is helpful for localizing the site of uptake.

Suggested Reading

Kanoh T, Uchino H, Yamamoto I, Torizuka K. Soft-tissue uptake of ^{99m}Tc MDP in multiple myeloma. Clin Nucl Med 1986;11(12):878–879

Lee VW, Caldarone AG, Falk RH, Rubinow A, Cohen AS. Amyloidosis of heart and liver: comparison of ^{99m}Tc pyrophosphate and ^{99m}Tc methylene diphosphonate for detection. Radiology 1983;148(1):239–242

VanAntwerp JD, O'Mara RE, Pitt MJ, Walsh S. ^{99m}Tc-diphosphonate accumulation in amyloid. J Nucl Med 1975;16(3):238–240

CASE 7

Clinical Presentation

An 82-year-old woman presents with a recent history of bilateral hearing loss (**Figs. 7.1** and **7.2**).

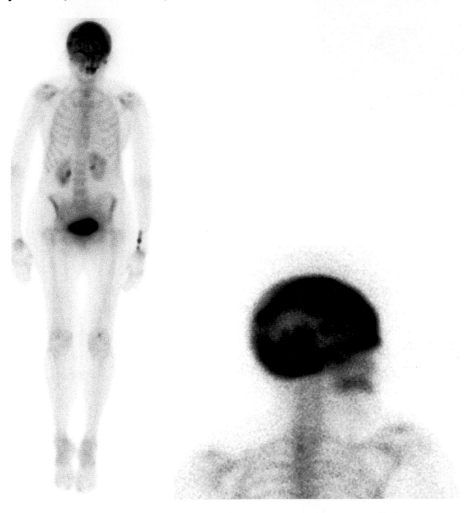

Fig. 7.1   **Fig. 7.2**

Technique

- A 20 mCi dose of ^{99m}Tc-HDP is administered intravenously.
- Whole-body and spot images are obtained 3 hours after tracer administration.
- Emphasize the importance of oral hydration to improve soft tissue and bladder clearance.

Image Interpretation

Anterior whole-body (**Fig. 7.1**) and lateral skull (**Fig. 7.2**) views show intense, abnormal uptake within the calvarium, with relatively faint visualization of the remainder of the axial skeleton and the appendicular portions of the skeleton. The injection site is seen in the left hand.

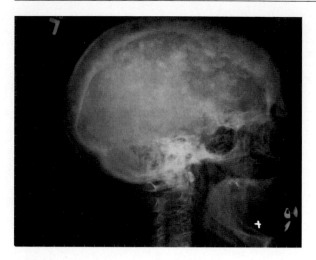

Fig. 7.3

Differential Diagnosis

(Diffuse increased uptake throughout a single bone)
- Paget disease
- Metastatic disease
- Acute inflammatory changes secondary to radiation therapy
- Inflammation in adjacent soft tissues (increased delivery of tracer to the bone)

Diagnosis and Clinical Follow-Up

Findings of mixed lytic and sclerotic lesions with calvarial thickening on a lateral skull radiograph (**Fig. 7.3**) are suggestive of the mixed phase of Paget disease. Paget disease was diagnosed based on the scintigraphic, radiographic, and clinical presentation, including alkaline phosphatase levels five times the upper limit of normal. The patient's recent hearing loss was attributed to involvement of the temporal bone.

Discussion

Paget disease is often an incidental finding on skeletal scintigraphy. The increased uptake is seen in both the early, resorptive (lucent) phase and the proliferative (sclerotic) phase. A mixed phase, in which the proliferative phase overlaps the resorptive phase, can also occur, as shown in this case on the skull radiographs. The incidence of malignant transformation in pagetoid bone is low. When the patient experiences pain in the involved bone, however, further evaluation for malignant transformation is warranted.

PEARLS AND PITFALLS

- If malignant change is suspected in a patient with known Paget disease, radiographic investigation is required.
- Sarcomatous changes in a bone already involved with Paget disease may show a relative absence of tracer localization. Gallium scintigraphy often shows increased tracer uptake in the areas of decreased tracer uptake on skeletal scintigraphy.
- Involvement of the temporal bone in Paget disease may cause hearing loss.

Suggested Reading

Serafini AN. Paget's disease of bone. Semin Nucl Med 1976;6(1):47–58

Smith J, Botet JF, Yeh SD. Bone sarcomas in Paget disease: a study of 85 patients. Radiology 1984;152(3):583–590

Smith SE, Murphey MD, Motamedi K, Mulligan ME, Resnik CS, Gannon FH. From the archives of the AFIP. Radiologic spectrum of Paget disease of bone and its complications with pathologic correlation. Radiographics 2002;22(5):1191–1216

CASE 8

Clinical Presentation

A 51-year-old woman with a diagnosis of breast carcinoma and cervical carcinoma who is undergoing chemotherapy and radiation therapy for cervical carcinoma presents for staging (**Figs. 8.1** and **8.2**).

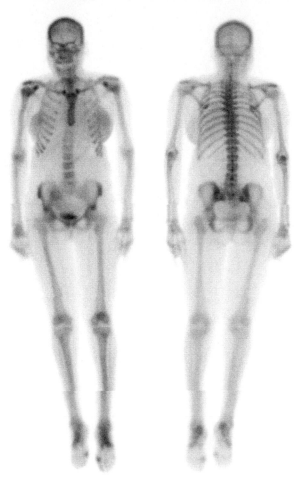

Fig. 8.1   **Fig. 8.2**

Technique

- A 20 mCi dose of ^{99m}Tc-MDP is administered intravenously.
- Whole-body images of the skeleton are obtained 3 hours after tracer administration.
- A 1024 × 256 matrix is used for whole-body images.
- Emphasize the importance of oral hydration to improve soft tissue and bladder clearance.

Image Interpretation

No native kidneys are seen on anterior (**Fig. 8.1**) and posterior (**Fig. 8.2**) whole-body images. Normal soft tissue clearance is seen with appropriate osseous uptake. Within the right lower quadrant, focal uptake is shown overlying the right ilium. A degenerative/arthritic type of uptake is shown in the ankles, midfeet, and both first metatarsophalangeal joints. Mild uptake in the breast soft tissue is shown bilaterally.

Differential Diagnosis

- Right lower quadrant uptake
  - Soft tissue metastasis
  - Soft tissue trauma
  - Retained tracer within bowel after recent radiopharmaceutical administration
  - Kidney transplant
- Bilateral absence of renal uptake within the renal beds
  - Superscan
  - End-stage renal disease (ESRD)
  - Ptotic/ectopic/transplanted kidneys

Diagnosis and Clinical Follow-Up

The patient had no scintigraphic evidence of metastatic disease. She had end stage renal disease secondary to hypertension, with a right lower quadrant renal transplant (**Fig. 8.3**), 15 years prior. The native kidneys were atrophic bilaterally, as shown on a CT (**Fig. 8.4**). She had a recent graft failure and resumed hemodialysis. Bilateral breast uptake can be a normal finding. The patient was to complete chemotherapy and radiation therapy for cervical carcinoma and then undergo a left mastectomy.

Discussion

Assessing the urinary bladder and kidneys on skeletal scintigraphy should be a routine practice. The absence of native kidney uptake should alert the clinician to consider a superscan, or to look for ptotic/ectopic/transplanted kidneys. An additional clue to the presence of a functioning kidney is normal clearance of tracer and uptake of tracer by the skeletal system 3 hours after tracer injection. Although soft tissue metastasis can show increased tracer uptake, in this particular case, the clinical history and correlative imaging studies confirmed the presence of a transplanted kidney and ESRD.

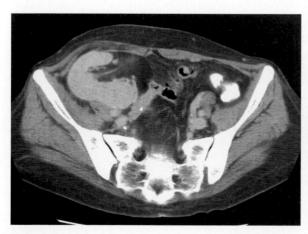

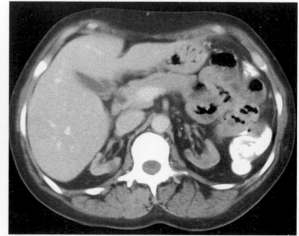

Fig. 8.3   **Fig. 8.4**

- The kidneys and urinary bladder should be assessed on skeletal scintigraphy studies.
- Nonvisualization of the native kidneys does not always imply a "superscan."
- Soft tissue metastasis can concentrate skeletal scintigraphy agents.

Suggested Reading

Pryma DA, Akhurst T. Hydronephrotic ectopic pelvic kidney simulates sacral metastasis from breast cancer. Clin Nucl Med 2005;30(4):244–245

Sy WM, Patel D, Faunce H. Significance of absent or faint kidney sign on bone scan. J Nucl Med 1975;16(6):454–456

CASE 9

Clinical Presentation

A 25-year-old woman without a significant past medical history presents with left hip pain and an elevated erythrocyte sedimentation rate (ESR; **Figs. 9.1, 9.2, 9.3, 9.4,** and **9.5**).

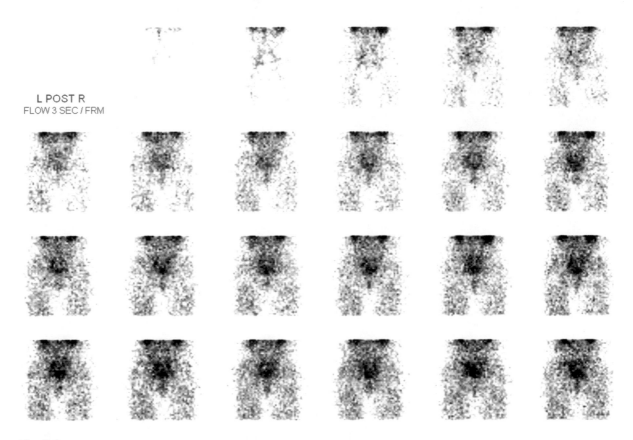

L POST R
FLOW 3 SEC / FRM

Fig. 9.1

Technique

- A 20 mCi dose of ^{99m}Tc-MDP is administered intravenously.
- Flow images of the pelvis are obtained for 1 second per frame at the time of tracer injection in the anterior and posterior projections. (For display purposes, images were summed at 3 seconds per frame.)
- A blood pool image is obtained for 3 minutes within 10 minutes of tracer injection.
- Whole-body images of the skeleton are obtained 3 hours after tracer administration.
- A 1024 × 256 matrix is used for whole-body images.
- Emphasize the importance of oral hydration to improve soft tissue and bladder clearance.

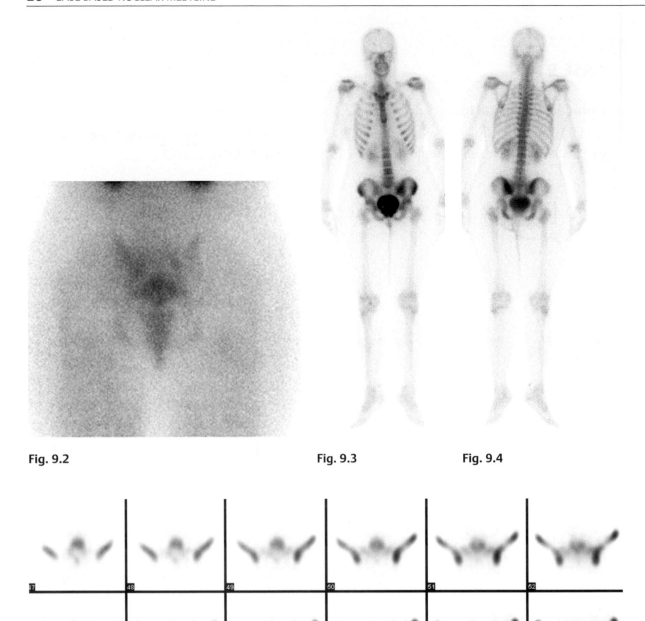

Fig. 9.2   Fig. 9.3   Fig. 9.4

Fig. 9.5

Image Interpretation

Posterior blood flow images (**Fig. 9.1**) are limited by vascular structures in the pelvis. Posterior blood pool images (**Fig. 9.2**) demonstrate mildly asymmetric findings (left > right tracer uptake over the sacroiliac [SI] joints). Delayed images (**Figs. 9.3** and **9.4**) show asymmetric tracer activity in the SI joints, with relatively increased tracer uptake in the left SI joint. No additional areas of abnormal tracer localization are seen.

SPECT images (**Fig. 9.5**) of the pelvis show increased tracer localization across the left SI joint in both the iliac bone and the sacrum.

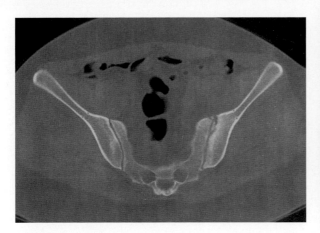

Fig. 9.6

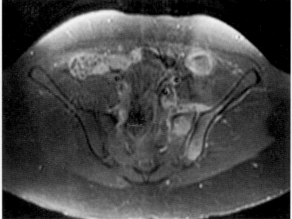

Fig. 9.7

Differential Diagnosis

- Septic arthritis
- Inflammatory arthritis
- Trauma
- Neoplastic disease (primary and metastatic)

Diagnosis and Clinical Follow-Up

The patient underwent CT and MRI follow-up after bone scintigraphy. The CT image (**Fig. 9.6**) showed sclerotic changes within the left SI joint and an osseous fragment within the joint space. MRI (**Fig. 9.7**) showed edema within the sacrum and iliac bones. There was enhancement and abnormal fluid collection within the SI joint space. The patient also underwent gallium whole-body scintigraphy (**Fig. 9.8**) with SPECT/CT imaging (**Fig. 9.9**), which showed abnormal tracer localization within the left SI joint slightly more prominent than the skeletal scintigraphy findings, suggestive of an active infectious process. The patient was taken to the operating room for surgical exploration. When the joint space was entered, purulent material was encountered. The joint was debrided, irrigated, and packed with antibiotics. Surgical cultures were positive for mycobacterial tuberculosis. The patient was treated with appropriate antibiotic therapy for tuberculous sacroiliitis.

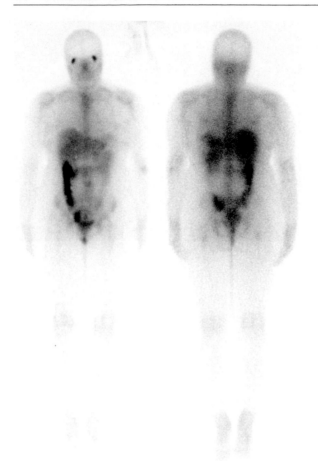

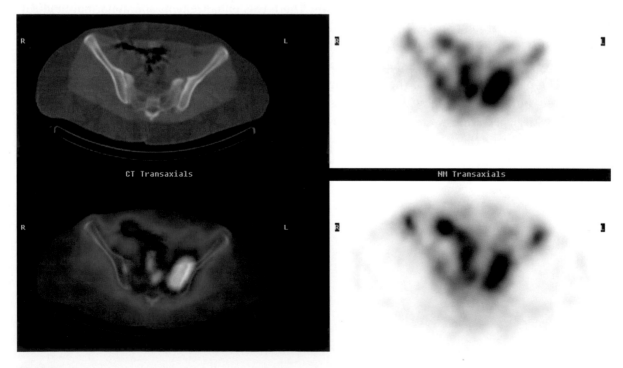

Fig. 9.8

Fig. 9.9

Discussion

Three-phase skeletal scintigraphy is highly sensitive and specific for osteomyelitis if the plain radiograph is normal. The pattern most commonly seen is increased activity in all three phases of the study. Flow images are more difficult to interpret when the area in question, such as the spine or pelvis, overlies major vessels or vascular structures. Increased tracer localization seen across a joint space suggests an arthritic process. In a case such as this one, in which infection was suspected, septic arthritis should be considered.

PEARLS AND PITFALLS

- The patient should be interviewed and examined before injection of the tracer to ensure that flow images are obtained in the optimal projection for detecting increased blood flow.
- Flow images over the spine or other bony structures adjacent to major arteries are of doubtful use because the normal arterial flow can obscure a more subtle area of increased flow to the bone.
- Septic arthritis appears as abnormal tracer localization across the joint space in question.

Suggested Reading

Mohana-Borges AV, Chung CB, Resnick D. Monoarticular arthritis. Radiol Clin North Am 2004;42 (1):135–149

Salomon CG, Ali A, Fordham EW. Bone scintigraphy in tuberculous sacroiliitis. Clin Nucl Med 1986;11(6):407–408

Schauwecker DS. The scintigraphic diagnosis of osteomyelitis. AJR Am J Roentgenol 1992;158(1):9–18

CASE 10

Clinical Presentation

History withheld (**Fig. 10.1**).

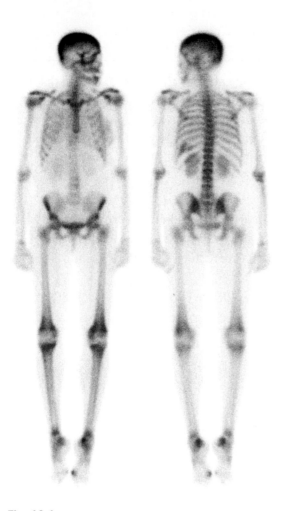

Fig. 10.1

Technique

- A 20 mCi dose of ^{99m}Tc-MDP is administered intravenously.
- Whole-body images of the skeleton are obtained 3 hours after tracer administration.
- A 1024 × 256 matrix is used for whole-body images.
- Emphasize the importance of oral hydration to improve soft tissue and bladder clearance.

Image Interpretation

Whole-body images in the anterior and posterior projections (**Fig. 10.1**) show relatively increased tracer concentration in the metaphyses of the long bones, particularly in the lower extremities. Also noted on the posterior whole-body image is tracer concentration just above the left kidney. Increased uptake within the calvarium and right orbit is best seen on the anterior view. Uptake in the left first metatarsophalangeal joint is related to post-traumatic/degenerative changes.

Differential Diagnosis

(Symmetric periarticular tracer uptake)
- Osteoarthritis
- Rheumatoid arthritis
- Other arthritides
- Marrow expansion, such as from the following:
  - Sickle cell disease
  - Myelofibrosis
  - Lupus

Diagnosis and Clinical Follow-Up

The patient had known sickle cell disease. No follow-up was obtained.

Discussion

Skeletal scintigraphy in patients with sickle cell disease can show several characteristic findings. In this patient, expansion of the red marrow resulted in increased tracer uptake in the metaphyseal regions of the long bones. Calvarial uptake was secondary to expansion of the marrow in the diploic space. Tracer uptake in an auto-infarcted spleen was also noted just above the kidney on the left. Uptake in the right orbit was likely related to infarct. Depending on the age of the patient, it is not uncommon to see tracer uptake in old infarcted areas and decreased uptake in acutely infarcted areas. Regions with active bone repair at sites of old infarcts, healing ischemic lesions, or osteomyelitis are difficult to distinguish on skeletal scintigraphy alone. Correlative imaging with ^{67}Ga-citrate scintigraphy or ^{111}In-WBC scintigraphy is often necessary to diagnose concurrent osteomyelitis. Avascular necrosis of the hip is a frequent complication of sickle cell disease, occurring in as many as 41% of patients.

PEARLS AND PITFALLS

- Tracer uptake in an infarcted spleen may be very slight and difficult to distinguish from the kidney below.
- Increased uptake on skeletal scintigraphy is not specific for infarct or osteomyelitis and may be caused by several conditions described in other cases. Correlative imaging with gallium, radioactively labeled white blood cells, or MRI is often needed.
- The appearance of bony lesions varies from decreased activity in an acute infarct to increased tracer activity in an infarct undergoing repair. Knowledge of the history of the disease is important in study interpretation.
- Small, acute infarcts in areas prone to avascular necrosis may not be seen adequately with skeletal scintigraphy. In doubtful cases, the patient should be referred for MRI.

Suggested Reading

Heck LL, Brittin GM. Splenic uptake of both ^{99m}Tc diphosphonate and ^{99m}Tc sulfur colloid in sickle cell beta (0) thalassemia. Clin Nucl Med 1989;14(8):557–563

Kahn CE Jr, Ryan JW, Hatfield MK, Martin WB. Combined bone marrow and gallium imaging: differentiation of osteomyelitis and infarction in sickle hemoglobinopathy. Clin Nucl Med 1988;13(6):443–449

Lonergan GJ, Cline DB, Abbondanzo SL. Sickle cell anemia. Radiographics 2001;21(4):971–994

Mandell GA. Imaging in the diagnosis of musculoskeletal infections in children. Curr Probl Pediatr 1996;26(7):218–237

CASE 11

Clinical Presentation

An elderly man with a history of prostate carcinoma presents for follow-up (**Fig. 11.1**).

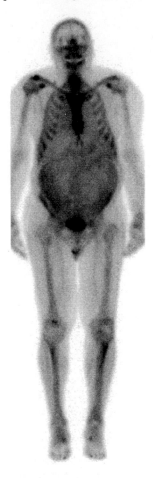

Fig. 11.1

Technique

- A 20 mCi dose of ^{99m}Tc-MDP is administered intravenously.
- Whole-body images of the skeleton are obtained 3 hours after tracer administration.
- A 1024 × 256 matrix is used for whole-body images.
- Emphasize the importance of oral hydration to improve soft tissue and bladder clearance.

Image Interpretation

A whole-body image in the anterior projection (**Fig. 11.1**) shows diffuse mild uptake of tracer throughout the peritoneal cavity, with more focal moderate uptake within the periphery. Other uptake within the right acromioclavicular joint, right knee, and both midfeet appears to be arthritic/post-traumatic/degenerative.

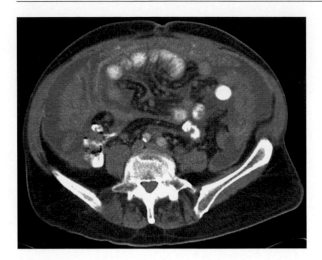

Fig. 11.2

Differential Diagnosis

- Ascites (or other exudative effusion)
- Peritoneal carcinomatosis
- Recent administration of other radiopharmaceutical

Diagnosis and Clinical Follow-Up

Peritoneal carcinomatosis secondary to metastatic prostate carcinoma was diagnosed. No additional follow-up is available.

Discussion

A correlative axial CT slice through the abdomen with intravenous and oral administration of contrast (**Fig. 11.2**) shows ascites, peritoneal wall thickening, and omental caking. In this case, the uptake within the peritoneal cavity is secondary to peritoneal carcinomatosis and includes uptake within the peritoneal nodular thickening and omental caking. The diffuse uptake seen throughout the peritoneal cavity is related to the malignant ascites. Although this case was proven to be prostate carcinoma, one should consider other gastrointestinal malignancies and ovarian carcinomas in female patients as the cause of peritoneal uptake, especially in the absence of osseous metastasis (**Fig. 11.2**).

PEARLS AND PITFALLS

- Evaluation of the soft tissue should always be part of the interpretation of skeletal scintigraphy.
- Although rare, prostate carcinoma can present as peritoneal carcinomatosis.
- The uptake of tracer within known ascites may reflect both inflammatory and malignant effusions.
- Prior administration of radiopharmaceutical with a biodistribution that includes the gastrointestinal tract may mimic nonosseous tracer uptake on bone scintigraphy.

Suggested Reading

Lapoile E, Bellaïche G, Choudat L, et al. [Ascites associated with prostate cancer metastases: an unusual localisation]. Gastroenterol Clin Biol 2004;28(1):92–94

Peller PJ, Ho VB, Kransdorf MJ. Extraosseous ^{99m}Tc MDP uptake: a pathophysiologic approach. Radiographics 1993;13(4):715–734

CASE 12

Clinical Presentation

A 22-year-old baseball pitcher presents with right shin pain (**Figs. 12.1, 12.2,** and **12.3**).

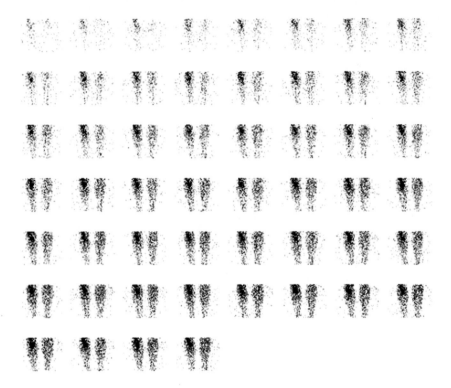

Fig. 12.1

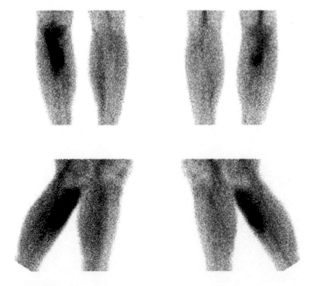

Fig. 12.2

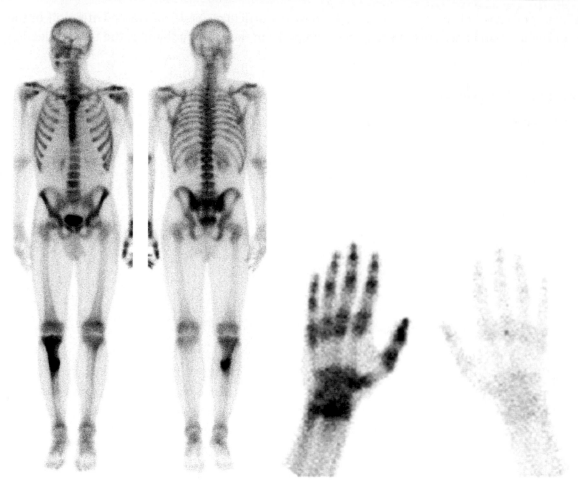

Fig. 12.3   **Fig. 12.4**

Technique

- A 20 mCi dose of ^{99m}Tc-MDP is administered intravenously.
- Flow images of the pelvis are obtained for 1 second per frame at the time of tracer injection in the anterior and posterior projections. (For display purposes, images are summed at 3 seconds per frame.)
- A blood pool image is obtained for 3 minutes within 10 minutes of tracer injection.
- Whole-body images of the skeleton are obtained 3 hours after tracer administration.
- A 1024 × 256 matrix is used for whole-body images.
- Emphasize the importance of oral hydration to improve soft tissue and bladder clearance.

Image Interpretation

Blood flow images (**Fig. 12.1**) show increased flow to the right proximal tibia. Blood pool images (**Fig. 12.2**) in multiple projections show increased tracer localization extending from the right tibial plateau into the proximal one-third of the diaphysis of the tibia. The uptake is predominantly in the anterior aspect of the right tibia. Delayed whole-body images in the anterior and posterior projections (**Fig. 12.3**) show findings similar to those in the blood pool images; however, additional abnormal uptake is shown within the left hand and wrist.

Palmar spot views of the hands (**Fig. 12.4**) show periarticular uptake of tracer within all of the joints of the left hand and wrist. A small focus of uptake in the right midhand is the tracer injection site.

Differential Diagnosis

- Tibia findings
  - Stress reaction
  - Fracture/stress fracture
  - Malignancy
  - Fibrous dysplasia
  - Paget disease
- Left hand findings
  - Complex regional pain syndrome (CRPS 1)
  - Arterial injection of tracer (if tracer injected in same extremity)
  - Soft tissue inflammation and hyperemia

Diagnosis and Clinical Follow-Up

The diagnosis for the tibial findings was stress fracture mimicking malignancy. Initial radiographs were negative. On directed questioning, the patient gave a prior history of a left-sided rotator cuff tear and subsequent surgical repair. The patient also reported some intermittent numbness and a warm sensation in the left hand without edema. Although three-phase bone scintigraphy of the hands was not performed, these findings were most consistent with CRPS 1, formerly known as reflex sympathetic dystrophy.

Discussion

The most common scintigraphic presentation of stress fracture is oval or fusiform tracer uptake parallel to the long axis of the involved bone. Diffuse or linear radioactive tracer uptake along the cortex is not uncommon, however.

CRPS 1, formerly known as reflex sympathetic dystrophy, has been described in patients who have undergone trauma, immobilization, surgery, myocardial infarction, or stroke. The exact mechanism of action of the various presenting signs and symptoms is not fully understood. The role of three-phase skeletal scintigraphy is also not widely accepted in the diagnosis of CRPS 1. The pattern of tracer uptake can vary with the three stages of the disease. The classic pattern seen on skeletal scintigraphy in adults is periarticular uptake of tracer within the affected limb on delayed imaging. The first two phases of a three-phase study may show increased flow and soft tissue uptake; however, this pattern is not always seen. Pediatric patients may show relatively decreased flow and uptake on soft tissue and delayed images, making the diagnosis even more difficult.

PEARLS AND PITFALLS _____

- An obvious finding may distract the reader from a careful review of the entire study, so that important additional findings are missed.
- The classic pattern of CRPS 1, formerly known as reflex sympathetic dystrophy, is increased periarticular tracer localization on delayed phase.
- Three-phase skeletal scintigraphy can vary in CRPS 1 during the flow and soft tissue phases in adults, and particularly in children.

- Stress fractures typically show a fusiform pattern of uptake along the long axis of the affected bone. Plain radiographs should be obtained to avoid missing an aggressive bone lesion that could mimic this pattern.

Suggested Reading

Davies AM, Carter SR, Grimer RJ, Sneath RS. Fatigue fractures of the femoral diaphysis simulating malignancy. Br J Radiol 1989;62(742):893–896

Fournier RS, Holder LE. Reflex sympathetic dystrophy: diagnostic controversies. Semin Nucl Med 1998;28(1):116–123

Holder LE, Mackinnon SE. Reflex sympathetic dystrophy in the hands: clinical and scintigraphic criteria. Radiology 1984;152(2):517–522

Intenzo CM, Kim SM, Capuzzi DM. The role of nuclear medicine in the evaluation of complex regional pain syndrome type I. Clin Nucl Med 2005;30(6):400–407

Laxer RM, Allen RC, Malleson PN, Morrison RT, Petty RE. ^{99m}Tc MDP bone scans in children with reflex neurovascular dystrophy. J Pediatr 1985;106(3):437–440

CASE 13

Clinical Presentation

A 64-year-old man with a history of prostate cancer diagnosed 2 years ago now has a prostate-specific antigen (PSA) level elevated to 25 ng/mL (**Fig. 13.1**).

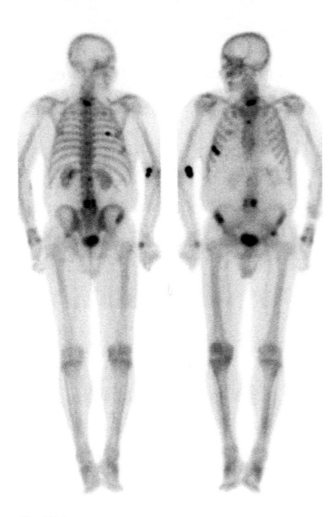

Fig. 13.1

Technique

- A 20 mCi dose of ^{99m}Tc-MDP is administered intravenously.
- Whole-body images of the skeleton are obtained 3 hours after tracer administration.
- A 1024 × 256 matrix is used for whole-body images.
- Emphasize the importance of oral hydration to improve soft tissue and bladder clearance.

Image Interpretation

Focally intense tracer uptake is seen at several sites, both articular and nonarticular. The injection site is seen at the right antecubital fossa.

Differential Diagnosis

- Metastatic disease
- Trauma

Diagnosis and Clinical Follow-Up

Radiographs showed blastic lesions, consistent with prostate cancer.

Discussion

If the initial workup of prostate cancer includes an elevated PSA level (> 8–20 ng/mL), bone pain, or a histologically aggressive tumor, the bone scan is the most cost-effective tool for the diagnosis of metastasis to bone. On the other hand, if the PSA level is less than 8 ng/mL and if other evidence of metastasis is lacking, the bone scan may not be warranted.

Prostate cancer is almost always associated with an aggressive osteoblastic response, causing obvious focal uptake in sites of metastatic disease. The tumor can initially spread through local lymphatics or hematogenously through Bateson's plexus to the pelvis and spine and throughout the axial skeleton. Spread to the appendicular skeleton outside regions occupied by red marrow is rare but not unheard of in cases of advanced metastatic disease.

Prostate cancer may also be associated with urinary tract obstruction by tumor at the prostate, unrelated prostatic hypertrophy, or local pelvic nodal metastases. Abnormal amounts of tracer retained in the ureters or renal pelves should be mentioned in the dictated report, and the patient should be questioned about symptoms of obstruction. It is not uncommon that back pain suspected to be caused by bony metastasis is subsequently found to be caused by urinary tract obstruction initially discovered on the bone scan.

PEARLS AND PITFALLS_____

- A discussion with the patient or the referring physician may help to determine the significance of equivocal lesions noted on the bone scan.
- Therapy with ^{153}Sm should be considered in patients with bone pain and avid tracer uptake in bony lesions. This therapy may be suggested in the written report.
- Local metastatic disease in the pelvis or sacrum may be obscured by tracer in the urinary bladder. If the bladder cannot be emptied completely, sitting-on-the-detector, SPECT, or lateral views may allow the separation of tracer activity concentrated in the urinary bladder from that in bony structures. Catheterization of the urinary bladder, particularly in patients with bladder outlet obstruction, can lead to urosepsis and therefore should not be done routinely.
- Hyperostosis frontalis in the skull may resemble metastatic disease without straight anteroposterior views demonstrating the bilateral, symmetric nature of the tracer uptake.
- Diffuse metastatic uptake in the hemipelvis or any other bone may resemble Paget disease. Radiographic correlation should always be obtained if this pattern of uptake is present.

- The utility of bone scans in patients with a PSA level of less than 8 ng/mL is unclear. It may serve as a useful baseline, particularly in patients with severe degenerative disease or other known bony disease.

Suggested Reading

Freitas JE, Gilvydas R, Ferry JD, Gonzalez JA. The clinical utility of prostate-specific antigen and bone scintigraphy in prostate cancer follow-up. J Nucl Med 1991;32(7):1387–1390

Harbert JC. The musculoskeletal system, 801–864. In: Harbert JC, Eckelman WC, Neumann RD, eds. Nuclear Medicine Diagnosis and Therapy. New York, NY: Thieme; 1996;801–864

Klein EA. An update on prostate cancer. Cleve Clin J Med 1995;62(5):325–338

Skeletal System. In: Mettler FA, Guiberteau MJ, eds. Essentials of Nuclear Medicine Imaging. 5th ed. New York, NY: Elsevier; 2006

CASE 14

Clinical Presentation

A 43-year-old woman with a history of breast cancer diagnosed 5 years earlier presents with elevated serum levels of calcium and alkaline phosphatase on routine follow-up (**Figs. 14.1, 14.2,** and **14.3**).

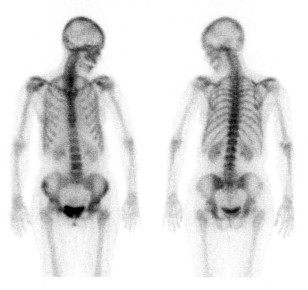

Fig. 14.1

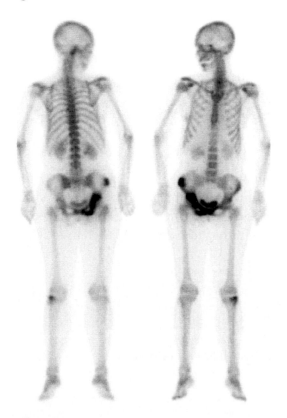

Fig. 14.2

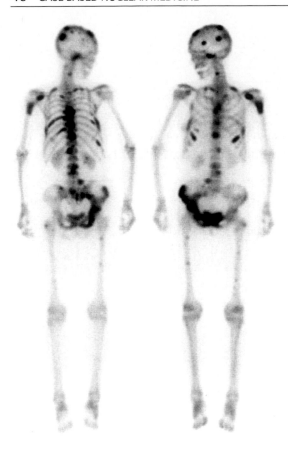

Fig. 14.3

Technique

- A 20 mCi dose of ^{99m}Tc-MDP is administered intravenously.
- Whole-body images of the skeleton are obtained 3 hours after tracer administration.
- A 1024 × 256 matrix is used for whole-body images.
- Emphasize the importance of oral hydration to improve soft tissue and bladder clearance.

Image Interpretation

The images show the progression of metastatic disease over approximately 3 years. **Figure 14.1**, from January 1995, shows right anterior iliac crest involvement and the possibility of pubic symphysis involvement. **Figure 14.2**, from April 1996, shows definite progression of the disease within the pelvis. **Figure 14.3**, from April 1997, shows disseminated metastases throughout the axial skeleton, with faint focal abnormalities in the femora as well.

Differential Diagnosis

- Metastatic breast cancer
- Other neoplastic disease
- Neoplastic disease with superimposed metabolic disease, such as Paget disease

Diagnosis and Clinical Follow-Up

The patient had progressive breast cancer.

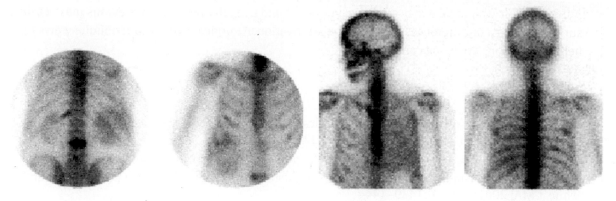

Fig. 14.4   **Fig. 14.5**

Discussion

Routine bone scanning during the primary workup of breast cancer is probably not warranted unless there are signs or symptoms to suggest the possibility of metastatic disease.

If the patient has a history of arthritis or other disease involving bone, but none of the signs or symptoms of bone metastasis, the benefit of a bone scan is more controversial. The low specificity of the bone scan makes it likely that abnormalities will be detected; a decision must then be made to determine to what extent these abnormalities are to be pursued. Plain film correlation is usually sufficient to diagnose changes secondary to arthritis or previous trauma. Although it is recognized that metastatic disease may be superimposed on arthritic changes, the number of missed lesions does not warrant more extensive testing of all sites of arthritis detected on bone scan.

The benefit of obtaining a bone scan, particularly in patients with known benign disease, is that a baseline study is available for comparison should signs or symptoms of metastatic disease arise. A lack of change in bony tracer uptake at sites of previously documented arthritis makes metastatic disease unlikely.

PEARLS AND PITFALLS

- Soft tissue should be carefully evaluated for the possibility of liver uptake (**Fig. 14.4**), which suggests metastatic spread to the liver, or hemithorax asymmetry (**Fig. 14.5**), which suggests malignant pleural effusion.
- Isolated sternal lesions may represent metastasis in up to 76% of patients with breast cancer.
- Focal lesions on adjacent ribs are most often caused by trauma, but chest wall invasion by locally recurrent disease should also be considered.
- Lesions noted in weight-bearing areas, such as the femora, should be imaged with radiography to rule out impending pathologic fracture.
- Therapy with ^{153}Sm should be considered in patients with bone pain and avid tracer uptake in bony lesions.
- Following therapy, particularly hormonal therapy, healing bony lesions noted on previous scans can demonstrate more intense tracer uptake. This "flare response" should not be mistaken for worsening disease.

- Anterior chest wall uptake may appear asymmetric and irregular because of previous mastectomy, surgical trauma, or differences in soft tissue attenuation. A surgical history and oblique views may help if rib lesions are being considered.

Suggested Reading

Kwai AH, Stomper PC, Kaplan WD. Clinical significance of isolated scintigraphic sternal lesions in patients with breast cancer. J Nucl Med 1988;29(3):324–328

Myers RE, Johnston M, Pritchard K, Levine M, Oliver T; Breast Cancer Disease Site Group of the Cancer Care Ontario Practice Guidelines Initiative. Baseline staging tests in primary breast cancer: a practice guideline. CMAJ 2001;164(10):1439–1444

Ohtake E, Murata H, Maruno H. Bone scintigraphy in patients with breast cancer: malignant involvement of the sternum. Radiat Med 1994;12(1):25–28

CASE 15

Clinical Presentation

A 65-year-old man with non–small-cell lung carcinoma undergoes bone scan for staging (**Fig. 15.1**).

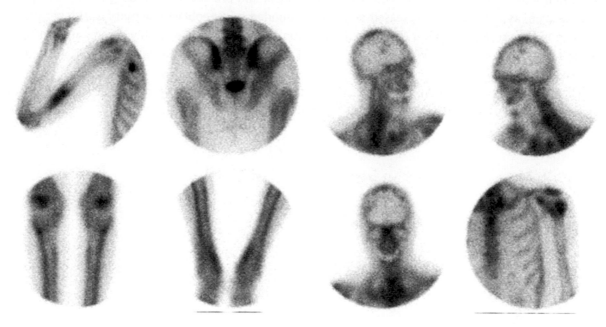

Fig. 15.1

Technique

- A 20 mCi dose of ^{99m}Tc-MDP is administered intravenously.
- Whole-body images of the skeleton are obtained 3 hours after tracer administration.
- A 1024 × 256 matrix is used for whole-body images.
- A 256 × 256 matrix is used for spot views.
- Emphasize the importance of oral hydration to improve soft tissue and bladder clearance.

Image Interpretation

Selected spot views show focally increased activity in the right distal humerus, the left proximal humerus, the skull, and a right upper rib anteriorly. Also noted is diffusely increased activity in the femora and tibiae bilaterally in a "tram track" cortical pattern, consistent with hypertrophic osteoarthropathy (HO).

Differential Diagnosis

- For the focal bony findings
  - Metastatic disease
  - Trauma

- For the leg uptake
  - HO
  - Venous stasis (usually only in tibiae)
  - Stress reaction (usually more focal)

Diagnosis and Clinical Follow-Up

The patient had metastatic lung cancer and HO. Lung cancer metastases in bone do not always show the intense osteoblastic response seen with breast cancer and prostate cancer. Irregular tracer uptake can be seen, as can areas of decreased activity surrounded by osteoblastic activity at the periphery, as seen in the skull in **Fig. 15.1.** Although osteoblastic activity almost invariably accompanies skeletal metastases, bone scans should always be surveyed for areas of decreased uptake as well as areas of increased uptake.

Like those of prostate and breast cancer, lung cancer metastases are likely to be seen in the central skeleton, but they can also be seen in the peripheral skeleton early in the disease.

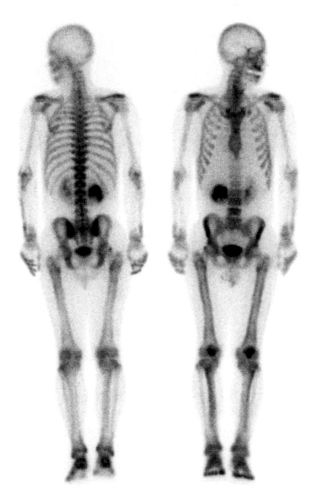

Fig. 15.2

- It is not uncommon to see HO associated with lung tumors (**Fig. 15.2**). In patients with known lung cancer or other malignancies known to have spread to the lung, the extremities should be surveyed for signs of HO.
- Look for asymmetric tracer uptake in the lung fields. Malignant pleural effusion or focal tumor uptake of tracer may be seen.
- Soft tissue uptake, as in all bone scans, should be carefully reviewed. Because of the frequency with which lung cancer metastasizes to the adrenal glands, the contour of both kidneys should especially be considered. The patient in **Fig. 15.2** had previously undetected hydronephrosis and horseshoe kidney, although these findings were not related to metastatic disease.
- Areas of decreased tracer uptake are more difficult to see than areas of increased uptake. Make sure you adequately review all areas of the bone scan for focally decreased activity.

Suggested Reading

Argiris A, Murren JR. Staging and clinical prognostic factors for small-cell lung cancer. Cancer J 2001;7(5):437–447

Knight SB, Delbeke D, Stewart JR, Sandler MP. Evaluation of pulmonary lesions with FDG-PET: comparison of findings in patients with and without a history of prior malignancy. Chest 1996;109(4):982–988

Sazon DA, Santiago SM, Soo Hoo GW, et al. Fluorodeoxyglucose-positron emission tomography in the detection and staging of lung cancer. Am J Respir Crit Care Med 1996;153(1):417–421

CASE 16

Clinical Presentation

A 31-year-old woman presents with back pain. The patient was referred to a neurologist after a chiropractor noted a spine lesion on plain films. CT and MRI demonstrate a large mass in the left kidney. A bone scan is obtained to demonstrate the extent of metastasis (**Fig. 16.1**).

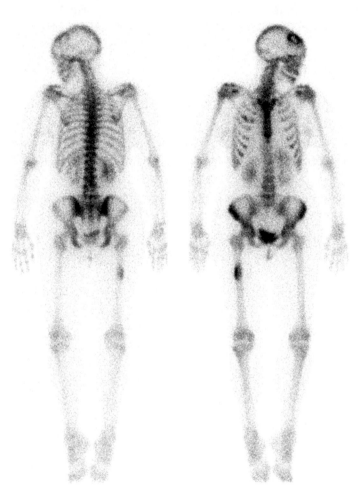

Fig. 16.1

Technique

- A 20 mCi dose of ^{99m}Tc-MDP is administered intravenously.
- Whole-body images of the skeleton are obtained 3 hours after tracer administration.
- A 1024 × 256 matrix is used for whole-body images.
- A 256 × 256 matrix is used for spot views.
- Emphasize the importance of oral hydration to improve soft tissue and bladder clearance.

Image Interpretation

Whole-body images show foci of increased tracer uptake in the skull and proximal right femur. A fainter area of increased uptake is noted in approximately the right third rib on the anterior image. The skull lesion suggests a central photopenic defect. There is also irregularity in the lower lumbar spine, with a possible focus of diminished tracer uptake at approximately L4–5. The left kidney, although faint, demonstrates an unusual contour, noted more readily on the anterior views.

Differential Diagnosis

- Metastatic disease
- Trauma or prior surgery
- Urine contamination
- Osteomyelitis (unusual to have multifocal osteomyelitis in an adult)

Diagnosis and Clinical Follow-Up

Metastatic renal cell carcinoma of the left kidney was diagnosed. The defect in the lower lumbar spine was the site of the lesion noted on the plain film. Like those from lung cancer, bone metastases from renal carcinoma may not demonstrate the marked osteoblastic response seen with breast and prostate metastases. It is common to see areas with little tracer uptake surrounded by a ring of osteoblastic response, as in the skull lesion of this patient. Fewer than 5% of bone scans done during the staging workup of patients with renal carcinoma are positive. Therefore, the bone scan is more likely to be obtained during the workup of a symptomatic patient or when a lesion is noted on another imaging study.

Many patients with renal cell carcinoma have already had a nephrectomy when the bone scan is obtained. A nephrectomy may or may not be accompanied by the removal of one of the lower ribs.

It should not be assumed that a missing kidney or rib is the result of surgery, however. The patient should be questioned about a surgical history to rule out a nonfunctioning kidney or an aggressive

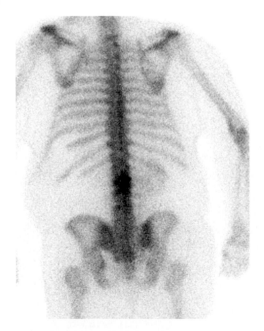

Fig. 16.2

metastatic lesion to the rib. Because renal cell carcinoma can be multifocal, careful attention should also be paid to the contour of the kidney contralateral to the one with the known primary tumor.

Figure 16.2 shows a patient with renal cell carcinoma and an absent left kidney and left lower rib, both removed surgically. The bony tracer uptake in the lumbar spine is the site of a metastatic lesion.

PEARLS AND PITFALLS_____

- Renal cell carcinoma is an excellent example of why soft tissue uptake should be carefully evaluated in all bone scans. In patients referred for bone pain who do not have a diagnosis, irregular uptake in the kidneys may direct the referring physician to the diagnosis.
- Radiographic correlation with lesions noted on bone scan is especially important because of the osteolytic nature of renal cell carcinoma. Treating sites of impending fracture with external beam therapy or orthopedic intervention may prevent a debilitating fracture.
- The less intense osteoblastic response may make some lesions difficult to see, as in the spine of the index case. Patients should be carefully questioned about symptomatic sites.

Suggested Reading

Jacobson AF. Bone scanning in metastatic disease. In: Collier DB, Fogelman I, Rosenthall L, eds. Skeletal Nuclear Medicine. St. Louis, MO: Mosby; 1996:87

CASE 17

Clinical Presentation

A 72-year-old man with a history of metastatic prostate cancer is referred for a bone scan because of pain in the left shoulder and lower neck (**Fig. 17.1**).

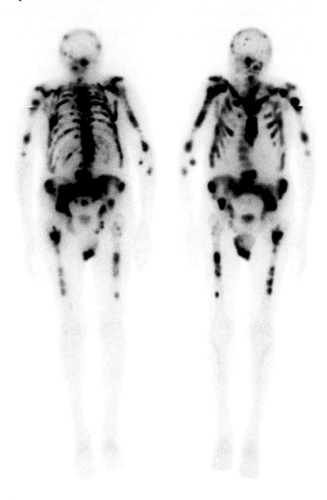

Fig. 17.1

Technique

- A 20 mCi dose of ^{99m}Tc-MDP is administered intravenously.
- Whole-body images of the skeleton are obtained 3 hours after tracer administration.
- A 1024 × 256 matrix is used.
- Emphasize the importance of oral hydration to improve soft tissue and bladder clearance.

Image Interpretation

Whole-body images show intense tracer uptake throughout the axial skeleton and proximal portions of the appendicular skeleton. Little uptake is noted in the soft tissues, including the kidneys. A small amount of tracer is noted in the urinary bladder.

Diagnosis and Clinical Follow-Up

- Disseminated prostate cancer. The patient had previously received ^{89}Sr therapy with little relief of his pain. He was therefore scheduled for external beam therapy to the neck and left shoulder.

Discussion

A bone scan with disseminated, intense uptake is often called a *superscan*. The definition of a superscan is not clearly established, however, and the term should not be considered as describing a specific set of findings on bone scintigraphy. Generally, a superscan is considered when markedly increased uptake in the skeleton is causing diminished soft tissue activity. Faint tracer activity may still be seen in the kidneys and bladder, even when confluent, intense uptake in the axial skeleton is present. As in this case, some superscans show tracer uptake that is heterogeneous enough to identify individual lesions.

Superscans caused by metastatic disease (usually prostate cancer) are characterized by involvement of the axial skeleton (red marrow) as opposed to the appendicular skeleton. Occasionally, these lesions are diffuse and confluent, and the scan may at first appear normal. The abnormally increased uptake can be identified by noting the unusually clear appearance of the axial bony structures, the paucity of soft tissue uptake, and the relatively abrupt cutoff of increased tracer uptake in the proximal versus the distal portions of the appendicular skeleton (**Fig. 17.2**).

Like metastatic disease, hyperparathyroidism or other metabolic disease causing rapid bone turnover may also result in a superscan. Metabolic disease, as distinguished from metastatic disease, affects

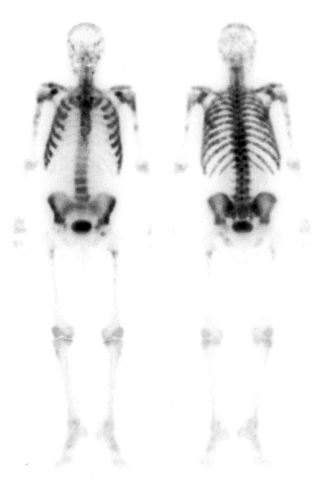

Fig. 17.2

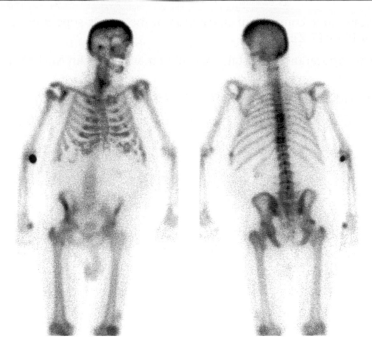

Fig. 17.3 Superscan caused by hyperparathyroidism. Although some soft tissue uptake is noted, very little tracer is seen in the urinary system. Also noted on this study is uptake in the costal cartilage and particularly intense uptake in the skull.

all the bones, resulting in an even distribution of increased tracer uptake throughout the axial and appendicular portions of the skeleton (**Fig. 17.3**).

PEARLS AND PITFALLS

- The term *superscan* does not represent a specific set of criteria expressed by the bone scan. In general, it means that there is diffuse, avid bony uptake of tracer with relatively decreased soft tissue uptake. It does not necessarily mean a complete lack of activity in the kidneys, urinary tract, or soft tissues, or confluent activity that is mistaken for a normal scan.
- Patients with a superscan may benefit from ^{89}Sr or ^{153}Sm therapy for the palliation of bone pain. The active osteoblastic activity results in a high radiation dose to the sites of metastasis.
- The most common pitfall in reading a bone superscan is mistaking the diffusely increased bony uptake for normal tracer uptake.
- Do not mistake a superscan caused by metabolic disease for one caused by metastatic disease. Metabolic disease most often involves the entire bony skeleton, whereas metastatic disease involves predominantly the axial skeleton.
- Confluent tracer uptake that can be mistaken for the normal distribution of tracer activity is not necessary for a study to be called a superscan. In older imaging systems, such as rectilinear scanners, resolution was poorer than in modern gamma cameras, and minor irregularities in tracer distribution were more difficult to detect. The resolution of today's gamma cameras results in less frequent appearances of confluent uptake mimicking normal tracer distribution.

Suggested Reading

Constable AR, Cranage RW. Recognition of the superscan in prostatic bone scintigraphy. Br J Radiol 1981;54(638):122–125

Massie JD, Sebes JI. The headless bone scan: an uncommon manifestation of metastatic superscan in carcinoma of the prostate. Skeletal Radiol 1988;17(2):111–113

Ohashi K, Smith HS, Jacobs MP. "Superscan" appearance in distal renal tubular acidosis. Clin Nucl Med 1991;16(5):318–320

Sy WM. Bone scan in primary hyperparathyroidism. J Nucl Med 1974;15(12):1089–1091

Sy WM, Patel D, Faunce H. Significance of absent or faint kidney sign on bone scan. J Nucl Med 1975;16(6):454–456

CASE 18

Clinical Presentation

A 50-year-old woman presents with a history of breast cancer (**Fig. 18.1**).

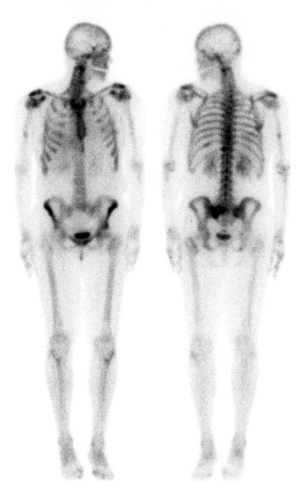

Fig. 18.1

Technique

- A 20 mCi dose of ^{99m}Tc-MDP is administered intravenously.
- Whole-body or spot images of the skeleton are obtained 3 hours after tracer administration.
- Emphasize the importance of oral hydration to improve soft tissue and bladder clearance.

Image Interpretation

Whole-body views (**Fig. 18.1**) demonstrate tracer uptake in the upper cervical spine, midshaft of the right humerus, and left sacroiliac joint, and a smaller focus in the adjacent sacrum. Also noted is uptake in the soft tissues of the right upper quadrant of the abdomen.

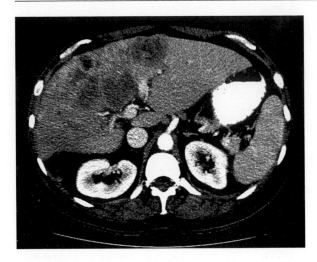

Fig. 18.2

Differential Diagnosis

(Uptake in the right upper quadrant of the abdomen)
- Hepatic metastasis
- Soft tissue tracer uptake secondary to metastatic calcification, superimposed on liver
- Prior radioactive colloid scan
- Colloid formation during radiopharmaceutical preparation
- Hepatic necrosis
- Metastatic calcification in the liver

Diagnosis and Clinical Follow-Up

The bony abnormalities were secondary to metastatic colon cancer. The uptake in the right upper quadrant was secondary to metastatic disease in the liver (**Fig. 18.2**).

Discussion

Bone scans are insensitive for soft tissue metastases, yet all scans should include a survey of the soft tissues, especially when the patient is referred for the staging of metastatic disease. Uptake noted in the soft tissues on bone scan can be the first indication of metastatic disease.

PEARLS AND PITFALLS

- The symmetry of tracer distribution in the soft tissues of the abdomen and chest should be reviewed on all studies. Faint uptake in the liver or in a pleural effusion may be caused by metastatic disease.
- The metastatic soft tissue uptake in this case could be mistaken for asymmetric renal uptake. Asymmetry of uptake in the region of the liver should be carefully reviewed before it is dismissed.

Suggested Reading

Peller PJ, Ho VB, Kransdorf MJ. Extraosseous [99mTc] MDP uptake: a pathophysiologic approach. Radiographics 1993;13(4):715–734

Petersen M. Radionuclide detection of primary pulmonary osteogenic sarcoma: a case report and review of the literature. J Nucl Med 1990;31(6):1110–1114

Pickhardt PJ, McDermott M. Intense uptake of [99mTc]-MDP in primary breast adenocarcinoma with sarcomatoid metaplasia. J Nucl Med 1997;38(4):528–530

CASE 19

Clinical Presentation

A 78-year-old man with a history of colon cancer presents with knee pain (**Figs. 19.1** and **19.2**).

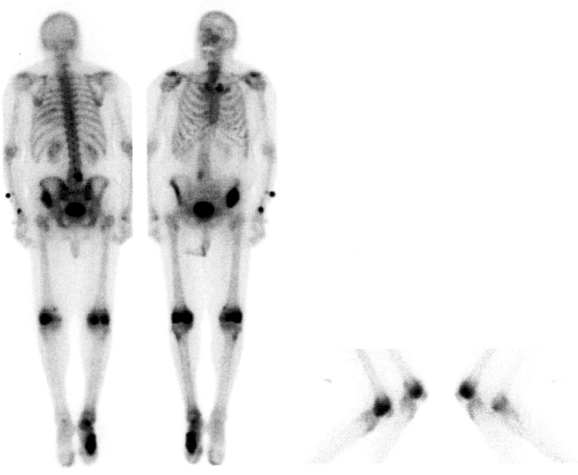

Fig. 19.1

Fig. 19.2

Technique

- A 20 mCi dose of ^{99m}Tc-MDP is administered intravenously.
- Whole-body or spot images of the skeleton are obtained 3 hours after tracer administration.
- Lateral spot views of the knees are obtained.
- Emphasize the importance of oral hydration to improve soft tissue and bladder clearance.

Image Interpretation

Whole-body images (**Fig. 19.1**) and spot views of the knees (**Fig. 19.2**) show mildly increased activity posteriorly in approximately the eighth left rib; in addition, intense, focally increased tracer uptake is seen in the lumbar spine at approximately L4 and L5, in the region of the anterior iliac crest on the left, in the distal femora bilaterally, and in the midfoot on the right. The injection site is noted at the intravenous access in the left distal forearm.

Differential Diagnosis

- Metastatic disease
- Trauma
- Degenerative joint disease
- Paget disease
- Fibrous dysplasia
- Avascular necrosis (of the knees)
- Skin contamination (particularly at the foot)

Diagnosis and Clinical Follow-Up

The rib abnormality was diagnosed as secondary to recent open thoracotomy and biopsy of a lung mass. CT showed that the left iliac crest uptake was in the soft tissues and consistent with myositis ossificans. (The patient had a history of a surgical procedure in this area.) On CT scan, the lumbar spine was read as degenerative disease. MRI of the lumbar spine later demonstrated marrow abnormalities, consistent with metastatic disease, in the same location as the bone scan abnormality. It is important to note that the knee findings were largely confined to the distal femora and did not involve the tibial surfaces, decreasing the likelihood of degenerative disease. On MRI, the knees showed osteonecrosis. The right foot lesion was biopsied and demonstrated to be secondary to metastatic colon cancer.

Discussion

Several important points are illustrated by this study. First, bone scans are very sensitive for abnormalities but not very specific. The rib abnormality was caused by trauma, the pelvis abnormality was benign, the knee abnormalities were secondary to ischemia, and the spine and foot abnormalities were secondary to malignant disease. The bone uptake at any of these sites could be caused by a variety of diseases. The pattern of bone uptake may suggest a particular disease, but the scintigraphic findings must be correlated with the results of other tests as well as with the history and physical examination findings.

Second, the CT scan directed at the bone scan finding in the lumbar spine was read as consistent with degenerative disease. It is clear from the intensity and focus of the uptake on bone scan, however, that the finding is not typical of degenerative disease. If the physician reading the CT scan had also looked at the bone scan, he or she might have been less likely to dismiss the reported bone scan findings when the CT scan showed changes typical of degenerative disease in the same region of the spine.

The final point is that, although it is always a good idea to try to relate all findings to one disease process, if there is any question of the cause of several abnormalities noted on a single bone scan, the examiner should pursue all the abnormalities individually rather than diagnose the cause of one abnormality and attribute the same disease process to the others.

- If a different physician is going to read the correlative imaging studies prompted by the bone scan findings, it is very helpful for the other physician to have a copy of the bone scan images. The dictated report of the scan does not convey as much information as the images do.
- Soft tissue uptake can be superimposed on bony structures and therefore mistaken as a bony abnormality. If soft tissue uptake is suspected, additional views, such as oblique views or SPECT or SPECT/CT images, can separate bony structures from soft tissue.
- Not all physicians believe all abnormalities noted on bone scan should be pursued with correlative imaging. Some findings may be typical for degenerative disease or for additional sites of metastasis in patients with known bony metastatic disease. The decision to pursue any abnormality should be made in light of the history, physical examination findings, and other test results.

Suggested Reading

Bordy Z, Pasztarak E, Bánsági G, Sik E. Soft-tissue involvement by adenocarcinoma imaged during bone scintigraphy. Clin Nucl Med 1997;22(7):508

Drane WE. Myositis ossificans and the three-phase bone scan. AJR Am J Roentgenol 1984;142(1):179–180

Nisolle JF, Delaunois L, Trigaux JP. Myositis ossificans of the chest wall. Eur Respir J 1996;9(1):178–179

Stuckey SL. Colonic adenocarcinoma metastatic to bone with gross heterotopic bone formation: bone scan appearance with correlative imaging. Clin Nucl Med 1996;21(5):396–397

Sud AM, Wilson MW, Mountz JM. Unusual clinical presentation and scintigraphic pattern in myositis ossificans. Clin Nucl Med 1992;17(3):198–199

CASE 20

Clinical Presentation

A 51-year-old woman presents with leiomyosarcoma (**Fig. 20.1**).

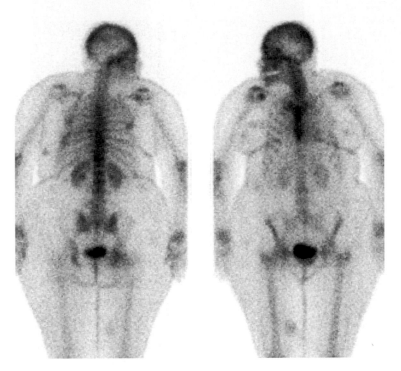

Fig. 20.1

Technique

- A 20 mCi dose of ^{99m}Tc-MDP is administered intravenously.
- Whole-body images of the skeleton are obtained 3 hours after tracer administration.
- A 1024 × 256 matrix is used for whole-body images.
- Emphasize the importance of oral hydration to improve soft tissue and bladder clearance.

Image Interpretation

Whole-body anterior and posterior views (**Fig. 20.1**) show tracer uptake in the right shoulder and also in the soft tissues of the right thigh medially and the right and left flanks.

Differential Diagnosis

- Soft tissue metastases
- Cellulitis
- Soft tissue trauma
- Primary soft tissue tumor

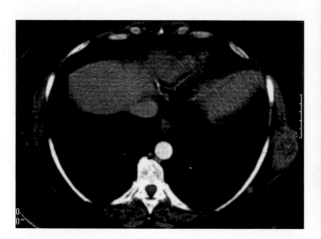

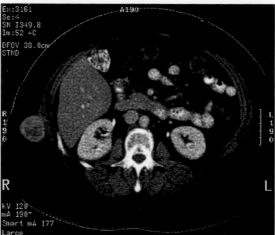

Fig. 20.2   **Fig. 20.3**

- Skin contamination
- Soft tissue abscess

Diagnosis and Clinical Follow-Up

CT scans (**Figs. 20.2** and **20.3**) demonstrate disseminated disease, including a 7 × 7 × 3-cm soft tissue mass in the posterior aspect of the left chest wall and in the soft tissues of the right flank, lateral to the kidney. There were also numerous nodules in the lungs and axillae (**Figs. 20.2** and **20.3**).

Discussion

The uptake of bone radiopharmaceuticals in soft tissue metastasis is important and should be reported when it is detected with bone scanning. In some cases, however, bone tracer uptake in soft tissues may not be very sensitive for soft tissue metastases as illustrated by this patient, in whom only the largest soft tissue metastases were noted. Most of the lesions in the lungs, abdomen, and axillae were not detected.

Suggested Reading

Peller PJ, Ho VB, Kransdorf MJ. Extraosseous 99mTc MDP uptake: a pathophysiologic approach. Radiographics 1993;13(4):715–734

CASE 21

Clinical Presentation

A 68-year-old man presents with low back pain (**Fig. 21.1**).

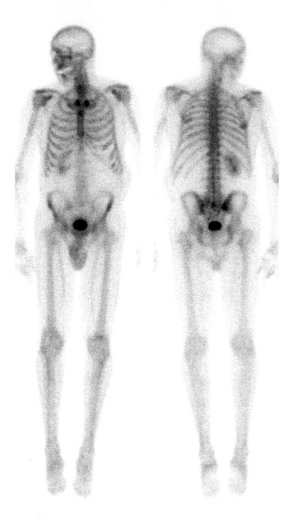

Fig. 21.1

Technique

- A 20 mCi dose of ^{99m}Tc-MDP is administered intravenously.
- Whole-body images of the skeleton are obtained 3 hours after tracer administration.
- A 1024 × 256 matrix is used for whole-body images.
- Emphasize the importance of oral hydration to improve soft tissue and bladder clearance.

Image Interpretation

Whole-body images demonstrate increased focal uptake in the sternoclavicular joints bilaterally and in the sternomanubrial joint. A focus of decreased uptake is noted in the sacrum with adjacent irregular activity in the sacroiliac joints.

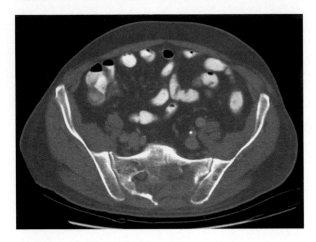

Fig. 21.2

Differential Diagnosis

- Metastatic disease (eg, lung, thyroid, or renal cancer or multiple myeloma; less likely to be seen with prostate or breast cancer)
- Attenuation artifact (metallic object in back pocket, belt)
- Prosthetic joint (hip, knee)
- Avascular necrosis
- Prior surgery (eg, bony resection)
- Early osteomyelitis
- Bone infarct from sickle cell disease
- Benign tumor (eg, hemangioma)
- Bone cyst
- Pixel overflow
- Camera defect (eg, crystal, photomultiplier tube, or collimator defect)

Diagnosis and Clinical Follow-Up

The diagnosis was metastatic renal cell carcinoma. CT scan showed a large sacral lytic lesion (**Fig. 21.2**).

Discussion

As noted before, focal cold defects noted on bone scans can have many causes, ranging from malignant to benign to artifactual. The malignancies that most commonly warrant bone scanning—prostate and breast cancer—rarely cause cold defects because of the intense osteoblastic response often associated with these tumors. Even if plain radiographs demonstrate "lytic" lesions (in tumors other than multiple myeloma), the bone scan is likely to demonstrate an area of increased tracer uptake caused by osteoblasts attempting to repair the bony injury.

- Identifying foci of decreased tracer uptake requires more attention than locating foci of increased activity.
- Metastatic lesions causing cold defects are frequently associated with increased uptake at the interface between the tumor (cold area) and adjacent normal bone. An isolated defect with no adjacent increased uptake should raise the suspicion of attenuation artifact.
- Before reporting a cold defect on a bone scan, make certain that the abnormality cannot be explained by an attenuation artifact such as a pacemaker, a prosthetic joint implant, barium in the colon, jewelry, or metallic items in pockets.
- The usefulness of bone scans in multiple myeloma is doubtful. The bone scan is not sensitive for the lytic lesions seen in multiple myeloma; as many as half of these lesions are not seen.

Suggested Reading

Bataille R, Chevalier J, Rossi M, Sany J. Bone scintigraphy in plasma-cell myeloma: a prospective study of 70 patients. Radiology 1982;145(3):801–804

Berruti A, Piovesan A, Torta M, et al. Biochemical evaluation of bone turnover in cancer patients with bone metastases: relationship with radiograph appearances and disease extension. Br J Cancer 1996;73(12):1581–1587

Kagan AR, Steckel RJ, Bassett LW. Diagnostic oncology case study: lytic spine lesion and cold bone scan. AJR Am J Roentgenol 1981;136(1):129–131

Otsuka N, Fukunaga M, Morita K, Ono S, Nagai K. Photon-deficient finding in sternum on bone scintigraphy in patients with malignant disease. Radiat Med 1990;8(5):168–172

Weingrad T, Heyman S, Alavi A. Cold lesions on bone scan in pediatric neoplasms. Clin Nucl Med 1984;9(3):125–130

CASE 22

Clinical Presentation

A 51-year-old man with a recent diagnosis of hepatoma presents with low back pain (**Fig. 22.1**).

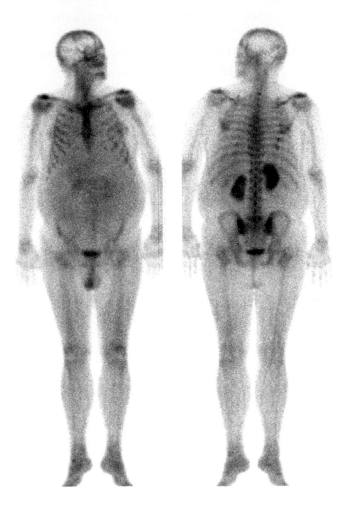

Fig. 22.1

Technique

- A 20 mCi dose of ^{99m}Tc-MDP is administered intravenously.
- Whole-body images of the skeleton are obtained 3 hours after tracer administration.
- A 1024 × 256 matrix is used for whole-body images.
- Emphasize the importance of oral hydration to improve soft tissue and bladder clearance.

Image Interpretation

Whole-body images demonstrate diffuse tracer uptake in the abdomen. Slightly more intense uptake is noted in the region of the left lobe of the liver. Also seen are two foci of increased activity in approximately the eighth and ninth right ribs posteriorly and uptake at approximately L5.

Differential Diagnosis

- Ascites (or other exudative effusion)
- Nonspecific uptake within a hepatic tumor (would not be likely to cause diffuse uptake throughout the abdomen)
- Renal failure (although this would also cause diffuse soft tissue uptake throughout the extremities)

Diagnosis and Clinical Follow-Up

The diagnosis was hepatoma with ascites. The diffuse uptake in the abdomen was secondary to ascites. Bony remodeling at L5 might have been related to the cause of the lower back pain. Follow-up radiographs were not obtained because the back pain abated spontaneously.

Discussion

Diffuse uptake of tracer in a body cavity, such as the pleural space or the abdominal cavity, is often secondary to tracer accumulation in an effusion. The tracer is more likely to accumulate in an exudative effusion caused by malignancy, but exudates can also be seen with inflammatory processes.

PEARLS AND PITFALLS

- The detection of faint, diffuse tracer uptake in an effusion is aided by comparing the tracer activity with that in adjacent normal areas, such as the opposite lung field in the case of a localized pleural effusion or, as in this case, the soft tissues of the lateral abdominal wall and the hips.
- Bilateral pleural effusions may be difficult to detect without an adjacent area of normal tracer distribution for comparison.
- Although tracer uptake in an effusion is often thought to be caused by malignancy, the finding is not specific and should not be automatically attributed to metastatic disease.

Suggested Reading

Kida T, Hujita Y, Sasaki M, Inoue J. Accumulation of ^{99m}Tc methylene diphosphonate in malignant pleural and ascitic effusion. Oncology 1984;41(6):427–430

Peller PJ, Ho VB, Kransdorf MJ. Extraosseous ^{99m}Tc MDP uptake: a pathophysiologic approach. Radiographics 1993;13(4):715–734

CASE 23

Clinical Presentation

A 71-year-old man with history of prostate cancer undergoes bone scan to assess bony metastasis (**Fig. 23.1**).

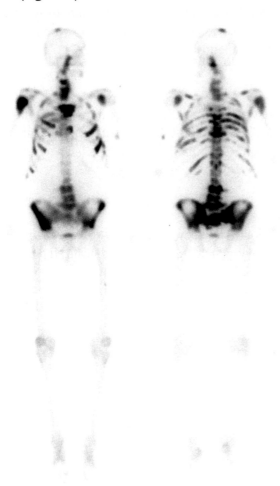

Fig. 23.1

Technique

- A 20 mCi dose of ^{99m}Tc-MDP is administered intravenously.
- Whole-body images of the skeleton are obtained 3 hours after tracer administration.
- A 1024 × 256 matrix is used for whole-body images.
- Emphasize the importance of oral hydration to improve soft tissue and bladder clearance.

Image Interpretation

Whole-body images of the skeleton demonstrate increased tracer uptake in many foci throughout the axial skeleton and in the vertex of the skull. There are also areas of decreased tracer activity from the midthoracic region down to approximately L3 and in the lower half of the pelvis.

Differential Diagnosis

(Region of decreased tracer uptake)
- Radiation therapy
- Prosthetic implant
- Attenuation artifact
- Electrical burn
- Severe vascular disease

Diagnosis and Clinical Follow-Up

CT and MRI demonstrated disseminated prostate cancer with metastases throughout the spine and ribs. The patient had previously received radiation therapy to the spine and pelvis.

Discussion

Radiation therapy should be considered as a cause of diminished bony tracer uptake, particularly when the pattern of diminished uptake approximates the size and location of a known radiation port. When one considers the frequency with which bone scans are obtained in patients who have had radiation therapy, however, it is interesting that diminished tracer uptake in the bony skeleton is not seen more often. In this patient, visualization of the radiation port was certainly enhanced by the surrounding disseminated disease. What we are seeing as an area of "diminished" activity may actually be one of the few skeletal regions where the bony metastatic disease has responded to therapy.

PEARLS AND PITFALLS

- Before diagnosing an area of abnormal decreased uptake, consider that the surrounding areas may alternatively have abnormal increased uptake.
- Radiation therapy changes do not always follow normal anatomic structures—they have a non-anatomic configuration that matches the radiation port.
- Radiation therapy can also cause areas of increased bony tracer uptake lasting for several months following therapy.
- Decreased uptake resembling a radiation therapy port can also be secondary to attenuation artifacts, such as overlying soft tissue or prosthetic implants (eg, breast implants).

Suggested Reading

Ahluwalia R, Morton KA, Whiting JH Jr, Menzel-Anderson C, Datz FL. Scintigraphic appearance of bone during external beam irradiation. Clin Nucl Med 1994;19(5):385–387

Cox PH. Abnormalities in skeletal uptake of ^{99m}Tc polyphosphate complexes in areas of bone associated with tissues which have been subjected to radiation therapy. Br J Radiol 1974;47(564):851–856

Israel O, Gorenberg M, Frenkel A, et al. Local and systemic effects of radiation on bone metabolism measured by quantitative SPECT. J Nucl Med 1992;33(10):1774–1780

King MA, Casarett GW, Weber DA. A study of irradiated bone, I: histopathologic and physiologic changes. J Nucl Med 1979;20(11):1142–1149

King MA, Weber DA, Casarett GW, Burgener FA, Corriveau O. A study of irradiated bone, II: Changes in ^{99m}Tc pyrophosphate bone imaging. J Nucl Med 1980;21(1):22–30

CASE 24

Clinical Presentation

A 63-year-old man with a history of prostate cancer presents with increasing alkaline phosphatase and pain in the left chest wall (**Fig. 24.1**).

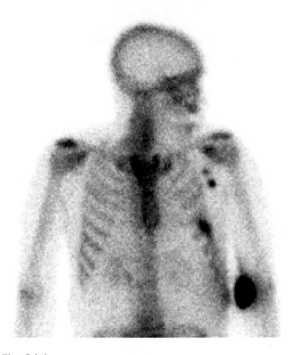

Fig. 24.1

Technique

- A 20 mCi dose of ^{99m}Tc-MDP is administered intravenously.
- Whole-body images of the skeleton are obtained 3 hours after tracer administration.
- A 1024 × 256 matrix is used for whole-body images.
- Emphasize the importance of oral hydration to improve soft tissue and bladder clearance.

Image Interpretation

The selected anterior view of the chest (**Fig. 24.1**) shows increased tracer uptake in the left axilla and in a left rib laterally. A large area of infiltrated tracer is seen in the left antecubital region.

Differential Diagnosis

(Focal soft tissue uptake of tracer)
- Accumulation of tracer in an axillary node secondary to infiltration at the injection site
- Contamination (clothing, skin surface, camera face, imaging table)
- Normal breast uptake
- Soft tissue injury (cellulitis, abscess, electrical burn)
- Adenocarcinoma metastatic to soft tissues (eg, colon, lung)

- Primary soft tissue tumor (benign or malignant)
- Vascular calcification
- Injection site (eg, meperidine, iron dextran)

Diagnosis and Clinical Follow-Up

There was infiltration of the tracer injection with subsequent tracer migration to the ipsilateral axillary lymph nodes. The rib abnormality was found to be a lytic metastatic lesion.

Discussion

Soft tissue uptake of tracer is occasionally seen in bone scans for several reasons, including metastatic disease. In one of the more common scenarios, the soft tissue uptake is axillary nodal uptake secondary to lymphatic drainage from an infiltrated tracer injection. This is usually easily identified when the injection site is imaged. If no infiltration is seen at the injection site or the injection site is in the contralateral arm, further investigation of the nodal uptake is warranted.

PEARLS AND PITFALLS

- Infiltration of the injected dose is easily diagnosed by imaging the injection site.
- If the infiltrated injection site is just out of the field of view, narrow-angle scatter from the high level of activity in the injection site can be mistaken for tracer concentration in the superficial soft tissues of the body adjacent to the injection site (as in the lower left ribs in **Fig. 24.1**).
- Focal uptake in the lateral portions of the breasts can also be mistaken for axillary nodal uptake.
- Nodal uptake can also be caused by malignancy. Uptake in axillary nodes should be definitively demonstrated to be proximal to an infiltrated injection site before it is discounted as unimportant.

Suggested Reading

Datz FL. Gamuts in Nuclear Medicine. 3rd ed. Chapter 3, 97–182. St. Louis, MO: Mosby; 1995

CASE 25

Clinical Presentation

A 73-year-old woman presents with pleuritic chest pain (**Figs. 25.1** and **25.2**).

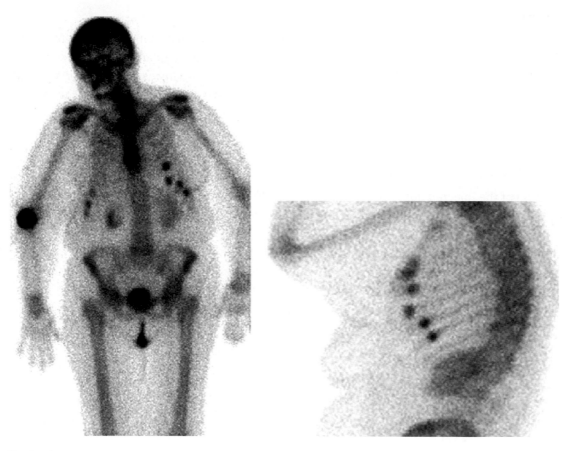

Fig. 25.1   **Fig. 25.2**

Technique

- A 20 mCi dose of ^{99m}Tc-MDP is administered intravenously.
- Whole-body images of the skeleton are obtained 3 hours after tracer administration.
- A 1024 × 256 matrix is used for whole-body images.
- Emphasize the importance of oral hydration to improve soft tissue and bladder clearance.

Image Interpretation

Figure 25.1 is an anterior view of the upper bony skeleton demonstrating intense tracer uptake at the costochondral junctions of several lower ribs bilaterally and in the midsternum. **Figure 25.2** is a left lateral view of the chest confirming the location of the abnormalities in the ribs and sternum.

Differential Diagnosis

(Adjacent focal abnormalities in adjacent ribs)

- Trauma
- Surgical resection
- Local extension of an invasive chest wall lesion (may be associated with destruction of adjacent portions of the ribs)
- Pooling of tracer in underlying renal calyces (for T11 and T12 ribs posteriorly)

Diagnosis and Clinical Follow-Up

The focal uptake in several adjacent ribs was most consistent with trauma. The symmetry of the abnormalities and the uptake in the sternum suggested that the trauma had been caused by a blow to the anterior aspect of the chest. This patient had a cardiorespiratory arrest in the emergency room several days before the study, and cardiopulmonary resuscitation had been performed in the emergency department.

Discussion

The pattern of uptake in bony abnormalities provides some information about the cause of the abnormalities. Focal uptake in several adjacent ribs in the absence of other findings suggests trauma.

PEARLS AND PITFALLS

- Isolated tracer uptake in one or several adjacent costochondral junctions is almost always associated with trauma or other benign conditions. Radiographic findings are often negative, and further workup is rarely necessary.
- Isolated sternal lesions should not be dismissed as readily as isolated rib lesions. More than 75% of isolated sternal lesions in one series were found to be secondary to malignancy.

Suggested Reading

Kwai AH, Stomper PC, Kaplan WD. Clinical significance of isolated scintigraphic sternal lesions in patients with breast cancer. J Nucl Med 1988;29(3):324–328

CASE 26

Clinical Presentation

A 55-year-old man with a history of benign prostatic hyperplasia presents with elevated prostate-specific antigen (**Fig. 26.1**).

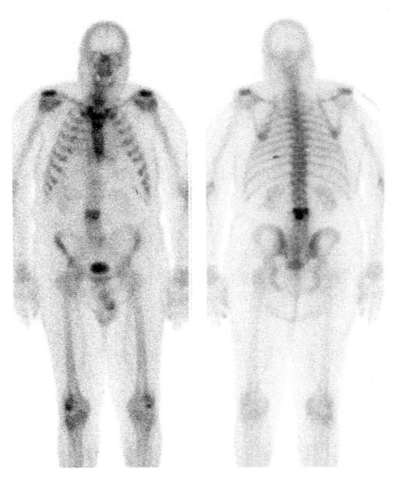

Fig. 26.1

Technique

- A 20 mCi dose of ^{99m}Tc-MDP is administered intravenously.
- Whole-body images of the skeleton are obtained 3 hours after tracer administration.
- A 1024 × 256 matrix is used for whole-body images.
- Emphasize the importance of oral hydration to improve soft tissue and bladder clearance.

Image Interpretation

Anterior and posterior views of the whole body (**Fig. 26.1**) demonstrate focally increased tracer uptake in the entire vertebral body of approximately L3. The left eighth rib also shows focal uptake posteriorly.

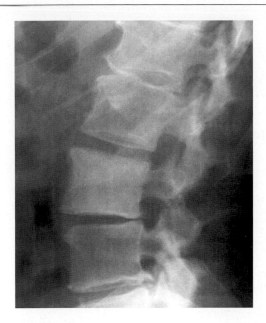

Fig. 26.2

Differential Diagnosis

- Paget disease
- Prostate cancer
- Osteomyelitis
- Primary bone tumor

Diagnosis and Clinical Follow-Up

A radiograph demonstrated Paget disease in a lumbar vertebra (**Fig. 26.2**).

Discussion

The appearance of the "Mickey Mouse" sign (also known as the "champagne glass" sign or T-sign) is consistent with the diagnosis of Paget disease. As with any abnormal bone uptake, however, a plain radiograph should be obtained to confirm the diagnosis.

PEARLS AND PITFALLS

- Bone scan findings should be correlated with history and physical examination findings. Signs or symptoms of infection or metastatic disease should raise suspicion that the bone scan finding is not related to Paget disease.
- Radiation to a spine with metastatic disease may cause a sharp transition between decreased uptake in irradiated bone and increased uptake in nonirradiated bone containing metastatic disease.

Suggested Reading

Estrada WN, Kim CK. Paget's disease in a patient with breast cancer [see comments]. J Nucl Med 1993;34(7):1214–1216

Van Heerden BB. Mickey Mouse sign in Paget's disease [letter]. J Nucl Med 1994;35(5):924–925

CASE 27

Clinical Presentation

A 41-year-old man presents with an abnormality in his head noted on gallium scan done 1 month prior (**Fig. 27.1**).

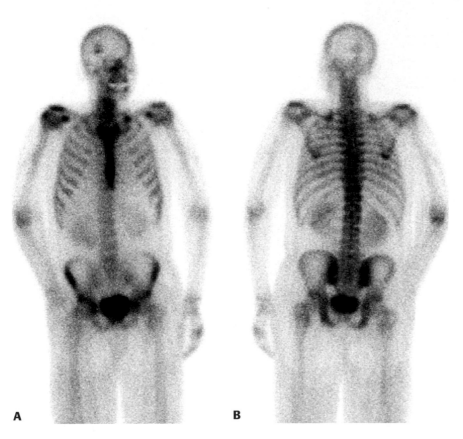

A   **B**

Fig. 27.1

Technique

- A 20 mCi dose of ^{99m}Tc-MDP is administered intravenously.
- Whole-body images of the skeleton are obtained 3 hours after tracer administration.
- A 1024 × 256 matrix is used for whole-body images.
- Emphasize the importance of oral hydration to improve soft tissue and bladder clearance.

Image Interpretation

Tracer uptake is noted in the right side of the skull in the right anterior oblique view (**Fig. 27.1A**). The posterior view of the skull (**Fig. 27.1B**) suggests a faint lesion that may be related to the occipital abnormality noted on the gallium scan or that may be shine-through of the lesion seen on the right in the anterior view.

Differential Diagnosis

(Focal uptake in the head)
- Skull metastasis
- Brain neoplasm (eg, meningioma)
- Cartilaginous rest
- Sinusitis
- Surface contamination
- Craniotomy site
- Brain abscess
- Fracture
- Brain infarct
- Bone island

Diagnosis and Clinical Follow-Up

CT demonstrated 3-cm enhancing abscesses in the left occipitoparietal region and the right subinsular region of the brain. No bone involvement was noted.

The results of this study suggested that the occipital lesion noted on the gallium scan and bone scan did not originate in the bone. They also revealed a second lesion that was likely to be on the right side of the head because it was seen better on the right anterior oblique view. The tracer uptake in this lesion was probably caused by the right insular lesion noted on the CT scan.

Discussion

The visualization of abscesses with bone radiopharmaceuticals is uncommon. In this case, the gallium and the bone radiopharmaceuticals seemed to favor different abscesses and therefore caused some confusion regarding the location of the two lesions. It is also possible that the two abscesses developed at different times, one before the gallium scan and the other just before the bone scan.

PEARLS AND PITFALLS

- Multiple views of a lesion are needed for the best localization.
- Focal uptake of bone radiopharmaceuticals in soft tissues may be mistaken for uptake in overlying or underlying bone.

Suggested Reading

Malley MJ, Holmes RA. Serendipitous detection of intrarenal abscesses on ^{99m}Tc MDP imaging while evaluating a foot ulcer. Clin Nucl Med 1988;13(2):127–128

Moallem A. Nonspecific tissue accumulation of diffusible radionuclide imaging agents in areas of inflammation. Clin Nucl Med 1992;17(1):4–6

Peller PJ, Ho VB, Kransdorf MJ. Extraosseous ^{99m}Tc MDP uptake: a pathophysiologic approach. Radiographics 1993;13(4):715–734

Tamgac F, Baillet G, Alper E, Delporte MP, Moretti JL. Extraskeletal accumulation of ^{99m}Tc HMDP in a tuberculous cold abscess. Clin Nucl Med 1995;20(12):1092

CASE 28

Clinical Presentation

A 29-year-old female runner presents with pain in her lower legs of 1 week's duration. Bone scan is requested to evaluate these symptoms (**Figs. 28.1** and **28.2**).

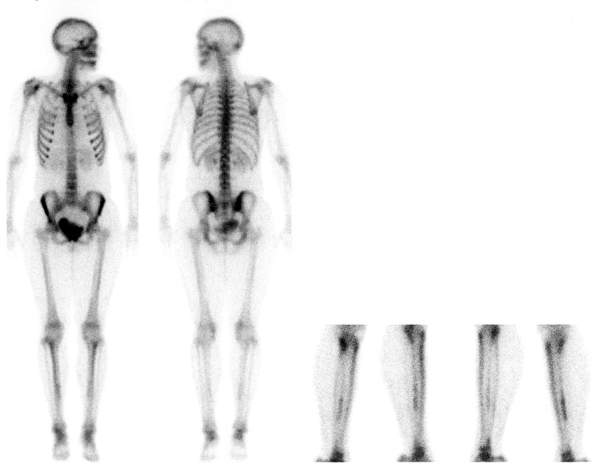

Fig. 28.1   **Fig. 28.2**

Technique

- A 20 mCi dose of ^{99m}Tc-MDP is administered intravenously.
- Whole-body images of the skeleton are obtained 3 hours after tracer administration.
- A 1024 × 256 matrix is used for whole-body images.
- Emphasize the importance of oral hydration to improve soft tissue and bladder clearance.

Image Interpretation

Anterior whole-body views (**Fig. 28.1**) show very mild, irregular tracer uptake at the midportion of the right and left tibiae. Spot lateral and medial views of the lower legs (**Fig. 28.2**) show moderately increased linear tracer uptake involving the middle to distal portions of the tibiae posteriorly.

Differential Diagnosis

- Shin splints
- Stress fracture
- Trauma

Diagnosis and Clinical Follow-up

The diagnosis was shin splints. No follow-up was available for this patient.

Discussion

The term *shin splint* is used to describe stress-related pain along the medial or posteromedial aspect of the tibia in athletes. It is often bilateral. The etiology is thought to be periosteal microtears at points of periosteal stress. The periosteal stress is likely mediated by Sharpey fibers through their connection to the bone. Bone scintigraphy is highly sensitive for the diagnosis of shin splints.

To help differentiate stress reaction from stress fracture, blood flow and blood pool images, in addition to orthogonal views, are often helpful. Blood flow and blood pool images are classically normal in stress reaction and positive in stress fracture. Orthogonal views are helpful to determine the depth of the increased uptake. If the increased uptake involves 50% or more of the bone diameter on all views, then stress fracture is more likely.

PEARLS AND PITFALLS

- It is important to obtain lateral views in patients with lower limb pain; otherwise, the diagnosis of shin splints may be missed on the anterior and posterior views.
- If a lateral view is not obtained, the differentiation between shin splints and stress fracture may be difficult.
- The scintigraphic pattern of shin splints is not predictive of further injury unless there is a focal component to the tracer uptake.
- The clinical significance of shin splints is quite different from that of a stress fracture because patients with shin splints can continue to exercise, whereas patients with stress fractures may need to refrain from exercising for at least 6 weeks to allow the fractures to heal.
- Conventional radiographs often do not show any abnormality with stress reaction.

Suggested Reading

Muthukumar T, Butt SH, Cassar-Pullicino VN. Stress fractures and related disorders in foot and ankle: plain films, scintigraphy, CT, and MR Imaging. Semin Musculoskelet Radiol 2005;9(3):210–226

Pavlov H. Athletic injuries. Radiol Clin North Am 1990;28(2):435–443

Spitz DJ, Newberg AH. Imaging of stress fractures in the athlete. Radiol Clin North Am 2002;40(2): 313–331

CASE 29

Clinical Presentation

A 79-year-old woman with a history of osteoporosis presents with persistent low back pain (**Fig. 29.1**).

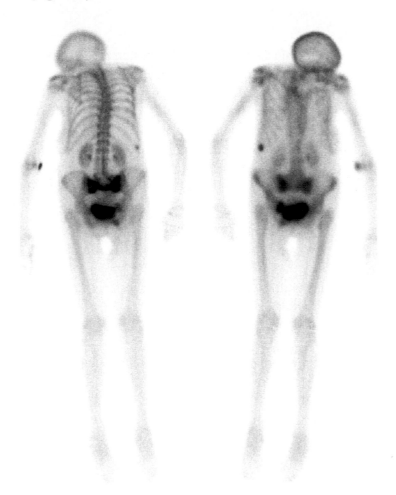

Fig. 29.1

Technique

- A 20 mCi dose of ^{99m}Tc-MDP is administered intravenously.
- Whole-body images of the skeleton are obtained 3 hours after tracer administration.
- A 1024 × 256 matrix is used for whole-body images.
- Emphasize the importance of oral hydration to improve soft tissue and bladder clearance.

Differential Diagnosis

- Fracture
- Metastatic disease
- Paget disease

Image Interpretation

Anterior and posterior whole-body images show increased tracer uptake across the body of the sacrum and increased uptake in the sacral alae bilaterally—an "H-type" insufficiency fracture (Honda sign).

Diagnosis and Clinical Follow-Up

The diagnosis was sacral insufficiency fracture. No follow-up was available for this patient.

Discussion

The term *insufficiency fracture* is used to describe a fracture that occurs when normal or physiologic stress is applied to abnormally weakened bones, as in patients with osteoporosis.

The presentation usually includes low back pain, and unless insufficiency fracture is considered, the problem may go undiagnosed for some time. Plain films are often the study initially performed in patients with low back pain. In elderly patients, plain films will often demonstrate degenerative disease; at the same time, they are very insensitive for insufficiency fracture, further delaying the diagnosis.

PEARLS AND PITFALLS

- CT, MRI, and scintigraphy may all be used for the diagnosis of insufficiency fracture. The advantages of scintigraphy include high sensitivity and the ability to detect other abnormalities, such as additional sites of fracture in the pelvic ring and other bony lesions.
- Oblique and lateral sacral views may be useful in the diagnosis of sacral and coccygeal insufficiency fractures.
- A full bladder can obscure the sacrum. If the patient is unable to empty the bladder, delayed imaging, up to 24 hours after tracer injection, is recommended.

Suggested Reading

Diel J, Ortiz O, Losada RA, Price DB, Hayt MW, Katz DS. The sacrum: pathologic spectrum, multimodality imaging, and subspecialty approach. Radiographics 2001;21(1):83–104

CASE 30

Clinical Presentation

A 37-year-old man who underwent a total left hip replacement with a noncemented prosthesis one year earlier presents with left hip pain (**Figs. 30.1** and **30.2**).

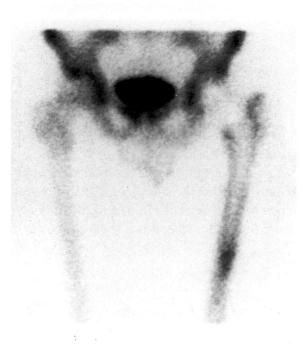

Fig. 30.1

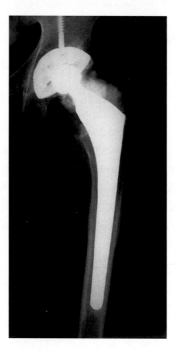

Fig. 30.2

Technique

- A 20 mCi dose of ⁹⁹ᵐTc-MDP is administered intravenously.
- A spot view of the left hip (0.5 million counts) is obtained 3 to 4 hours after tracer injection.
- A 256 × 256 matrix is used for the spot image.
- Emphasize the importance of oral hydration to improve soft tissue and bladder clearance.

Image Interpretation

The anterior view of the left hip and proximal left femur (**Fig. 30.1**) shows a focus of increased tracer uptake at the tip of the femoral component of a total hip prosthesis. An arthrogram of the left hip (**Fig. 30.2**) shows a contiguous collection of contrast over the posterosuperior aspect of the greater trochanter, most likely indicating pseudocapsule formation. Sclerosis at the tip of the prosthesis laterally indicates a normal pressure response, correlating with the focal tracer uptake in this region. There is no radiographic evidence of loosening of the prosthesis.

Differential Diagnosis

- Loosening
- Infection
- Postsurgical remodeling

Diagnosis and Clinical Follow-Up

The diagnosis was normal bony remodeling around a noncemented prosthesis. No other evidence of loosening of the prosthesis was found.

Discussion

The differentiation of loosening from the post-surgical remodeling of bone in a patient with a surgically implanted prosthesis is often a difficult task. Persistent tracer uptake on the bone scan may be seen for up to one year after surgery and even longer in the region of the greater trochanter when this area has sustained significant trauma.

PEARLS AND PITFALLS

- Focal uptake at the tip of the femoral component of a cemented prosthesis when accompanied by clinical symptoms raises the possibility of loosening.
- Focal tracer uptake at the tip of the femoral component of a noncemented prosthesis can be due to osteoblastic remodeling of the native bone in contact with the prosthesis. It may persist for years after surgery and is not always a sign of loosening.

Suggested Reading

Weissman BN. Imaging of total hip replacement. Radiology 1997;202(3):611–623

CASE 31

Clinical Presentation

A 17-year-old male adolescent presents with a history of low back pain of 5 months' duration. A bone scan is requested (**Figs. 31.1, 31.2,** and **31.3**).

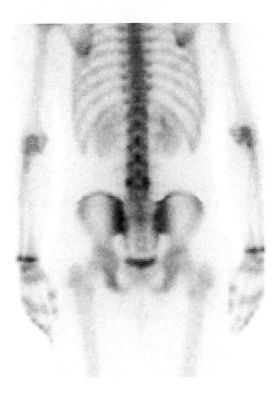

Fig. 31.1

Technique

- A 20 mCi dose of ^{99m}Tc-MDP is administered intravenously.
- Whole-body images of the skeleton are obtained 3 hours after tracer administration.
- A 1024 × 256 matrix is used for whole-body images.
- Emphasize the importance of oral hydration to improve soft tissue and bladder clearance.
- SPECT of the lumbar spine is obtained 4 hours after tracer injection: 64 stops, 25 seconds per stop, and a 360-degree rotation.

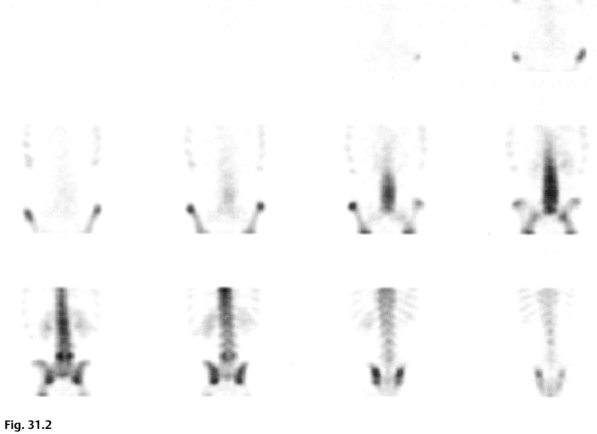

Fig. 31.2

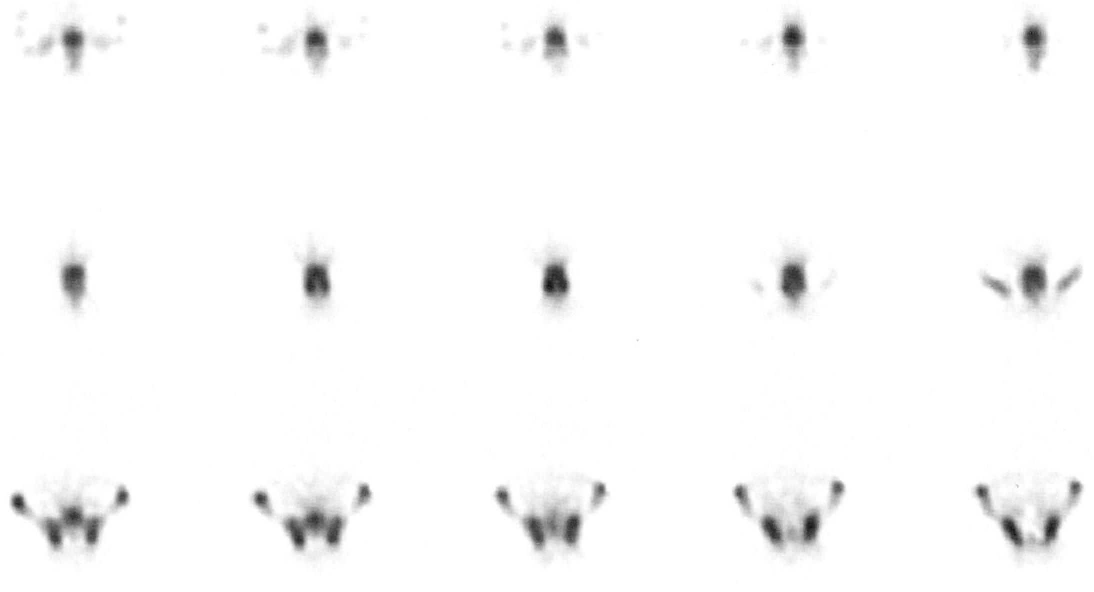

Fig. 31.3

Image Interpretation

A posterior whole-body view of the lumbar spine (**Fig. 31.1**) shows focally increased tracer uptake in the region of the pars interarticularis of the L4 vertebra. Coronal reconstructions of SPECT imaging of the lumbar spine (**Fig. 31.2**) show bilateral pars interarticularis defects at L4. Transverse reconstructions also show abnormal tracer uptake (**Fig. 31.3**).

Differential Diagnosis

*   Spondylolysis
*   Trauma
*   Osteomyelitis (unlikely to be bilateral)

Diagnosis and Clinical Follow-Up

The CT scan findings were diagnostic of pars interarticularis defects. No other follow-up was obtained.

Discussion

A defect in the pars interarticularis of a vertebra can often be seen on oblique radiographs of the spine. Bone scan, however, has a higher sensitivity for early diagnosis of spondylolysis, particularly when SPECT is used. It is not uncommon for the planar scintigraphic images to be normal and the SPECT images to show the site of an abnormality.

PEARLS AND PITFALLS

*   It is not uncommon to see focal tracer uptake on the side opposite a unilateral pars defect, presumably in response to the increased stress placed on the intact side.
*   If the planar images are normal, SPECT can often be helpful in detecting the pars defect.

Suggested Reading

Standaert CJ. The diagnosis and management of lumbar spondylolysis. Oper Tech Sports Med 2005;13:101–107

Section II

Cardiac Scintigraphy

Marcelo F. DiCarli and Mouaz H. Al-Mallah

CASE 32

Clinical Presentation

An 85-year-old woman with no known coronary artery disease (CAD) is referred for an exercise myocardial perfusion single-photon emission tomography (SPECT) study to evaluate for nonanginal chest pain. Her cardiac risk factors include hypertension. The resting electrocardiogram (ECG) shows normal sinus rhythm and nonspecific T-wave abnormalities. She is on lisinopril and hydrochlorothiazide at the time of testing.

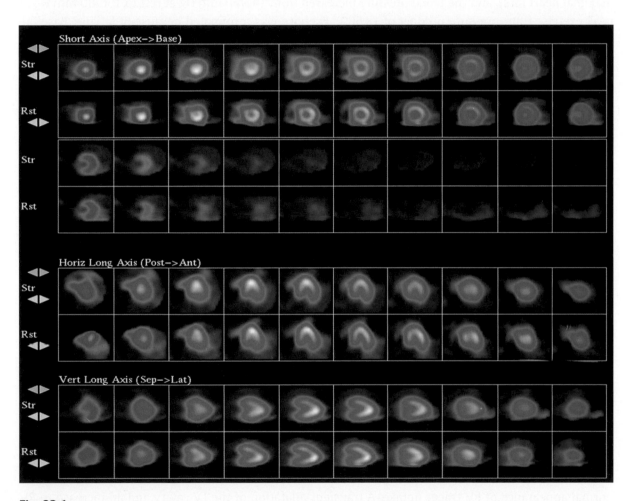

Fig. 32.1

Technique

- The patient had nothing to eat within 4 hours of the test.
- Rest images were acquired 40 minutes after the intravenous injection of 10 mCi of ^{99m}Tc-sestamibi. Images were acquired in the supine position with a two-headed gamma camera with step-and-shoot rotation, 32 projections over a 90-degree arc for each head (64 projections over a 180-degree arc), 30 seconds per projection, and a 64 × 64 matrix.
- Exercise: 9 minutes, 0 second on a Bruce protocol (10.1 METs [metabolic workloads]).

- Heart rate, blood pressure, and 12-lead ECG were recorded at baseline and every minute thereafter during stress.
- A 33 mCi dose of ^{99m}Tc-sestamibi was injected during peak stress.
- At 45 minutes after the exercise injection of radiotracer, image data were acquired with settings similar to those used for rest imaging. Gated images were acquired at 8 frames per cardiac cycle.
- Transverse images were reconstructed with a Butterworth filter (order of 5 and cutoff frequency of 0.792 cycles per pixel) for the rest and stress studies.

Image Interpretation

The heart rate increased from 59 beats/min at rest to a peak of 116 beats/min (86% of the age-predicted maximal heart rate), and the blood pressure increased from 140/60 mm Hg at rest to 160/80 mm Hg at peak exercise (rate-pressure product of 18,560). Exercise was terminated because of fatigue. Baseline ECG was normal. There were no symptoms of ischemia.

The perfusion images are shown in **Fig. 32.1.** No regional perfusion defect is seen on the stress or rest images. Gated SPECT demonstrates a post-stress left ventricular (LV) ejection fraction of more than 70% with normal LV volumes. There are no regional wall motion abnormalities.

Differential Diagnosis

- Normal perfusion scan
- Noncardiac chest pain

Diagnosis and Clinical Follow-Up

Normal stress test. The patient had no further clinical events.

Discussion: Systematic Approach to Interpreting SPECT Images

The systematic approach to interpreting cardiac SPECT images begins with a careful inspection of the projection images. These provide important information regarding patient motion, body habitus, gastrointestinal and hepatic uptake, breast and diaphragm position, and potential gating artifacts. The magnitude of radiotracer retention in the lungs can also be evaluated from the raw projections. Excessive retention of radiotracer in the lungs may be a sign of extensive myocardial ischemia (even in the absence of extensive perfusion defects). The projection images are also a source of potentially relevant extracardiac findings.

The first step in the interpretation of cardiac SPECT images is to make sure that the corresponding tomographic slices are well aligned. The LV and right ventricular (RV) sizes, both at rest and during stress, are then evaluated, as is the magnitude of tracer uptake in the RV free wall. This case shows the normal appearance of RV tracer uptake. A transient dilatation of the LV cavity and an increase in RV tracer uptake are generally associated with multiple-vessel CAD and therefore are important ancillary markers of increased risk.

It is recommended that the interpretation and semiquantification of regional tracer uptake follow the American Heart Association 17-segment model (**Fig. 32.2**). The LV apex is evaluated from the midvertical long-axis views, and the other LV segments are interpreted from the short-axis images, with use of the vertical long-axis and horizontal long-axis views to confirm, localize, and quantify the extent and severity of hypoperfusion. The American Society of Nuclear Cardiology/Society of Nuclear Medicine guidelines recommend that a visual scoring system be used to provide a semiquantitative

17-Segment Model of Left Ventricular Perfusion

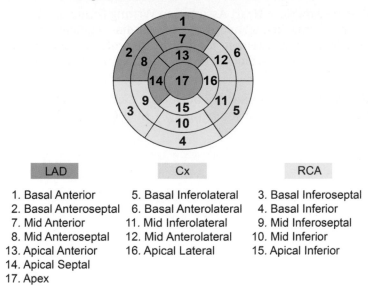

LAD	Cx	RCA
1. Basal Anterior	5. Basal Inferolateral	3. Basal Inferoseptal
2. Basal Anteroseptal	6. Basal Anterolateral	4. Basal Inferior
7. Mid Anterior	11. Mid Inferolateral	9. Mid Inferoseptal
8. Mid Anteroseptal	12. Mid Anterolateral	10. Mid Inferior
13. Apical Anterior	16. Apical Lateral	15. Apical Inferior
14. Apical Septal		
17. Apex		

Fig. 32.2

assessment of the extent of scar and ischemia. The recommended 4-point scoring system is as follows: normal, 0; mild defect, 1; moderate defect, 2; severe defect, 3; and defect equal to background activity, 4. These regional scores are then summed into global scores as follows: summed stress score (SSS, total perfusion defect during stress reflecting scar plus ischemia); summed rest score (SRS, total perfusion defect at rest reflecting scar); and summed difference score (SDS, difference between stress and rest reflecting ischemia). The global scores can also be expressed as percentage of myocardium abnormal, scarred, or ischemic by dividing the corresponding summed scores by 68, which is the maximum possible score (17 segments × 4). These semiquantitative scores are helpful to define the subsequent risk for death or myocardial infarction (see Cases 37 and 38).

Regional and global LV function is then evaluated from the gated images. The gated images are also useful to troubleshoot fixed perfusion defects and differentiate attenuation artifacts from myocardial scar. Finally, the report should clearly state whether the study result is normal or abnormal, describe the extent and severity of perfusion deficit, and provide a semiquantitative measure of the extent of abnormality (scar and/or ischemia). The conclusions should also include a brief discussion of the significance of the results in the context of the clinical history and results of the stress test.

PEARLS AND PITFALLS_____

- It is important to systematically review nuclear perfusion images and report perfusion and gated findings.
- The gated images are also useful to troubleshoot fixed perfusion defects and differentiate attenuation artifacts from myocardial scar.

Suggested Reading

Cerqueira MD, Weissman NJ, Dilsizian V, et al.; American Heart Association Writing Group on Myocardial Segmentation and Registration for Cardiac Imaging. Standardized myocardial segmentation and nomenclature for tomographic imaging of the heart: a statement for healthcare professionals from the Cardiac Imaging Committee of the Council on Clinical Cardiology of the American Heart Association. Circulation 2002;105(4):539–542

Hansen CL, Goldstein RA, Akinboboye OO, et al.; American Society of Nuclear Cardiology. Myocardial perfusion and function: single photon emission computed tomography. J Nucl Cardiol 2007;14(6): e39–e60

CASE 33

Clinical Presentation

A 60-year-old man is referred for the evaluation of atypical chest pain. There is no known prior cardiac history. The only risk factor for coronary artery disease is obesity. He is not on cardiac medications.

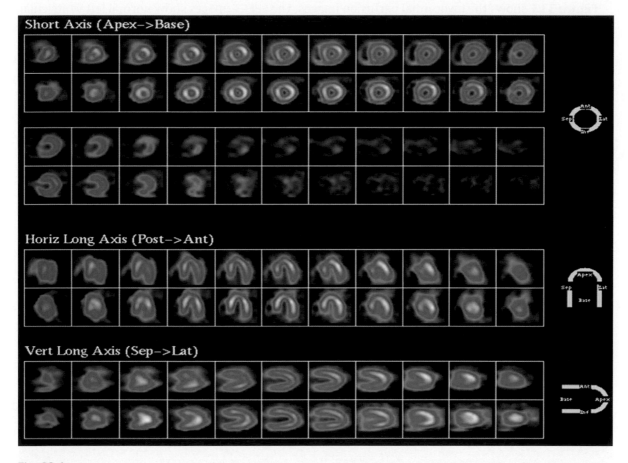

Fig. 33.1

Technique

- The patient had nothing to eat within 4 hours of the test.
- Rest images were acquired 40 minutes after the intravenous injection of 10 mCi of ^{99m}Tc-sestamibi.
- Images were acquired in the supine position with a two-headed gamma camera with step-and-shoot rotation, 32 projections over a 90-degree arc for each head (64 projections over a 180-degree arc), 30 seconds per projection, and a 64 × 64 matrix.
- Exercise: 10 minutes, 40 seconds on a Bruce protocol (12.8 METs [metabolic workloads]).
- Heart rate, blood pressure, and 12-lead ECG were recorded at baseline and every minute thereafter during stress.
- A 33 mCi dose of ^{99m}Tc-sestamibi was injected during peak stress.

- At 45 minutes after the exercise injection of radiotracer, stress images were acquired in a manner similar to that used for rest imaging. Gated images were acquired at 8 frames per cardiac cycle.
- Transverse images were reconstructed with a Butterworth filter (order of 5 and cutoff frequency of 0.792 cycles per pixel) for the rest and stress studies.

Image Interpretation

A hypertensive blood pressure response (increase from 130/75 to 230/90 mm Hg) was noted, and 96% of the age-predicted maximal heart rate was attained. Baseline ECG was normal. There were no symptoms of ischemia.

Figure 33.1 shows the myocardial perfusion images. The SPECT images show normal left ventricular (LV) and right ventricular size. There is a medium-size perfusion defect in the inferior and inferolateral walls, with complete reversibility. The gated images show normal regional and global LV function, suggesting no prior myocardial infarction.

Differential Diagnosis

- Inferior and inferolateral ischemia
- Artifact secondary to motion

Diagnosis and Clinical Follow-Up

Artifact secondary to motion. Careful inspection of the projection images (not shown) revealed patient motion during acquisition of the stress images. Repeated acquisition of the stress images (**Fig. 33.2**)

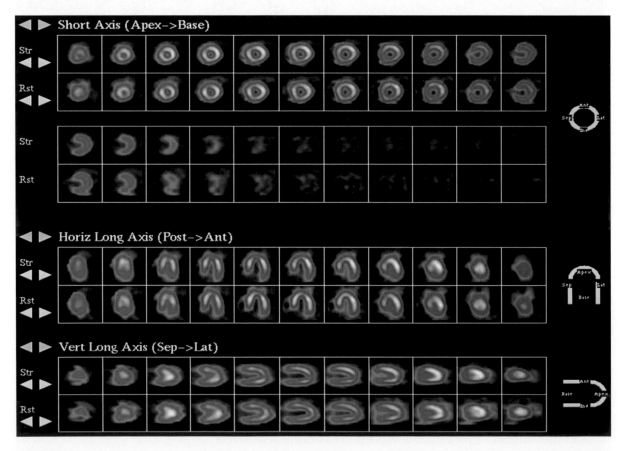

Fig. 33.2

demonstrated nearly complete resolution of the previously noted reversible defect. The repeated scan changed the study interpretation from abnormal to probably normal.

Discussion

When pronounced, patient motion frequently results in artifacts that may show as transient perfusion defects and apparent ischemia, changes in LV shape, and/or "hot spots." Sources of motion artifacts include exaggerated physiologic motion of the heart along its own axis, respiratory motion, and simple patient motion. Review of cine projection images will show patient motion and, as previously discussed, should be a routine and critical component of the quality control process. Patient motion in the Z axis can sometimes be corrected with motion correction software. More complex motion, however, often requires repeated acquisition of the images.

PEARLS AND PITFALLS

- Patient motion or isolated cardiac motion can cause focal areas of apparently decreased or increased tracer activity during image reconstruction.
- A review of cine projection images is critical in identifying motion artifact.

Suggested Reading

Cooper JA, Neumann PH, McCandless BK. Effect of patient motion on tomographic myocardial perfusion imaging. J Nucl Med 1992;33(8):1566–1571

Friedman J, Berman DS, Van Train K, et al. Patient motion in ^{201}Tl myocardial SPECT imaging: an easily identified frequent source of artifactual defect. Clin Nucl Med 1988;13(5):321–324

CASE 34

Clinical Presentation

A 56-year-old woman is referred for the evaluation of atypical chest pain. There is no known prior cardiac history. Risk factors include hypercholesterolemia and postmenopausal status. Medications are aspirin and simvastatin.

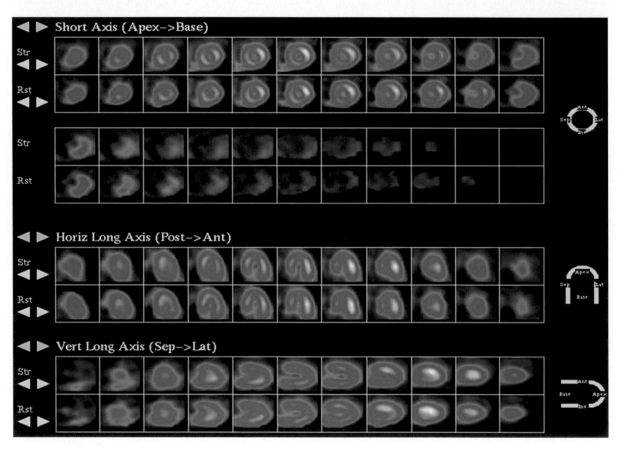

Fig. 34.1

Technique

- The patient had nothing to eat within 4 hours of the test.
- Rest images were acquired 40 minutes after the intravenous injection of 10 mCi of ^{99m}Tc-sestamibi. Images were acquired in the supine position with a two-headed gamma camera with step-and-shoot rotation, 32 projections over a 90-degree arc for each head (64 projections over a 180-degree arc), 30 seconds per projection, and a 64 × 64 matrix.
- Exercise: 10 minutes, 40 seconds on a Bruce protocol (12.8 METs [metabolic workloads]).
- Heart rate, blood pressure, and 12-lead ECG were recorded at baseline and every minute thereafter during stress.
- A 29 mCi dose of ^{99m}Tc-sestamibi was injected during peak stress.

- At 45 minutes after the exercise injection of radiotracer, images were acquired in a manner similar to that used for rest imaging. Gated images were acquired at 8 frames per cardiac cycle.
- Transverse images were reconstructed with a Butterworth filter (order of 5 and cutoff frequency of 0.792 cycles per pixel) for the rest and stress studies.

Image Interpretation

The blood pressure response (increase from 120/80 to 172/86 mm Hg) was appropriate, and 75% of the age-predicted maximal heart rate was obtained. Baseline ECG was normal. There were no symptoms of ischemia.

The raw images (not shown) revealed breast tissue overlying the heart. The myocardial perfusion images (**Fig. 34.1**) demonstrate a medium-size defect involving the mid and apical anterior and anteroseptal walls, which is fixed at rest. The gated images (not shown) demonstrate normal regional wall motion and thickening. The presence of normal regional wall motion and thickening in an area of fixed perfusion defect suggests an attenuation artifact, which in this case corresponds to breast tissue attenuation.

Differential Diagnosis

- Anterior myocardial infarction
- Artifact secondary to breast attenuation

Diagnosis and Clinical Follow-Up

Breast attenuation artifact. The patient had no further symptoms.

Discussion

See the discussion and suggested reading for Case 36.

PEARLS AND PITFALLS

- Breast attenuation may cause a fixed defect in the left anterior descending (LAD) coronary artery territory. Raw data and wall motion images should be carefully reviewed when LAD coronary artery defects are noted.
- Attenuation correction image processing may be helpful.

CASE 35

Clinical Presentation

A 58-year-old man presents with a history of coronary artery disease and prior percutaneous coronary intervention and stent placement in the right coronary artery. He has no chest pain or shortness of breath. Medications are aspirin, clopidogrel, β-blockers, and calcium channel blockers.

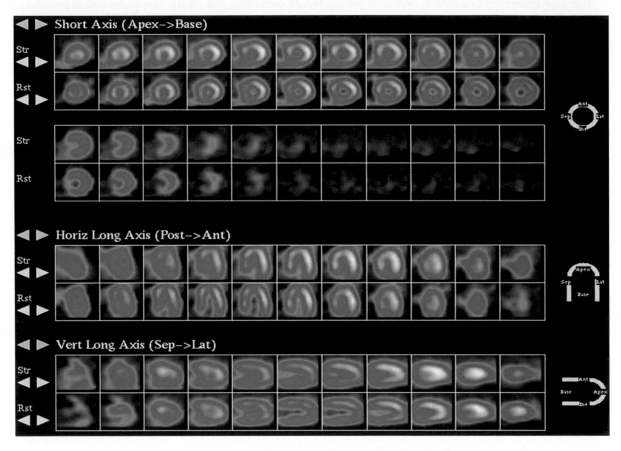

Fig. 35.1

Technique

- The patient had nothing to eat within 4 hours of the test.
- Rest images were acquired 40 minutes after the intravenous injection of 10 mCi of ^{99m}Tc-sestamibi. Images were acquired in the supine position with a two-headed gamma camera with step-and-shoot rotation, 32 projections over a 90-degree arc for each head (64 projections over a 180-degree arc), 30 seconds per projection, and a 64 × 64 matrix.
- Exercise: 9 minutes, 4 seconds on a Bruce protocol (12.8 METs [metabolic workloads]).
- Heart rate, blood pressure, and 12-lead ECG were recorded at baseline and every minute thereafter during stress.
- A 32 mCi dose of ^{99m}Tc-sestamibi was injected during peak stress.

- At 45 minutes after the exercise injection of radiotracer, stress images were acquired. A dual-head camera was used to acquire post-stress images in the supine position with 32 projections at 25 seconds per projection.
- Following post-stress supine imaging, post-stress prone imaging was obtained with 32 projections per head at 15 seconds per projection.
- Gated images were acquired at 8 frames per cardiac cycle.

Image Interpretation

The patient had symptoms of chest pain at peak exercise. A hypertensive blood pressure response (increase from 128/90 to 183/100 mm Hg) was recorded, and 69% of the age-predicted maximal heart rate was attained. The baseline ECG was normal, and the ECG response to exercise was nonischemic.

The myocardial perfusion images are shown in **Fig. 35.1**. The SPECT images show a medium-size perfusion defect of moderate intensity throughout the inferior and inferoseptal walls, which is essentially fixed. The gated images (not shown) demonstrated normal regional wall motion and thickening, making an inferior scar less likely.

Differential Diagnosis

- Inferior myocardial infarction
- Artifact secondary to diaphragmatic attenuation

Diagnosis and Clinical Follow-Up

Diaphragmatic attenuation artifact. Repeated imaging in the prone position (**Fig. 35.2**) shows complete resolution of the inferior and inferoseptal defects noted on images acquired in the supine position. The prone images also demonstrate a new mid and apical anterior defect, which is likely caused by attenuation by the imaging table.

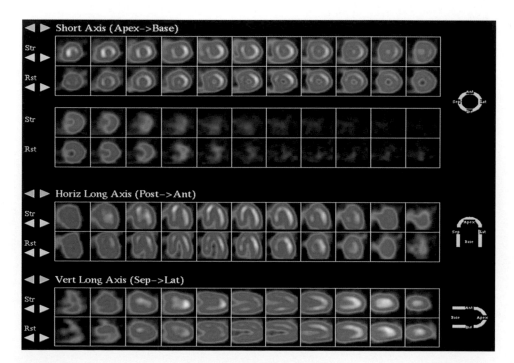

Fig. 35.2

Discussion

See discussion and suggested reading for Case 36.

PEARLS AND PITFALLS

- Diaphragmatic attenuation artifact usually results in a fixed inferior defect with normal inferior wall motion.
- Prone imaging helps to correct for this artifact in the inferior wall but may cause fixed anterior defects.

CASE 36

Clinical Presentation

A 68-year-old man is referred for the evaluation of atypical chest pain. The patient denies shortness of breath. His past medical history includes hypertension, atrial fibrillation, and diabetes. He is on aspirin, insulin, metoprolol, and a calcium channel blocker.

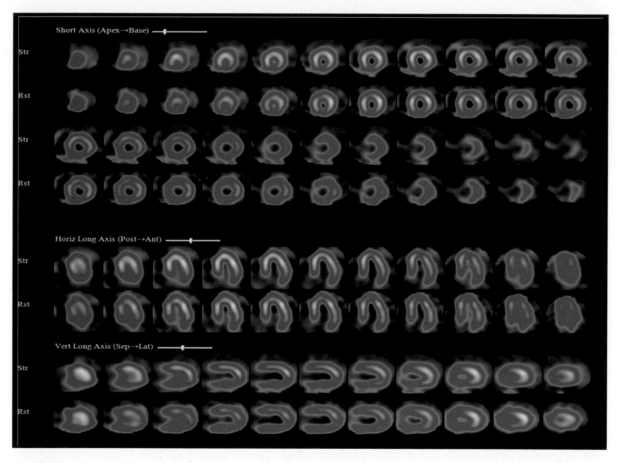

Fig. 36.1

Technique

- The patient had nothing to eat within 4 hours of the test. The β-blocker (metoprolol) was withheld on the day of the test. Caffeinated beverages were withheld for 24 hours before the test.
- Rest images were acquired 40 minutes after the intravenous injection of 10 mCi of ^{99m}Tc-sestamibi. Images were acquired in the supine position with a two-headed gamma camera with step-and-shoot rotation, 32 projections over a 90-degree arc for each head (64 projections over a 180-degree arc), 30 seconds per projection, and a 64 × 64 matrix.
- A 6-minute adenosine infusion was done.
- Heart rate, blood pressure, and 12-lead ECG were recorded at baseline and every minute thereafter during stress.
- A 28 mCi dose of ^{99m}Tc-sestamibi was injected during peak stress (at minute 3).

- Images were acquired 45 minutes after tracer injection. Acquisition protocols for post-stress supine imaging used 32 stops at 25 seconds per stop and a dual-head camera.
- The study was not gated because of the irregular heart rate caused by atrial fibrillation.
- CT images were obtained with a SPECT/CT system. A low-dose nongated CT scan of the chest was obtained for attenuation correction (AC) with the following parameters: scan length, 15 cm; rotation time, 0.5 second; total scan time, 3.9 seconds; tube voltage, 140 kV; and slice thickness, 5 mm. Attenuation correction was performed with the standard reconstruction software.

Image Interpretation

Chest pain was noted with adenosine. No ischemic ECG changes were seen. **Figure 36.1** shows perfusion images without AC. The SPECT images without AC show a perfusion defect throughout the inferior left ventricular (LV) wall, which is fixed. In this case, gated images were not available because of atrial fibrillation.

Differential Diagnosis

- Inferior myocardial infarction
- Artifact secondary to diaphragmatic attenuation

Diagnosis and Clinical Follow-Up

Images reprocessed (**Fig. 36.2**) with AC show complete resolution of the inferior wall defect. The study is considered normal.

Discussion

Cases 34 through 36 are typical examples of attenuation artifacts. Attenuation artifacts caused by breast tissue are related to a combination of breast size and degree of overlap over the LV, as well as breast tissue density. Breast attenuation can also be seen in male patients.

Diaphragmatic attenuation can be seen in men or women. It is more frequently seen in obese patients when elevation of the left hemidiaphragm causes the heart to adopt a more horizontal position within the chest. Acute gastric dilatation can occasionally cause a similar artifact. Diaphragmatic attenuation usually (although not always) causes a fixed perfusion defect.

Gated images are extremely helpful for differentiating attenuation artifacts from scar. In patients with marked diaphragmatic attenuation, prone imaging can also be helpful. In the prone position, the heart moves anteriorly, so that the inferior wall moves away from the diaphragm. The disadvantages of prone imaging are that the imaging table may cause anterior or apical defects and that additional image acquisition is required if it is done in combination with supine imaging.

Attenuation correction with the use of an external radionuclide source or CT is an effective way to troubleshoot attenuation artifacts. Numerous clinical studies during the past 10 years have shown increased diagnostic accuracy for detecting and localizing coronary artery disease in comparison with non-AC SPECT, particularly increasing test specificity and normalcy rate.

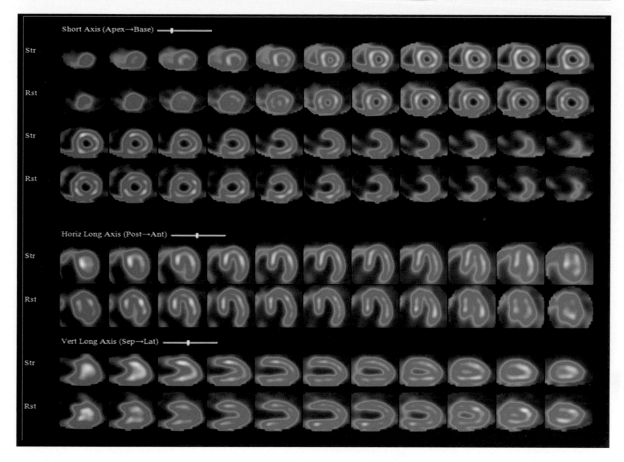

Fig. 36.2

PEARLS AND PITFALLS

- A fixed inferior defect caused by diaphragmatic attenuation artifact should be suspected if inferior wall motion is normal.
- Gating may not be possible in patients with an irregular heart rhythm, such as atrial fibrillation.
- Attenuation correction increases test specificity and normalcy rate.

Suggested Reading

Bateman TM, Cullom SJ. Attenuation correction single-photon emission computed tomography myocardial perfusion imaging. Semin Nucl Med 2005;35(1):37–51

Berman DS, Kang X, Nishina H, et al. Diagnostic accuracy of gated 99mTc sestamibi stress myocardial perfusion SPECT with combined supine and prone acquisitions to detect coronary artery disease in obese and nonobese patients. J Nucl Cardiol 2006;13(2):191–201

Choi JY, Lee KH, Kim SJ, et al. Gating provides improved accuracy for differentiating artifacts from true lesions in equivocal fixed defects on 99mTc tetrofosmin perfusion SPECT. J Nucl Cardiol 1998;5(4):395–401

Garcia EV. SPECT attenuation correction: an essential tool to realize nuclear cardiology's manifest destiny. J Nucl Cardiol 2007;14(1):16–24

Garver PR, Wasnich RD, Shibuya AM, Yeh F. Appearance of breast attenuation artifacts with thallium myocardial SPECT imaging. Clin Nucl Med 1985;10(10):694–696

Hansen CL, Goldstein RA, Akinboboye OO, et al; American Society of Nuclear Cardiology. Myocardial perfusion and function: single photon emission computed tomography. J Nucl Cardiol 2007;14(6): e39–e60

Nishina H, Slomka PJ, Abidov A, et al. Combined supine and prone quantitative myocardial perfusion SPECT: method development and clinical validation in patients with no known coronary artery disease. J Nucl Med 2006;47(1):51–58

Segall GM, Davis MJ. Prone versus supine thallium myocardial SPECT: a method to decrease artifactual inferior wall defects. J Nucl Med 1989;30(4):548–555

CASE 37

Clinical Presentation

A 56-year-old woman without a known cardiac history is referred for the evaluation of exertional chest pain. Her risk factors include hypertension and obesity. She is being treated with atenolol and amlodipine.

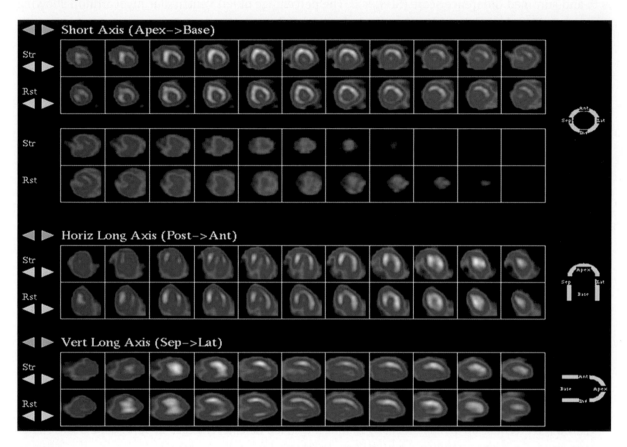

Fig. 37.1

Technique

- The patient had nothing to eat within 4 hours of the test. The β-blocker was withheld on the day of the test.
- On day 1, the patient exercised for 4 minutes on a Bruce protocol and achieved 96% of the age-predicted maximal heart rate. Heart rate, blood pressure, and 12-lead ECG were recorded at baseline and every minute thereafter during exercise.
- A 32 mCi dose of ^{99m}Tc-sestamibi was injected during peak stress.
- At 45 minutes after the exercise injection of radiotracer, supine images were obtained with a two-headed gamma camera with step-and-shoot rotation, 32 projections over a 90-degree arc for each head (64 projections over a 180-degree arc), 30 seconds per projection, and a 64 × 64 matrix. Gated images were acquired at 8 frames per cardiac cycle.
- On day 2, a 32 mCi dose of ^{99m}Tc-sestamibi was injected at rest. Rest images were acquired 40 minutes after injection with the imaging settings previously specified.

Image Interpretation

The blood pressure response was blunted (from 100/65 to 120/60 mm Hg). There were no ischemic symptoms during exercise. Baseline ECG was normal. There were no ischemic ECG changes with exercise.

Figure 37.1 shows the myocardial perfusion images. There is a severe, medium-size perfusion defect throughout the inferior and basal inferolateral walls, showing significant but not complete reversibility at rest. The finding is consistent with a moderate amount of exercise-induced ischemia in the posterior descending coronary artery territory. Her summed stress score (SSS) is 10, summed rest score (SRS) is 5, and summed difference score (SDS) is 5. The percentage of left ventricular myocardium showing ischemia is 7%, which is considered moderately abnormal.

Differential Diagnosis

- Inferior myocardial ischemia secondary to right coronary artery stenosis
- Inferior myocardial ischemia secondary to left circumflex coronary artery stenosis
- Attenuation artifact

Diagnosis and Clinical Follow-Up

The patient continued to have symptoms and underwent coronary angiography, which showed 90% stenosis in the left circumflex coronary artery.

Discussion

See discussion and suggested reading in Case 38.

PEARLS AND PITFALLS

- Inferior ischemia results from obstructive disease in the right coronary artery or left circumflex coronary artery.
- Patients with mildly or moderately abnormal scans generally fare better with medical therapy (unless their symptoms are poorly controlled).
- Although attenuation artifacts usually manifest as fixed defects, changes in soft tissue position between rest and stress studies can mimic reversible perfusion abnormalities.

CASE 38

Clinical Presentation

A 61-year-old man with known coronary artery disease (CAD), prior myocardial infarction, and revascularization is referred for myocardial perfusion imaging to evaluate risk before thoracic surgery. The patient denies any chest pain or shortness of breath. His risk factors include diabetes and hypertension. His medications include metoprolol, enalapril, atorvastatin, aspirin, clopidogrel, and insulin.

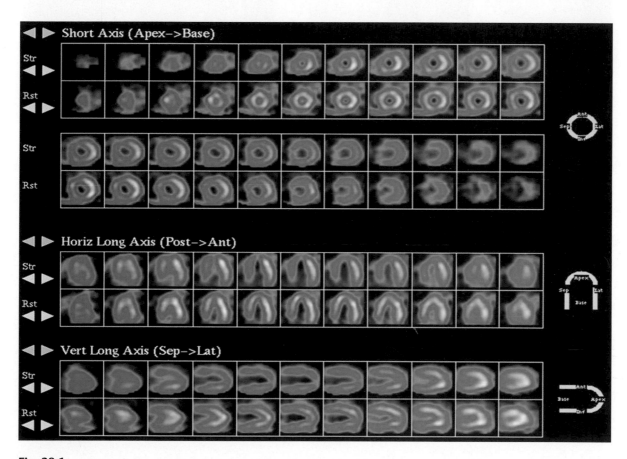

Fig. 38.1

Technique

- The patient had nothing to eat within 4 hours of the test. The β-blocker (metoprolol) was withheld the day of the test. Caffeine-containing beverages were withheld for 24 hours before the test.
- Rest images were acquired 40 minutes after the intravenous injection of 11 mCi of ^{99m}Tc-sestamibi. Images were acquired in the supine position with a two-headed gamma camera with step-and-shoot rotation, 32 projections over a 90-degree arc for each head (64 projections over a 180-degree arc), 30 seconds per projection, and a 64 × 64 matrix.
- Vasodilator stress was done with adenosine infused over 4 minutes.

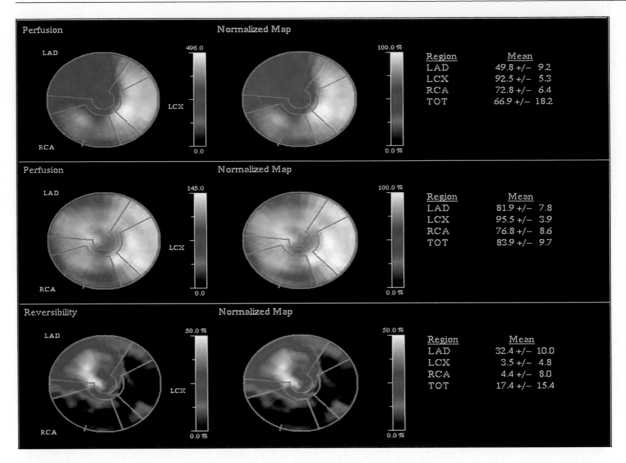

Fig. 38.2

- Heart rate, blood pressure, and 12-lead ECG were recorded at baseline and every minute thereafter during stress.
- A 32 mCi dose of ^{99m}Tc-sestamibi was injected during peak stress (at minute 2).
- At 45 minutes after tracer injection, images were obtained with 32 projections over a 90-degree arc for each head of the gamma camera (64 projections over a 180-degree arc), 30 seconds per projection, and a 64 × 64 matrix. Gated images were acquired at 8 frames per cardiac cycle.

Image Interpretation

There were no symptoms of chest pain or shortness of breath. The blood pressure decreased from 156/67 to 142/66 mm Hg during stress. The baseline ECG was normal. There were no ischemic ECG changes during stress. Transient atrioventricular block was noted.

Figure 38.1 shows the myocardial perfusion images. There is evidence of transient left ventricular (LV) dilatation during adenosine stress. There is a large, severe perfusion defect throughout the anterior and anteroseptal walls and the LV apex, which shows complete reversibility at rest. The summed stress score (SSS) is 23, the summed rest score (SRS) is 0, and the summed difference score (SDS) is 23. The percentage of LV myocardium showing ischemia is 34% (see discussion in Case 36), which is considered severely abnormal and is seen easily in the polar plots in **Fig. 38.2**. This finding is consistent with extensive stress-induced ischemia throughout the left anterior descending (LAD) coronary territory.

Differential Diagnosis

•   Proximal anterior myocardial ischemia secondary to LAD coronary artery stenosis

Diagnosis and Clinical Follow-Up

The patient underwent coronary angiography, which showed 90% stenosis in the LAD coronary artery.

Discussion

The importance of using global scores (ie, SSS, SRS, and SDS; see earlier) derived from a detailed segmental analysis of the perfusion images, rather than simply categorizing scan results as normal or abnormal, to assess clinical risk is supported by a wealth of clinical evidence. Indeed, it is well established that the percentage of myocardium with abnormality or ischemia is linearly related to the risk for subsequent death or myocardial infarction and is thus a powerful marker of prognosis. There is consistent evidence that a normal myocardial perfusion scan is generally associated with an excellent prognosis. In risk-adjusted analysis, patients with mild or moderate ischemia (see Case 37) have a low to intermediate clinical risk, whereas patients with severe scar and/or ischemia (Case 38) are at high risk for death or myocardial infarction. In addition, ancillary findings, including transient ischemic cavity dilatation, increased right ventricular (RV) tracer uptake, and increased pulmonary uptake, are also markers of increased clinical risk. In a risk-based approach to management, patients with mildly or moderately abnormal scans generally fare better with medical therapy (unless their symptoms are poorly controlled), whereas patients with severely abnormal scans showing extensive ischemia have improved outcomes with revascularization. This risk-based approach to the management of CAD based on myocardial perfusion results is also cost-effective.

PEARLS AND PITFALLS_____

•   Patients with severe scar and/or ischemia are at high risk for death or myocardial infarction
•   Transient ischemic cavity dilatation, increased RV tracer uptake, and increased pulmonary uptake are also markers of increased clinical risk.

Suggested Reading

Chouraqui P, Rodrigues EA, Berman DS, Maddahi J. Significance of dipyridamole-induced transient dilation of the left ventricle during thallium-201 scintigraphy in suspected coronary artery disease. Am J Cardiol 1990;66(7):689–694

DePace NL, Iskandrian AS, Hakki AH, Kane SA, Segal BL. Value of left ventricular ejection fraction during exercise in predicting the extent of coronary artery disease. J Am Coll Cardiol 1983;1(4):1002–1010

Gill JB, Ruddy TD, Newell JB, Finkelstein DM, Strauss HW, Boucher CA. Prognostic importance of thallium uptake by the lungs during exercise in coronary artery disease. N Engl J Med 1987;317(24):1486–1489

Hachamovitch R, Hayes SW, Friedman JD, Cohen I, Berman DS. Comparison of the short-term survival benefit associated with revascularization compared with medical therapy in patients with no prior coronary artery disease undergoing stress myocardial perfusion single photon emission computed tomography. Circulation 2003;107(23):2900–2907

Shaw LJ, Hachamovitch R, Berman DS, et al; Economics of Noninvasive Diagnosis (END) Multicenter Study Group. The economic consequences of available diagnostic and prognostic strategies for the evaluation of stable angina patients: an observational assessment of the value of precatheterization ischemia. J Am Coll Cardiol 1999;33(3):661–669

Weiss AT, Berman DS, Lew AS, et al. Transient ischemic dilation of the left ventricle on stress thallium-201 scintigraphy: a marker of severe and extensive coronary artery disease. J Am Coll Cardiol 1987;9(4):752–759

CASE 39

Clinical Presentation

A 57-year-old man with no known coronary artery disease is referred for a dobutamine myocardial perfusion PET/CT study to evaluate for atypical chest pain and dyspnea. His risk factors include hypertension and diabetes. He also has asthma and uses an albuterol inhaler daily. A resting ECG shows normal sinus rhythm and a right bundle branch block. He is also on aspirin at the time of testing.

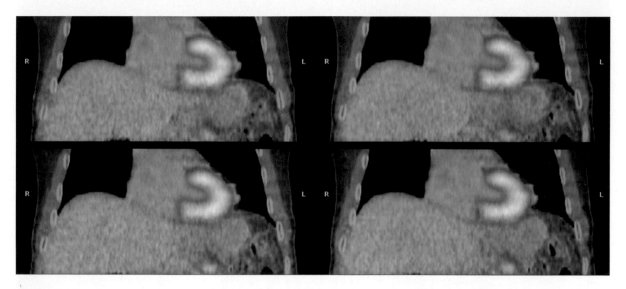

Fig. 39.1

Technique

- The patient had nothing to eat within 4 hours of the study.
- After a scout CT acquisition (120 kVp, 10 mA) for patient positioning, a CT transmission scan (140 kVp, 30 mA, pitch of 1.35) was acquired for attenuation correction. Commercial software was used for coregistration of the transmission and emission images.
- Rest emission images were obtained after the intravenous administration of 55 mCi of ^{82}Rb at rest. Imaging began 90 seconds after completion of the radionuclide infusion for a total imaging time of 5 minutes.
- Gated images were acquired with 8-frame gating.
- Images were reconstructed with ordered subsets expectation maximization (OSEM; 2 iterations and 30 subsets), and a three-dimensional PET filter was used (Butterworth filter cutoff frequency of 10, order of 5).
- After the rest image acquisition, a standard infusion of dobutamine (to a peak of 40 mcg/kg per minute) was done with an additional 0.2 mg of atropine. The heart rate increased from 46 beats/min at rest to a peak of 139 beats/min (85% of the age-predicted maximal heart rate), and the blood pressure increased from 110/63 mm Hg at rest to 138/63 mm Hg at peak stress. The infusion was terminated after 4 minutes.
- A 55 mCi dose of ^{82}Rb was injected during peak stress.

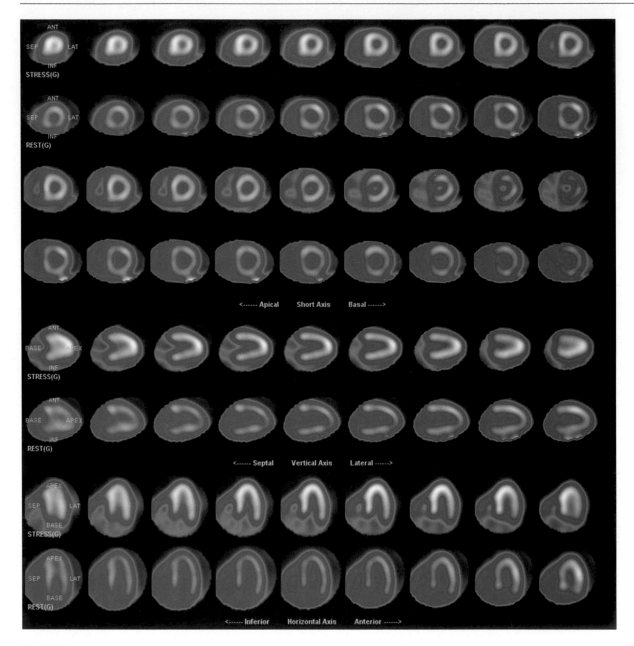

Fig 39.2

- Similarly, stress emission images were begun 90 seconds after completion of the radionuclide infusion and continued for 5 minutes.
- Another CT scan was obtained after completion of the stress PET emission scan. A CT transmission scan of the chest area was done with the following parameters: scan length, 15 cm; rotation time, 0.5 second; total scan time, 3.9 seconds; tube voltage, 140 kV; tube current, 30 mA; and slice thickness, 5 mm.

Image Interpretation

The clinical response to dobutamine was nonischemic. The blood pressure response was normal. The ECG response to dobutamine was nonischemic.

Figure 39.1 shows the fused CT and perfusion images to evaluate the quality of image coregistration and attenuation correction. **Figure 39.2** shows myocardial perfusion. The quality of the registration between the CT and perfusion images is excellent. The myocardial perfusion images demonstrate normal left ventricular (LV) and right ventricular (RV) size and normal RV tracer uptake. There are no regional perfusion defects seen on the stress or rest images. The gated PET images demonstrate a post-stress LV ejection fraction of more than 70% with normal LV volumes.

Differential Diagnosis

- Normal perfusion PET scan
- Nonischemic chest pain

Diagnosis and Clinical Follow-Up

Normal stress PET test. The patient had no further clinical evidence of ischemia.

Discussion

The PET images should be interpreted with the same systematic approach described in Case 34. In the interpretation of cardiac PET/CT studies, however, it is critical to review the quality of the transmission-emission image alignment to maintain the accuracy of the interpretation of the reconstructed images. When misalignment is present, proper correction should be performed before interpretation of the reconstructed images.

PEARLS AND PITFALLS

- Patients with normal PET scans have a good prognosis.
- When cardiac PET/CT studies are interpreted, it is critical to review the quality of the transmission-emission image alignment.

Suggested Reading

Bengel FM, Higuchi T, Javadi MS, Lautamäki R. Cardiac positron emission tomography. J Am Coll Cardiol 2009;54(1):1–15

Di Carli MF, Dorbala S, Meserve J, El Fakhri G, Sitek A, Moore SC. Clinical myocardial perfusion PET/CT. J Nucl Med 2007;48(5):783–793

CASE 40

Clinical Presentation

A 60-year-old man with no known coronary artery disease is referred for a dipyridamole myocardial perfusion PET study to evaluate for atypical chest pain. Cardiac risk factors include hypertension. The resting ECG is normal. Medications include atenolol and aspirin.

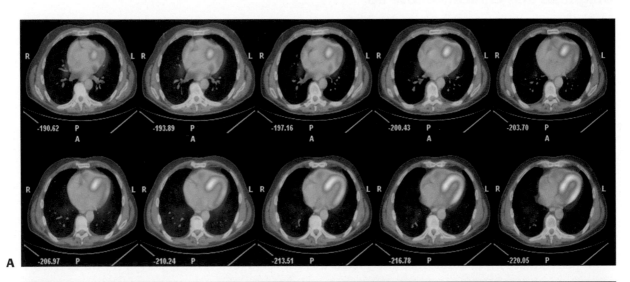

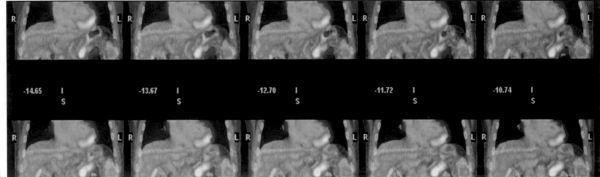

Fig. 40.1

Technique

- The patient had nothing to eat within 4 hours of the test. The β-blocker (atenolol) was withheld on the day of the test. Caffeinated beverages were withheld for 24 hours before the test.
- After a scout CT acquisition (120 kVp, 10 mA) for patient positioning, a CT transmission scan (140 kVp, 30 mA, pitch of 1.35) was acquired for attenuation correction. Commercial software was used for coregistration of the transmission and emission images.
- Rest emission images were obtained after the intravenous administration of 50 mCi of ^{82}Rb at rest. Imaging began 90 seconds after completion of the radionuclide infusion for a total imaging time of 5 minutes.

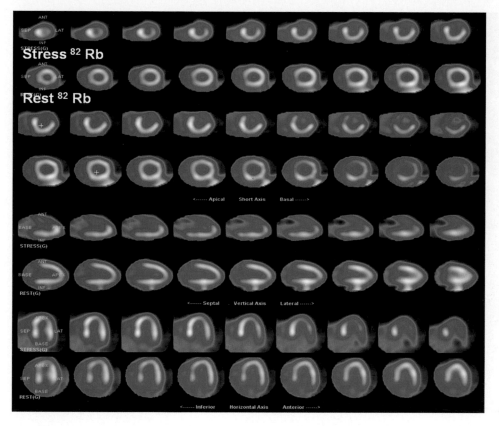

Fig. 40.2

- Gated images were acquired at 8 frames per cardiac cycle.
- Images were reconstructed with ordered subsets expectation maximization (OSEM; 2 iterations and 30 subsets), and a three-dimensional PET filter was used (Butterworth filter cutoff frequency of 10, order of 5).
- After rest image acquisition, vasodilator stress was achieved with a standard intravenous infusion of dipyridamole (0.14 mg/kg per minute) for 4 minutes.
- At 7 minutes after the start of the dipyridamole infusion, 50 mCi of ^{82}Rb was injected.
- Stress emission images were obtained for 5 minutes in a fashion similar to that used for the exercise images beginning 90 seconds after completion of the radionuclide infusion. Another CT scan was obtained after completion of the stress PET emission scan. A CT transmission scan of the heart was done with the following parameters: scan length, 15 cm; rotation time, 0.5 second; total scan time, 3.9 seconds; tube voltage, 140 kV; tube current, 30 mA; and slice thickness, 5 mm.

Image Interpretation

The heart rate increased from 61 beats/min at rest to a peak of 68 beats/min, and the blood pressure decreased from 182/82 mm Hg at rest to 175/90 mm Hg at peak stress. The clinical and ECG responses to dipyridamole were nonischemic.

Figure 40.1 shows the fused CT and perfusion images to evaluate the quality of the registration and attenuation correction. **Figure 40.2** shows myocardial perfusion. The CT transmission and emission images (**Fig. 40.1**) demonstrate a clear misalignment between the two data sets, with the anterolateral wall of the emission images overlapping the lung field. An apparently reversible perfusion deficit is shown on the myocardial perfusion images (**Fig. 40.2**).

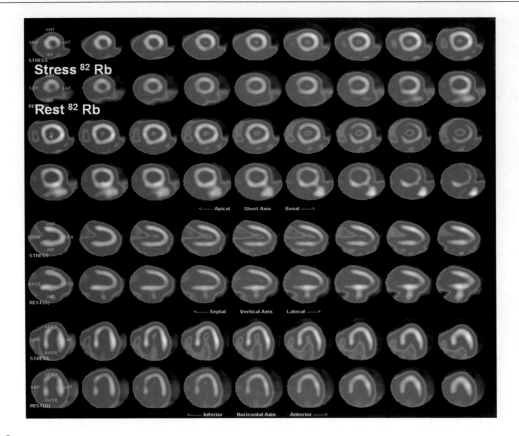

Fig. 40.3

Differential Diagnosis

- Abnormal perfusion PET scan with anterior ischemia
- Misregistration artifact

Diagnosis and Clinical Follow-Up

After proper correction of the misalignment, there is complete resolution of the defect, with a clearly normal study (**Fig. 40.3**). The gated PET study demonstrated a rest left ventricular (LV) ejection fraction of 60%, and the LV ejection fraction during peak stress was 76%.

Discussion

Misregistration of transmission and emission images is usually the result of differences in breathing patterns during CT and PET imaging. This misregistration can lead to an undercorrection of the anterior or anterolateral LV segments. When this occurs on the stress images, it can result in an inaccurate study interpretation (false-positive defects). In a study of 1,177 consecutive diagnostic myocardial perfusion PET studies, 252 (21.4%) had artifactual defects due to attenuation-emission misregistration. Misregistration can produce anterior, anterolateral, or inferolateral fixed or reversible defects. Most commercial PET/CT systems now include software tools to correct for transmission-emission misalignments.

PEARLS AND PITFALLS

- Misregistration of transmission and emission images can result in false-positive defects.
- When misalignment is present, proper correction should be performed before interpretation of the perfusion images.

Suggested Reading

Di Carli MF, Dorbala S, Meserve J, El Fakhri G, Sitek A, Moore SC. Clinical myocardial perfusion PET/CT. J Nucl Med 2007;48(5):783–793

Gould KL, Pan T, Loghin C, Johnson NP, Guha A, Sdringola S. Frequent diagnostic errors in cardiac PET/CT due to misregistration of CT attenuation and emission PET images: a definitive analysis of causes, consequences, and corrections. J Nucl Med 2007;48(7):1112–1121

CASE 41

Clinical Presentation

A 72-year-old woman with known coronary artery disease (CAD) and prior myocardial infarction is referred for a dipyridamole myocardial perfusion PET study to evaluate nonanginal chest pain. Her cardiac risk factors include hypertension and known CAD. The resting ECG shows normal sinus rhythm, poor R-wave progression, and nonspecific T-wave abnormalities. She is on diltiazem, hydrochlorothiazide, and aspirin at the time of testing.

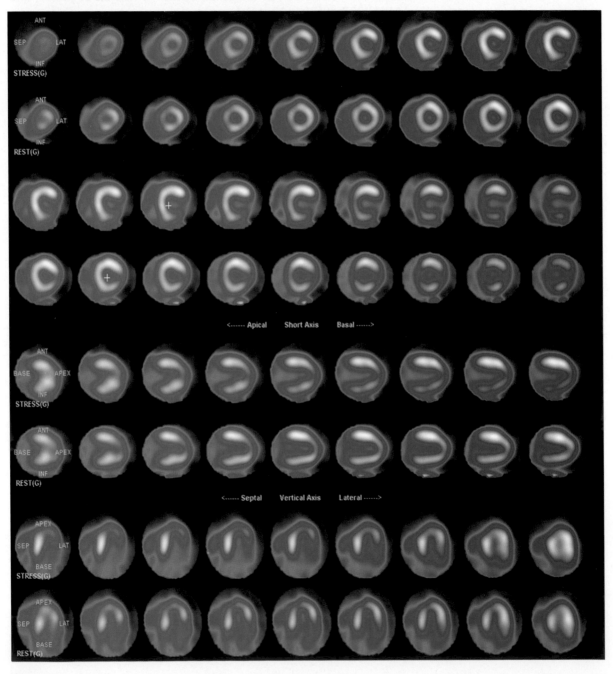

Fig. 41.1

Technique

- The patient had nothing to eat within 4 hours of the test. Caffeinated beverages were withheld for 24 hours before the test.
- After a scout CT acquisition (120 kVp, 10 mA) for patient positioning, a CT transmission scan (140 kVp, 30 mA, pitch of 1.35) was acquired for attenuation correction. Commercial software was used for coregistration of the transmission and emission images.
- A 60 mCi dose of ^{82}Rb was administered at rest.
- Resting images were obtained 90 seconds after completion of the radionuclide infusion for a total of 5 minutes. Resting gated images were acquired at 8 frames per cycle.
- PET images were reconstructed with ordered subsets expectation maximization (OSEM; 2 iterations and 30 subsets), and a three-dimensional PET filter was used (Butterworth filter cutoff frequency of 10, order of 5).
- Vasodilator stress was achieved with a standard intravenous infusion of dipyridamole (0.14 mg/kg per minute) for 4 minutes.
- A 60 mCi dose of 82Rb was injected 7 minutes after the start of the dipyridamole infusion. Stress emission images were obtained for 5 minutes beginning 90 seconds after completion of the radionuclide infusion. Stress gated images were acquired at 8 frames per cycle.
- A CT scan was obtained after completion of the stress PET emission scan. The CT transmission scan of the heart was done with the following parameters: scan length, 15 cm; rotation time, 0.5 second; total scan time, 3.9 seconds; tube voltage, 140 kV; tube current, 30 mA; and slice thickness, 5 mm.

Image Interpretation

The heart rate increased from 73 beats/min at rest to a peak of 86 beats/min, and the blood pressure decreased from 114/64 mm Hg at rest to 110/65 mm Hg at peak infusion of the vasodilator. There were no symptoms or ischemic ECG findings.

The perfusion images shown in **Fig. 41.1** demonstrate a normal left ventricular (LV) size and normal tracer uptake in the lungs. A medium-to-large defect of severe intensity throughout the inferolateral wall and the basal anterolateral wall is nearly completely reversible at rest. The combined extent and severity of ischemia plus scar during stress is severely abnormal (summed stress score [SSS], 14). The magnitude of reversible ischemia from stress to rest is also severely abnormal (summed difference score [SDS], 11). Gated PET demonstrates a left ventricular ejection fraction (LVEF) of 63% at rest and 55% at peak stress (images not shown). There is akinesis of the basal inferolateral, midinferolateral, and basal anterolateral ventricular walls during peak stress that resolves at rest.

Differential Diagnosis

- Abnormal perfusion PET scan with lateral ischemia
- Misregistration artifact

Diagnosis and Clinical Follow-Up

Because of the large area of ischemia and other high-risk features, a cardiac catheterization was done, which showed three-vessel disease: an 80% lesion in the mid-left anterior descending coronary artery, a 100% lesion in the mid-circumflex coronary artery, and 95% lesion in the distal right coronary artery. The patient underwent angioplasty to her right coronary artery and left circumflex coronary artery.

Discussion

This scan demonstrates a large, severe dipyridamole-induced perfusion abnormality in the distribution of the proximal left circumflex coronary artery, consistent with the presence of flow-limiting coronary stenosis. This study also shows a drop in the ejection fraction at peak vasodilation, another high-risk finding. ECG gating provides a unique opportunity to assess LV function at rest and *during peak stress* (as opposed to *after stress* with gated SPECT). Recent data suggest that in normal subjects, the LVEF increases during peak vasodilator stress. In the presence of CAD, however, changes in the LVEF (from baseline to peak stress) are inversely related to the magnitude of perfusion abnormalities during stress (reflecting myocardium at risk) and the extent of angiographic CAD.

PEARLS AND PITFALLS

*   The drop in ejection fraction at peak vasodilation is a high-risk feature on PET.
*   In patients with three-vessel or left main CAD, the LVEF during peak stress can decrease, even in the absence of apparent perfusion abnormalities.

Suggested Reading

Dorbala S, Vangala D, Sampson U, Limaye A, Kwong R, Di Carli MF. Value of vasodilator left ventricular ejection fraction reserve in evaluating the magnitude of myocardium at risk and the extent of angiographic coronary artery disease: a 82Rb PET/CT study. J Nucl Med 2007;48(3):349–358

CASE 42

Clinical Presentation

A 74-year-old man with known coronary artery disease (CAD) and prior myocardial infarction (MI) is referred for a dipyridamole myocardial perfusion PET study for post-MI evaluation. Cardiac risk factors include hypertension and dyslipidemia. The resting ECG shows normal sinus rhythm and anterior and lateral Q waves. Medications include a β–blocker, an angiotensin-converting enzyme inhibitor, aspirin, a statin, and clopidogrel.

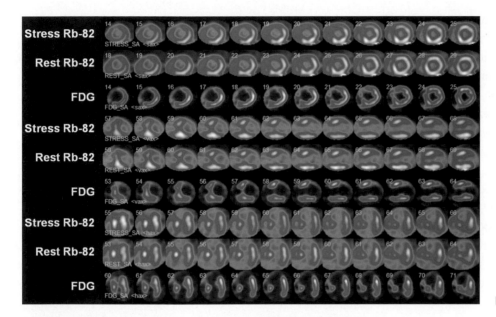

Fig. 42.1

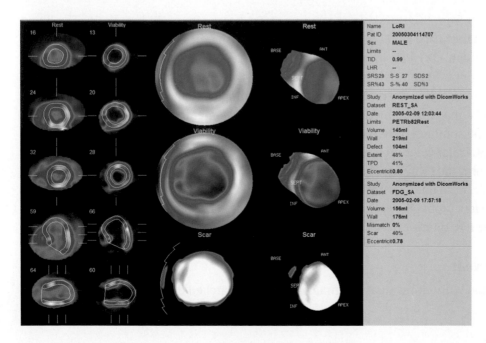

Fig. 42.2

Technique

- The patient had nothing to eat within 4 hours of the test. The β–blocker was withheld on the day of the test. Caffeinated beverages were withheld for 24 hours before the test.
- After a scout computed tomographic (CT) acquisition (120 kVp, 10 mA) for patient positioning, a CT transmission scan (140 kVp, 30 mA, pitch of 1.35) was acquired for attenuation correction. Commercial software was used for coregistration of the transmission and emission images.
- Rest emission images were obtained for 5 minutes after the intravenous administration of 60 mCi of ^{82}Rb at rest, with imaging starting 120 seconds (given the low ejection fraction) after completion of the radionuclide infusion. Rest gated images were acquired at 8 frames per cycle.
- PET images were reconstructed with ordered subsets expectation maximization (OSEM; 2 iterations and 30 subsets), and a three-dimensional PET filter was used (Butterworth filter cutoff frequency of 10, order of 5).
- Vasodilator stress was achieved with a standard intravenous infusion of dipyridamole (0.14 mg/kg per minute) for 4 minutes.
- The patient was injected with 60 mCi of ^{82}Rb during peak stress 7 minutes after the start of the dipyridamole infusion. Stress emission images were then obtained and processed in a manner similar to that used for the rest images.
- Another CT scan was obtained after completion of the stress PET scan. The CT transmission scan of the chest area was done with the following parameters: scan length, 15 cm; rotation time, 0.5 second; total scan time, 3.9 seconds; tube voltage, 140 kV; tube current, 30 mA; and slice thickness, 5 mm.
- The patient received 50 g of oral Trutol (glucose tolerance beverage) and a total of 20 U of regular insulin intravenously to optimize the myocardial utilization of glucose. The patient was then injected with 9.5 mCi of FDG, and 30 minutes later (to allow FDG trapping in the myocardium), gated PET imaging was acquired with 8-frame gating.
- A third CT scan was obtained after completion of the FDG PET scan. A CT transmission scan of the chest area was done with the same parameters as those previously described.

Image Interpretation

The heart rate decreased from 86 beats/min at rest to a stress heart rate of 74 beats/min. The blood pressure remained unchanged at 133/72 mm Hg. There were no ischemic changes on the ECG.

Rest-stress perfusion and FDG PET images are shown in **Fig. 42.1**. The polar maps are shown in **Fig. 42.2**. There is a large perfusion defect of severe intensity in the mid anterior wall, septum, and left ventricular (LV) apex, which is fixed at rest. This defect is completely matched on the FDG images (reduced perfusion and a matched reduction in myocardial glucose metabolism). The summed stress score (SSS) is 27, and the summed difference score (SDS) is 0. Gated PET images (not shown) demonstrate a resting left ventricular ejection fraction (LVEF) of 40%. The LVEF during peak stress is 41%. The mid anterior wall, septum, and LV apex are akinetic, with reduced wall thickening. The right ventricular (RV) function is normal. These findings are consistent with a region of myocardial scar without residual ischemia and suggest a low probability of significant improvement in regional wall motion if successful revascularization of the left anterior descending (LAD) coronary artery territory can be performed.

Differential Diagnosis

- Myocardial infarction without residual ischemia or viability (matched defect).

Diagnosis and Clinical Follow-Up

Given the lack of viability in the anterior wall, the patient was continued on medical therapy, with no revascularization planned.

Discussion

^{18}F-FDG-PET is an important diagnostic tool for detecting myocardial viability in patients with CAD and LV dysfunction. Normal myocardium utilizes fatty acids for its energy requirements. Insulin is needed to enhance the myocardial utilization of FDG. This is achieved by giving the patient a sugar load. Once the insulin level peaks (as suggested by a drop in the serum sugar level), the patient is injected with ^{18}F-FDG. A mismatch pattern with reduced perfusion and enhanced FDG uptake indicates viable myocardium. Conversely, a matched pattern with concordant reduction in FDG uptake and myocardial perfusion is indicative of scar tissue.

PEARLS AND PITFALLS

- Patients with matched defects have a low probability of significant improvement in regional wall motion following revascularization.

Suggested Reading

Di Carli MF, Davidson M, Little R, et al. Value of metabolic imaging with positron emission tomography for evaluating prognosis in patients with coronary artery disease and left ventricular dysfunction. Am J Cardiol 1994;73(8):527–533

Di Carli MF, Asgarzadie F, Schelbert HR, et al. Quantitative relation between myocardial viability and improvement in heart failure symptoms after revascularization in patients with ischemic cardiomyopathy. Circulation 1995;92(12):3436–3444

Schinkel AF, Poldermans D, Elhendy A, Bax JJ. Assessment of myocardial viability in patients with heart failure. J Nucl Med 2007;48(7):1135–1146

Sheikine Y, Di Carli MF. Integrated PET/CT in the assessment of etiology and viability in ischemic heart failure. Curr Heart Fail Rep 2008;5(3):136–142

CASE 43

Clinical Presentation

A 68-year-old woman presents with a 1-week history of exertional chest pain and shortness of breath. She is found to have heart failure, with an ejection fraction of 20%. The troponin level is elevated to 0.16 ng/mL, with lateral T-wave inversions on ECG. She is referred for PET to assess for myocardial viability and potential coronary revascularization.

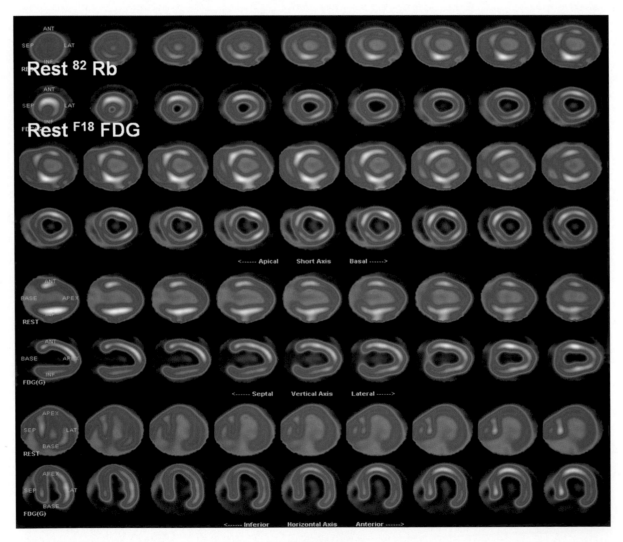

Fig. 43.1

Technique

- The patient had nothing to eat within 4 hours of the test.
- After a scout CT acquisition (120 kVp, 10 mA) for patient positioning, a CT transmission scan (140 kVp, 30 mA, pitch of 1.35) was acquired for attenuation correction. Commercial software was used for coregistration of the transmission and emission images.
- The patient underwent a rest myocardial perfusion PET study. Rest emission images were obtained after the intravenous administration of 60 mCi of ^{82}Rb, with imaging starting at 120 seconds (given the low ejection fraction) after completion of the radionuclide infusion and continued for 5 minutes. Rest gated images were acquired at 8 frames per cycle.
- PET images were reconstructed with ordered subsets expectation maximization (OSEM; 2 iterations and 30 subsets), and a three-dimensional PET filter was used (Butterworth filter cutoff frequency of 10, order of 5).
- After the rest image acquisition, the patient received 25 g of oral Trutol (glucose tolerance beverage) and a total of 9 U of regular insulin intravenously to optimize myocardial utilization of glucose.
- An 11 mCi dose of FDG was injected, with imaging 30 minutes later (to allow FDG trapping in the myocardium).
- Gated PET imaging was acquired at 8 frames per cycle.
- A second CT was obtained after completion of the FDG PET scan. A CT transmission scan of the chest area was done with the same parameters as those previously described.

Image Interpretation

The ^{82}Rb rest perfusion and ^{18}F-FDG-PET images, shown in **Fig. 43.1**, demonstrate severe left ventricular (LV) dilatation. The ^{82}Rb perfusion images demonstrate a large, severe perfusion defect involving the mid and apical anterior, anteroseptal, anterolateral, and apical inferior walls, where FDG uptake is preserved (PET mismatch). In addition, there is a moderately sized, severe ^{82}Rb perfusion defect throughout the lateral wall, also showing preserved FDG uptake (PET mismatch). This is consistent with a large area of viable but hibernating myocardium throughout the mid left anterior descending (LAD) coronary artery and left circumflex coronary artery territories. Gated PET demonstrates a rest LV ejection fraction of 21% and severely enlarged LV volumes (images not shown). There is severe global LV systolic dysfunction, with akinesis of the apical LV segments and LV apex.

Differential Diagnosis

- Abnormal perfusion PET scan with anterior and apical hibernating myocardium

Diagnosis and Clinical Follow-Up

The patient underwent cardiac catheterization, which showed left main, LAD, and circumflex coronary artery obstructive disease. She underwent bypass surgery two times: a left internal mammary artery graft to the LAD coronary artery and a saphenous vein graft to the obtuse marginal artery (OM1), as well as a mitral valve repair. A repeated echocardiogram 4 months after the surgery showed normal LV chamber size and wall thickness. There was mild global hypokinesis, and the estimated ejection fraction was 40%.

Discussion

Studies of patients with coronary artery disease and LV dysfunction have shown that preoperative quantification of myocardial viability is useful to identify those who will benefit most from revascularization. Clinically meaningful changes in global LV function can be expected after revascularization only in patients with relatively large areas of hibernating and/or stunned myocardium. Patients with large areas of PET mismatch (≥18% of the LV), in particular those located in the territory served by the LAD coronary artery, had the greatest clinical benefit.

PEARLS AND PITFALLS_____

- Contractile dysfunction is likely reversible after revascularization in regions with poor perfusion and increased FDG uptake, a perfusion-metabolism mismatch. Contractile dysfunction is more often irreversible in areas with poor perfusion and reduced FDG uptake (matched pattern).

Suggested Reading

Di Carli MF, Davidson M, Little R, et al. Value of metabolic imaging with positron emission tomography for evaluating prognosis in patients with coronary artery disease and left ventricular dysfunction. Am J Cardiol 1994;73(8):527–533

Di Carli MF, Asgarzadie F, Schelbert HR, et al. Quantitative relation between myocardial viability and improvement in heart failure symptoms after revascularization in patients with ischemic cardiomyopathy. Circulation 1995;92(12):3436–3444

Schinkel AF, Poldermans D, Elhendy A, Bax JJ. Assessment of myocardial viability in patients with heart failure. J Nucl Med 2007;48(7):1135–1146

Sheikine Y, Di Carli MF. Integrated PET/CT in the assessment of etiology and viability in ischemic heart failure. Curr Heart Fail Rep 2008;5(3):136–142

Section III

Pulmonary Scintigraphy

J. Anthony Parker

CASE 44

Clinical Presentation

A 26-year-old man presents with shortness of breath and chest discomfort.

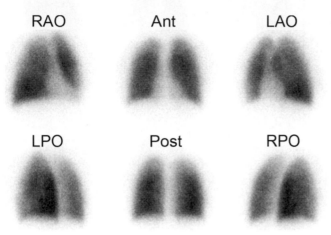

RAO Ant LAO

LPO Post RPO

Fig. 44.1

Technique

- A 3.0-mCi dose of ^{99m}Tc-MAA is administered intravenously with the patient supine.
- The patient should cough and take several deep breaths before administration of the MAA to clear any areas of resting atelectasis.
- The patient should breathe normally during tracer injection.
- Use a low-energy, all-purpose collimator.
- Energy window 20% centered at 140 keV.
- Imaging time is 500,000 counts per view.
- Matrix size is 128 × 128.
- Views are anterior, right anterior oblique, left anterior oblique, posterior, right posterior oblique, and left posterior oblique. Lateral views can also be obtained, although it is important to remember that counts from the contralateral lung will contribute to these views.

Image Interpretation

Homogeneous tracer distribution is seen throughout both lung fields (**Fig. 44.1**). The lungs are of normal contour. The cardiac silhouette is noted in the left lung field in the anterior projection.

Differential Diagnosis

- No evidence of pulmonary embolism. There are many causes of shortness of breath or chest pain other than pulmonary embolism. A normal lung scan rules out recent pulmonary embolism.

Diagnosis and Clinical Follow-Up

The lung perfusion pattern was normal. Shortness of breath and chest discomfort in this patient were felt to be secondary to anxiety and gastritis. No further follow-up was obtained.

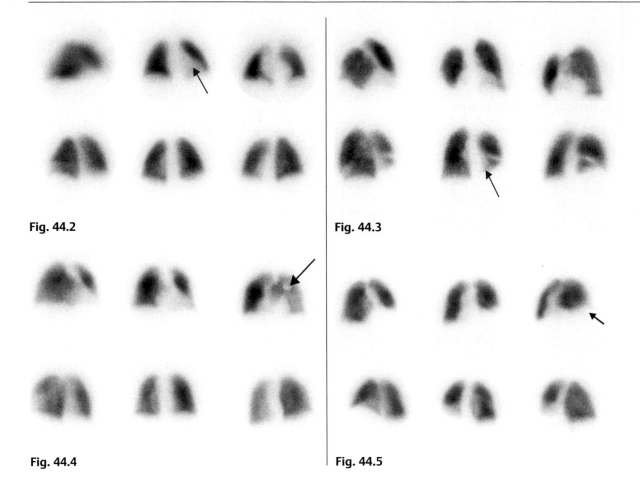

Fig. 44.2

Fig. 44.3

Fig. 44.4

Fig. 44.5

Discussion

Lung perfusion scans provide a method for the diagnosis of pulmonary embolism that is noninvasive and effective. A normal lung scan rules out recent pulmonary embolism.

When a perfusion defect is identified, one must first determine the size and anatomic extent of the defect(s) (**Table 44.1**). Nonsegmental defects do not occupy known vascular distributions and are therefore less likely to be caused by a thromboembolus. Nonsegmental defects include cardiomegaly (**Fig. 44.2**, *arrow*), pleural effusion (**Fig. 44.3**, *arrow*), a cardiac pacemaker superimposed on the chest wall (**Fig. 44.4**, *arrow*), and an elevated hemidiaphragm (**Fig. 44.5**, *arrow*; **Table 44.1**).

Once it has been determined that the defect respects segmental boundaries, its size must be determined. A small subsegmental defect occupies less than 25% of a lung segment, a moderate-size subsegmental defect occupies 25 to 75% of a lung segment, and a large subsegmental defect occupies more than 75% of a lung segment. Two moderate defects are equivalent to one large defect. Any number of small defects do not add up to a moderate or a large defect.

An experienced nuclear medicine physician's "gestalt" impression of a lung scan may provide the most accurate interpretation. However, the best way to become experienced is to learn and apply both standard criteria, such as the revised Prospective Investigation of Pulmonary Embolic Disease (PIOPED) criteria (Gottschalk et al., 1993), and the many ancillary scintigraphic signs that have been developed over the years (Freeman et al., 2001).

Table 44.1   Lung Scan Findings: Likelihood Ratio for Pulmonary Embolism

High-likelihood ratio
Clear chest radiograph
> 2 mismatched segmental equivalents*
2 mismatched segmental equivalents*: borderline between high- and intermediate-likelihood ratio
Intermediate-likelihood ratio
Clear chest radiograph
½–1½ mismatched segmental equivalents*
1 matched defect: borderline between intermediate- and low-likelihood ratio
Abnormal chest radiograph
Other perfusion patterns difficult to categorize as low- or high-likelihood ratio
Low-likelihood ratio
Clear chest radiograph
> 1 matched defect
> 3 small subsegmental perfusion defects
Abnormal chest radiograph
Perfusion defect substantially smaller than chest radiograph infiltrate
Nonsegmental defects (eg, cardiomegaly, enlarged aorta, enlarged hila, elevated diaphragm)
Very low-likelihood ratio
Clear chest radiograph
≤ 3 small subsegmental perfusion defects, matched or unmatched
Normal
Clear chest radiograph
Normal perfusion scan

* Segmental equivalents:
1, large subsegment (> 75% of a segment)
½, moderate subsegment (25–75% of a segment)
0, small subsegment (< 25% of a segment)

The revised PIOPED criteria have prospectively been shown to be more accurate than the original criteria (Sostman et al., 1994). However, the revised criteria exclude the very low category, which identifies a group of patients who have a much lower likelihood of pulmonary emboli than those in the low category do. **Table 44.1** shows the criteria for lung scan interpretation retaining the very low category. **Table 44.1** uses the likelihood ratio, a more accurate descriptor for a test outcome than probability.

In the PIOPED study, about one-third of patients had pulmonary embolism. With this prior probability of disease, the approximate posterior probability of disease is less than 5% for very low-likelihood ratio scans, less than 20% for low-likelihood ratio scans, 20 to 80% for intermediate-likelihood ratio scans, and more than 80% for high-likelihood ratio scans.

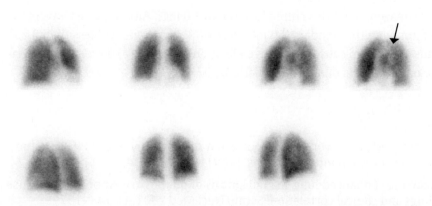

Fig. 44.6

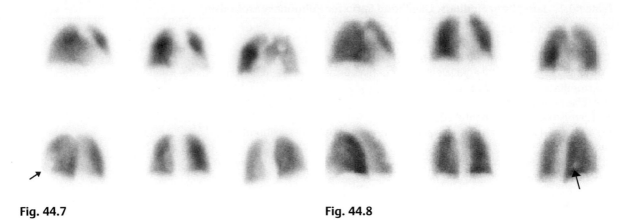

Fig. 44.7   **Fig. 44.8**

PEARLS AND PITFALLS

- The likelihood ratio for pulmonary embolism based on the lung scan must be combined with the clinical probability of pulmonary embolism to determine the overall (or posterior) probability of pulmonary embolism. Patients with an intermediate posterior probability should often undergo additional testing, such as pulmonary CT angiography or leg ultrasonography.

- The physical half-life of ^{99m}Tc is 6 hours, and the biological half-life of MAA in the lungs is variable, usually 1.5 to 3 hours. As a result, if a patient has another episode of acute shortness of breath 24 hours after a normal lung scan, a second lung scan can be performed with little contribution from the prior scan.

- An oblique band of relative photopenia oriented superomedially to inferolaterally is often seen on the left anterior oblique view (**Fig. 44.6**, *arrow*). This is a normal variant and corresponds to the aortic arch. The cardiac apex may cause another normal variant. This is seen as an area of photopenia in the region of the junction of the lateral basal segment of the left lower lobe and the inferior lingular segment on the left posterior oblique view (**Fig. 44.7**, *arrow*). This defect is characteristically of an intensity that gradually fades in comparison with the surrounding, normally perfused lung.

- Defects due to pulmonary embolism classically extend all the way to the lung periphery. When normally perfused lung surrounds a defect (the stripe sign), the defect is nonsegmental and unlikely to be due to acute pulmonary embolism (**Fig. 44.8**, *arrow*).

- Pregnancy is not a contraindication to lung scintigraphy. The theoretical risk to the fetus from the small radiation dose required for the lung scan is minimal in comparison with the risk to the fetus of undiagnosed pulmonary embolism in the mother.

- When pregnant patients are imaged, the dose is often lowered to 1.0 mCi. Although this lowers the fetal dose, the dose to the fetus from the standard 3.0 mCi dose of ^{99m}Tc-MAA is still less than 0.25% of the minimal effective dose known to cause an adverse effect on the fetus (~10 rads; United Nations Scientific Committee on the Effects of Atomic Radiation, 1977).

Suggested Reading

Gottschalk A, Sostman HD, Coleman RE, et al. Ventilation-perfusion scintigraphy in the PIOPED study, II: Evaluation of the scintigraphic criteria and interpretations. J Nucl Med 1993;34(7):1119–1126

Freeman LM, Krynyckyi B, Zuckier LS. Enhanced lung scan diagnosis of pulmonary embolism with use of anciliary scintigraphic findings and clinical correlation. Semin Nucl Med 2001;31:143–157

Sostman HD, Coleman RE, DeLong DM, Newman GE, Paine S. Evaluation of revised criteria for ventilation-perfusion scintigraphy in patients with suspected pulmonary embolism. Radiology 1994;193(1): 103–107

United Nations Scientific Committee on the Effects of Atomic Radiation. Sources and Effects of Ionizing Radiation. New York, NY: United Nations; 1977

CASE 45

Clinical Presentation

A 54-year-old man presents with acute shortness of breath and chest pain.

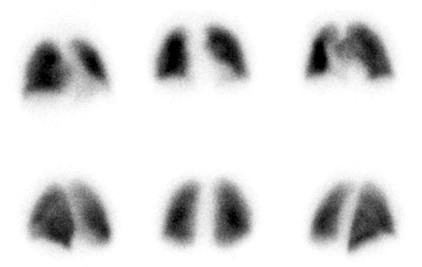

Fig. 45.1

Technique

- A 3.0 mCi dose of ^{99m}Tc-MAA is administered intravenously with the patient supine.
- The patient should cough and take several deep breaths before administration of the MAA to clear any areas of resting atelectasis.
- The patient should breathe normally during tracer injection.
- Use a low-energy, all-purpose collimator.
- Energy window 20% centered at 140 keV.
- Imaging time is 500,000 counts per view.
- Matrix size is 128 × 128.
- The views are anterior, right anterior oblique, left anterior oblique, posterior, right posterior oblique, and left posterior oblique. Lateral views can also be obtained, although it is important to remember that counts from the contralateral lung will contribute to these views.

Image Interpretation

There is a small subsegmental defect involving the anterior basal segment of the right lower lobe abutting the expected location of the right major fissure, best seen on the right posterior oblique view **(Fig. 45.1)**. No other segmental defects are identified. The chest radiograph was clear.

Differential Diagnosis

A small subsegmental perfusion defect is nonspecific and can have many causes, including the following:

- Atelectasis
- Bronchitis
- Asthma, chronic obstructive pulmonary disease (COPD)
- Pleural effusion
- Pneumonia
- Unresolved previous pulmonary embolism
- Previous surgery
- Attenuation artifact

Diagnosis and Clinical Follow-Up

Given the small size of this defect, the scan was read as very low likelihood ratio for recent pulmonary embolism. Chest pain was due to bronchitis.

Discussion

If only small subsegmental defects are noted on a lung perfusion scan, the study is read as very low likelihood ratio for recent pulmonary embolism (The PIOPED Investigators, 1990), given a clear chest radiograph. The ventilation findings will not alter this diagnosis.

The revised PIOPED criteria (Gottschalk et al., 1993) eliminated the very low likelihood ratio category; however, some nuclear medicine physicians still find this category useful because the incidence of pulmonary embolism is much lower in this category than in the low-likelihood ratio category.

PEARLS AND PITFALLS

- Perfusion abnormalities noted on lung scan are not specific for pulmonary embolism and may be caused by a large number of other diseases. Communication between the referring physician and the physician reading the lung scan can provide a great deal of useful information about potential alternative diagnoses.
- In general, patients with a **low likelihood** ratio lung scan are often managed as if they do not have a pulmonary embolism. If the clinical suspicion of pulmonary embolism is strong, however, it may be necessary to perform other diagnostic tests. Ancillary tests include Doppler ultrasonography to detect deep venous thrombus and pulmonary CT angiography. By contrast, patients with a **very low likelihood** ratio lung scan can almost always be followed without further testing.
- The resolution with xenon 133 ventilation is not as good as that with ^{99m}Tc-MAA, so that small ventilation defects (corresponding to small perfusion defects) may not be seen. Therefore, small perfusion abnormalities in these patients should not be thought of as mismatched.

Suggested Reading

Gottschalk A, Sostman HD, Coleman RE, et al. Ventilation-perfusion scintigraphy in the PIOPED study. Part II. Evaluation of the scintigraphic criteria and interpretations. J Nucl Med 1993;34(7):1119–1126

The PIOPED Investigators. Value of the ventilation/perfusion scan in acute pulmonary embolism. Results of the prospective investigation of pulmonary embolism diagnosis (PIOPED). JAMA 1990;263(20):2753–2759

CASE 46

Clinical Presentation

A 70-year-old woman presents with chest pain following a total hip replacement.

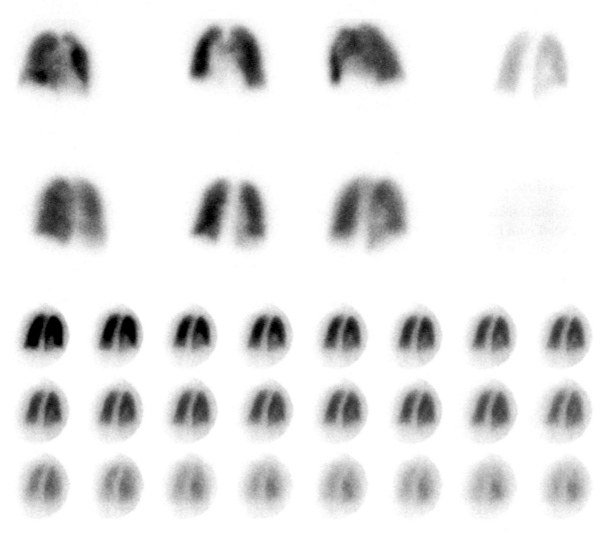

Fig. 46.1

Technique

Lung Perfusion Scan

- A 3.0 mCi dose of ^{99m}Tc-MAA is administered intravenously with the patient supine.
- The patient should cough and take several deep breaths before administration of the MAA to clear any areas of resting atelectasis.
- The patient should breathe normally during tracer injection.
- Use a low-energy, all-purpose collimator.
- Energy window 20% centered at 140 keV.

- Imaging time is 500,000 counts per view.
- Matrix size is 128 × 128.
- Views are anterior, right anterior oblique, left anterior oblique, posterior, right posterior oblique, and left posterior oblique. Lateral views can also be obtained, although it is important to remember that counts from the contralateral lung will contribute to these views.

Lung Ventilation Scan

- The view that best demonstrates the significant perfusion defects is chosen.
- A 20.0 mCi dose of xenon 133 is breathed in via mask with the patient sitting up.
- Use a low-energy, all-purpose collimator.
- Energy window 20% centered at 80 keV.
- Matrix is 128 × 128.
- Imaging sequence
  - Initial breath image: one 15-second image
  - Equilibrium phase: 15 images, 15 seconds per image
  - Washout phase: 15 images, 15 seconds per image
  - Trapping image: one 60-second image

Image Interpretation

The lung perfusion images demonstrate a large defect involving the posterior basal, lateral basal, and superior segments of the right lower lobe (**Fig. 46.1**). No other segmental defects are identified. On the ventilation images, these defects are completely matched by defects on the initial breath images. On washout and trapping images, there is delayed washout from this region. The chest radiograph was clear.

Differential Diagnosis

(Large, matching defects with clear chest radiograph)
- Chronic obstructive pulmonary disease (COPD)
- Acute exacerbation of asthma
- Pneumonia
- Congestive heart failure (defects usually smaller)
- Adult respiratory distress syndrome
- Mucous plugging of the airways
- Foreign body aspiration
- Neoplasm obstructing the airway
- Pneumonectomy

Diagnosis and Clinical Follow-Up

The scan was read as low-likelihood ratio for acute pulmonary embolism. Chest pain was caused by gastroesophageal reflux.

Discussion

If the chest radiograph is normal, segmental defects on a lung perfusion scan that are completely matched by ventilation abnormalities have a low-likelihood ratio for recent pulmonary embolism. Some criteria use the low-likelihood ratio category only for matched defects that involve less than 50%

of both lungs. If more than 50% of both lungs are involved, the scan is intermediate-likelihood ratio (Freitas et al., 1995).

If the chest radiograph has a corresponding opacity that is significantly larger than the perfusion defect, the scan is low-likelihood ratio. If the chest radiograph has a corresponding opacity that is the same size as the perfusion defect, the scan is intermediate-likelihood ratio.

PEARLS AND PITFALLS

- A ventilation equilibrium phase of at least 4 minutes is helpful to allow the xenon to penetrate obstructed airways.
- Small areas of washout abnormality are better seen if the ventilation portion of the study is done before perfusion imaging.
- The cardiac silhouette on chest radiograph is often less prominent than that on perfusion images because the former is obtained during maximal inspiration and the latter during tidal breathing. A left lingular defect on perfusion images is often caused by the normal position of the cardiac apex, even though it may not appear to extend that far laterally on the chest radiograph.
- Some imaging centers perform the ventilation scan after the perfusion scan, as in this case. The advantage of this method is that it allows one to select the optimal view in which to perform the ventilation scan and to avoid the ventilation study completely when perfusion images are normal. The disadvantage is that the 140-keV photons from the ^{99m}Tc-MAA perfusion scan will be "down-scattered" into the 80-keV window of the ^{133}Xe image, making interpretation of the ventilation study slightly more difficult. It is important to acquire an MAA down-scatter image with the 80-keV window before the ventilation scan is performed. This helps to distinguish tracer activity caused by trapping from that caused by down-scatter. Trapping, a sign of severe airway obstruction, is generally considered to be present if tracer activity persists in the lungs until the end of the washout phase.

Suggested Reading

Freitas JE, Sarosi MG, Nagle CC, Yeomans ME, Freitas AE, Juni JE. Modified PIOPED criteria used in clinical practice. J Nucl Med 1995;36(9):1573–1578

CASE 47

Clinical Presentation

A 50-year-old man with a productive cough presents with atypical chest pain. Cardiac catheterization is negative, and a chest radiograph shows bilateral patchy opacities in both lungs.

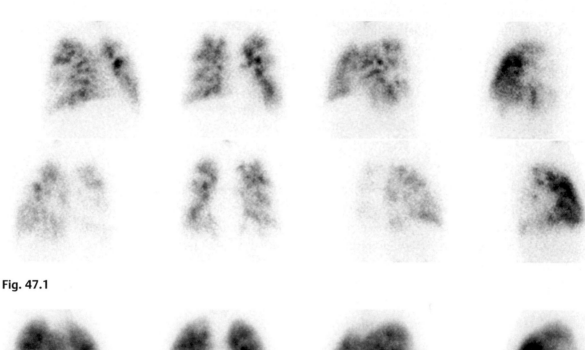

Fig. 47.1

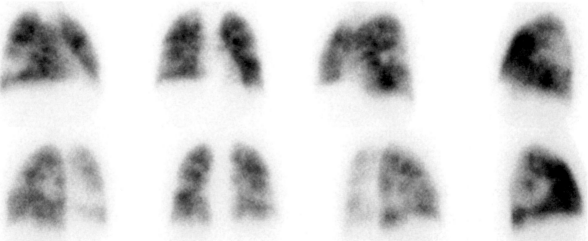

Fig. 47.2

Technique

Lung Ventilation Scan

- A 40.0 mCi dose of ^{99m}Tc-DTPA is placed in the aerosolizer (delivers < 1 mCi to the lungs).
- Use a low-energy, all-purpose collimator.
- Energy window 20% centered at 80 keV.

- Matrix size is 128 × 128.
- Views are anterior, right anterior oblique, left anterior oblique, posterior, right posterior oblique, left posterior oblique, right lateral view, and left lateral.

Lung Perfusion Scan

- A 3.0 mCi dose of ^{99m}Tc-MAA is administered intravenously with the patient supine.
- The patient should cough and take several deep breaths before administration of the MAA to clear any areas of resting atelectasis.
- The patient should breathe normally during tracer injection.
- Use a low-energy, all-purpose collimator.
- Energy window 20% centered at 140 keV.
- Imaging time is 500,000 counts per view.
- Matrix size is 128 × 128.
- Views are anterior, right anterior oblique, left anterior oblique, posterior, right posterior oblique, left posterior oblique, right lateral view, and left lateral.

Image Interpretation

The lung ventilation images demonstrate large defects that do not appear to correspond to the segmental anatomy of the lung (**Fig. 47.1**). The lung perfusion images demonstrate similar defects, although the degree of abnormality is less severe (**Fig. 47.2**). Given the patchy abnormalities on the chest radiograph and the extensive matched defects on the ventilation and perfusion scans, this study, which does not fall into either the low- or the high-likelihood category, is intermediate-likelihood ratio for pulmonary embolism.

Differential Diagnosis

(Large, matching defects; abnormal chest radiograph)
- Chronic obstructive pulmonary disease (COPD)
- Acute exacerbation of asthma
- Pneumonia
- Congestive heart failure
- Adult respiratory distress syndrome
- Possible pulmonary embolism

Diagnosis and Clinical Follow-Up

A pulmonary CT angiogram was negative for pulmonary embolism but showed a tree-in-bud infiltrative pattern typical of air space disease (**Fig. 47.3**).

Discussion

Pulmonary CT angiography, which shows clots within the lumina of the pulmonary arteries, provides more direct evidence of pulmonary embolism. Lung scintigraphy shows the physiologic effect of the embolism on the perfusion of the pulmonary parenchyma. Lung perfusion can be affected by a long list of other disease processes, especially diseases that affect pulmonary ventilation. Thus, lung scintigra-

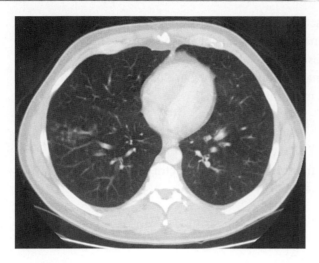

Fig. 47.3

phy is less specific than CT angiography. Lung scintigraphy does provide a physiologic assessment of the extent of embolization, which may be useful in understanding the severity of the disease process.

Pulmonary CT angiography has an advantage compared with lung scintigraphy in patients who have known chest disease or in whom other chest disease is likely. In this patient, the finding of a tree-in-bud pattern helped confirm the diagnosis of pneumonia. When technically adequate, pulmonary CT angiography has been confirmed to have a high sensitivity (83%) and a high specificity (96%) for the diagnosis of pulmonary embolism (Stein et al., 2006). In that study, only 6% of patients had technically inadequate studies.

Lung scintigraphy will be most likely to provide a firm diagnosis in patients who have normal chest radiographs and who are unlikely to have other chest disease. A high-likelihood ratio lung scan or, especially, a normal lung scan is very valuable diagnostic information. In patients with other lung disease, particularly those with pulmonary infiltrates, lung scan outcomes (low- or intermediate-likelihood ratio) are frequently less useful. The advantage of lung scintigraphy compared with pulmonary angiography is that the complication rates are lower because iodinated intravenous contrast does not have to be administered.

PEARLS AND PITFALLS

- The chance of obtaining an intermediate-likelihood ratio scan is considerably higher in a patient with an abnormal chest radiograph than in a patient with a normal chest radiograph. In a patient with evidence of pulmonary parenchymal disease on chest radiograph, pulmonary CT angiography is more likely to give a definitive diagnosis.
- An additional advantage of pulmonary CT angiography over lung scintigraphy is that it can provide information about lung diseases other than pulmonary embolism.
- Pulmonary disease (eg, pneumonia) is often a cause of nonsegmental matched ventilation and perfusion abnormalities. The ventilatory defects are frequently more prominent than the associated perfusion defects.

- Aerosol ventilation scans have the advantage that all of the views can be obtained for comparison with the perfusion scan. Washout and trapping information is not available with aerosol ventilation scans.
- Central deposition occurs frequently with aerosol scans, particularly when there is airway turbulence. Central deposition provides some information about the presence of turbulence, but it often makes interpretation of the ventilation images more difficult.

Suggested Reading

Stein PD, Fowler SE, Goodman LR, et al. PIOPED II Investigators. Multidetector computed tomography for acute pulmonary embolism. N Engl J Med 2006;354(22):2317–2327

CASE 48

Clinical Presentation

A 31-year-old man presents with increasing oxygen requirements. The chest radiograph is clear.

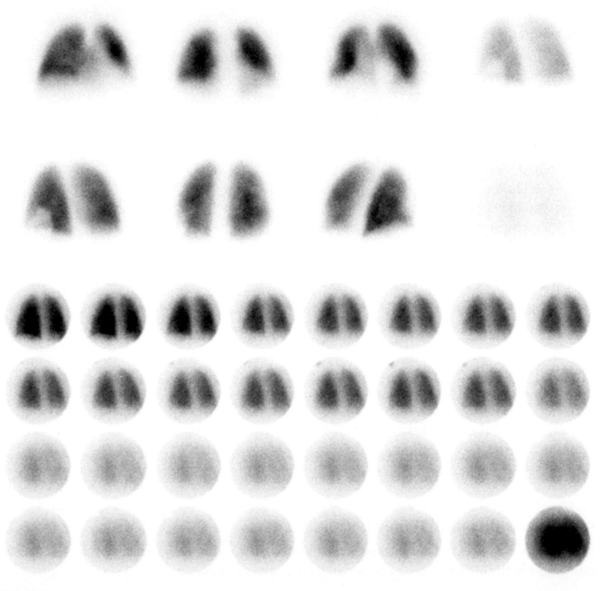

Fig. 48.1

Technique

Lung Perfusion Scan

- A 3.0 mCi dose of ^{99m}Tc-MAA is administered intravenously with the patient supine.
- The patient should cough and take several deep breaths before administration of the MAA to clear any areas of resting atelectasis.

- The patient should breathe normally during tracer injection.
- Use a low-energy, all-purpose collimator.
- Energy window 20% centered at 140 keV.
- Imaging time is 500,000 counts per view.
- Matrix size is 128 × 128.
- Views are anterior, right anterior oblique, left anterior oblique, posterior, right posterior oblique, and left posterior oblique. Lateral views can also be obtained, although it is important to remember that counts from the contralateral lung will contribute to these views.

Lung Ventilation Scan

- The view that best demonstrates the significant perfusion defects is chosen.
- Radiopharmaceutical is 20.0 mCi of xenon 133 breathed in via mask with the patient sitting up.
- Use a low-energy, all-purpose collimator.
- Energy window 20% centered at 80 keV.
- Matrix size is 128 × 128.
- Imaging time
  - Initial breath image: approximately 15 seconds
  - Equilibrium phase: 15 images, 15 seconds per image
  - Washout phase: 15 images, 15 seconds per image
  - Trapping image: one 60-second image

Image Interpretation

The lung perfusion images demonstrate a large defect involving the anteromedial basal segment of the left lower lobe and a moderate defect involving the lateral basal segment of the left lower lobe (**Fig. 48.1**). No other segmental defects are identified. The ventilation images are normal.

Differential Diagnosis

- Pulmonary embolism (acute)
- Pulmonary embolism (previous)
- Lung cancer (primary or metastatic)
- Histoplasmosis
- Pneumonia
- Sarcoidosis

Diagnosis and Clinical Follow-Up

The scan was read as indicating an intermediate-likelihood ratio for pulmonary embolism. The patient was treated with anticoagulants for presumed pulmonary embolism.

Discussion

When the chest radiograph is normal, if the mismatched defects on a lung perfusion scan are moderate, large, or both, then the defects should be summed by using 1 for each large segmental defect and ½ for each moderate subsegmental defect. Small defects are not counted (Freitas et al., 1995). In this case, the sum, 1½, is less than 2, so the interpretation is intermediate-likelihood ratio.

PEARLS AND PITFALLS_____

- Ventilation imaging is usually performed with the patient upright after practice ventilatory maneuvers, whereas perfusion imaging is usually performed with the patient supine (Parker et al., 2004). The change in position should be taken into account when the studies are compared. The practice maneuvers before the ventilation scan can clear the bronchi, resulting in an altered ventilation scan compared with the perfusion scan.
- The perfusion scan is performed with tidal breathing. By comparison, the initial breath image is at maximal inspiration. During equilibrium and washout, the breathing pattern may be altered when the patient breathes through the ventilation machine.
- If the lung scan is compromised by differences between ventilation and perfusion, it may be more difficult to categorize the study as high- or low-likelihood ratio.
- Pulmonary segments involved with obstructive disease may take several minutes to equilibrate with the ventilatory tracer. If the patient cannot tolerate the ventilation phase of the study (typically 4 minutes), sufficient time for equilibration with the obstructed lung segments may not have elapsed. Thus, on washout images, a delay in washout from the obstructed segments may not be demonstrated.

Suggested Reading

Freitas JE, Sarosi MG, Nagle CC, Yeomans ME, Freitas AE, Juni JE. Modified PIOPED criteria used in clinical practice. J Nucl Med 1995;36(9):1573–1578

Parker JA, Coleman RE, Siegel BA, et al. Society of Nuclear Medicine Procedure Guideline for Lung Scintigraphy Version 3.0, approved February 7, 2004. http://interactive.snm.org/docs/Lung%20Scintigraphy_v3.0.pdf. Accessed April 15, 2010

CASE 49

Clinical Presentation

A 74-year-old woman presents with the acute onset of chest pain and shortness of breath after a 2-day car ride. The chest radiograph is clear.

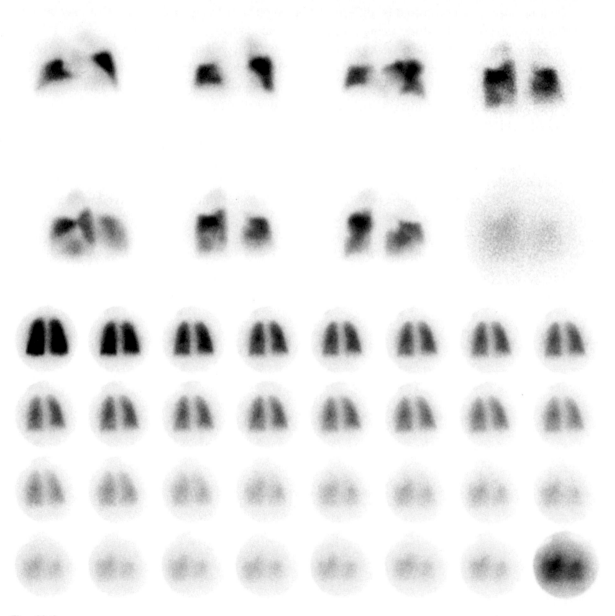

Fig. 49.1

Technique

Lung Perfusion Scan

- A 3.0 mCi dose of ^{99m}Tc-MAA is administered intravenously with the patient supine.
- The patient should cough and take several deep breaths before administration of the MAA to clear any areas of resting atelectasis.
- The patient should breathe normally during tracer injection.
- Use a low-energy, all-purpose collimator.
- Energy window 20% centered at 140 keV.
- Imaging time is 500,000 counts per view.
- Matrix size is 128 × 128.
- Views are anterior, right anterior oblique, left anterior oblique, posterior, right posterior oblique, and left posterior oblique. Lateral views can also be obtained, although it is important to remember that counts from the contralateral lung will contribute to these views.

Lung Ventilation Scan

- A 20.0 mCi dose of ^{133}Xe is breathed in via mask with the patient sitting up.
- Use a low-energy, all-purpose collimator.
- Energy window 20% centered at 80 keV.
- Matrix is 128 × 128.
- Imaging time
  - Initial breath image: one 15-second image
  - Equilibrium phase: 15 images, 15 seconds per image
  - Washout phase: 15 images, 15 seconds per image
  - Trapping image: one 60-second image
- The view that best demonstrates the significant perfusion defects is chosen.

Image Interpretation

The lung perfusion images demonstrate large defects involving all three segments of the right upper lobe, the superior segment of the right lower lobe, the anterior and apicoposterior segments of the left upper lobe, and the posterior basal and anteromedial basal segments of the left lower lobe (**Fig. 49.1**). The ventilation images are normal.

Differential Diagnosis

- Acute pulmonary thromboembolism
- Previous pulmonary thromboembolism

Diagnosis and Clinical Follow-Up

The scan was read as indicating a high-likelihood ratio for pulmonary embolism. The patient was treated for pulmonary embolism with thrombolysis and anticoagulation.

Discussion

If the segmental defects on a lung perfusion scan are moderate, large, or both; if they sum to at least two large segmental equivalents; and if they are not matched by a ventilation abnormality, then the scan interpretation is high-likelihood ratio for pulmonary embolism (Freitas et al., 1995). The reading will change only if a corresponding chest radiograph opacity is noted in a distribution similar to that of the perfusion defects, in which case the reading becomes indeterminate-likelihood ratio.

PEARLS AND PITFALLS

- The advantages of ventilation-perfusion scans are that they are relatively noninvasive, are easily performed, expose the patient to a low level of radiation, and have good interobserver agreement for normal and high-likelihood ratio scans.
- In the PIOPED study, 39% of the scans were intermediate-likelihood ratio (The PIOPED Investigators, 1990). With modified criteria, the incidence of intermediate-probability scans is approximately 17% (Freitas et al., 1995). The incidence should be even lower now that many patients who are likely to have an intermediate-likelihood ratio result go directly to pulmonary CT angiography.

Suggested Reading

Freitas JE, Sarosi MG, Nagle CC, Yeomans ME, Freitas AE, Juni JE. Modified PIOPED criteria used in clinical practice. J Nucl Med 1995;36(9):1573–1578

The PIOPED Investigators. Value of the ventilation/perfusion scan in acute pulmonary embolism: results of the prospective investigation of pulmonary embolism diagnosis (PIOPED). JAMA 1990;263(20):2753–2759

CASE 50

Clinical Presentation

A 61-year-old woman presents with acute shortness of breath.

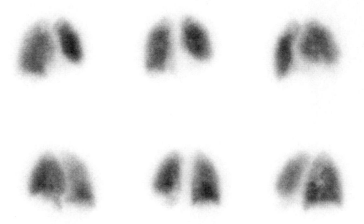

Fig. 50.1

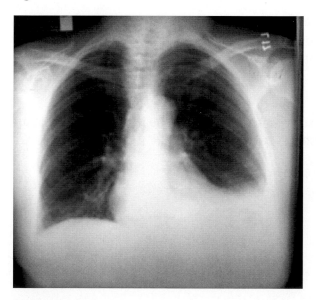

Fig. 50.2

Technique

- A 3.0 mCi dose of ^{99m}Tc-MAA is administered intravenously with the patient supine.
- The patient should cough and take several deep breaths before administration of the MAA to clear any areas of resting atelectasis.
- The patient should breathe normally during tracer injection.
- Use a low-energy, all-purpose collimator.

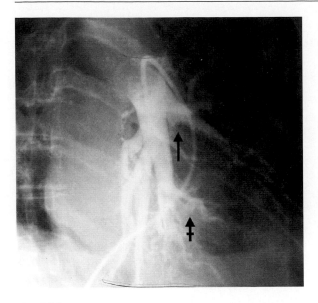

Fig. 50.3

- Energy window 20% centered at 140 keV.
- Imaging time is 500,000 counts per view.
- Matrix is 128 × 128.
- Views are anterior, right anterior oblique, left anterior oblique, posterior, right posterior oblique, and left posterior oblique. Lateral views can also be obtained, although it is important to remember that counts from the contralateral lung will contribute to these views.

Image Interpretation

The lung perfusion scan (**Fig. 50.1**) demonstrates subsegmental defects in the left lower lobe that are matched by the opacity on chest radiograph (**Fig. 50.2**).

Differential Diagnosis

- Pulmonary embolism (acute)
- Pulmonary embolism (previous)
- Lung cancer (primary or metastatic)
- Histoplasmosis
- Pneumonia
- Sarcoidosis

Diagnosis and Clinical Follow-Up

A perfusion defect in the area of chest radiograph abnormality is consistent with intermediate-likelihood ratio for pulmonary embolism. Pulmonary arteriogram (**Fig. 50.3**) demonstrates filling defects consistent with emboli in the left lower lobe vessels (*arrow*) as well as the inferior lingual segment (*crossed arrow*).

Discussion

When the perfusion defect on lung scan matches the opacity on chest radiograph, the scan is inter-mediate-likelihood ratio for pulmonary embolism (Freitas et al., 1995). A ventilation scan is not needed. A perfusion defect in the area of chest opacity can be due to a pulmonary parenchymal process like pneumonia with secondary pulmonary vasoconstriction, or it can be due to a pulmonary embolus with secondary infarction. If the clinical suspicion of pulmonary embolism is not strong enough to warrant treatment, these patients are usually further evaluated, in this case with selective pulmonary arteriography.

PEARLS AND PITFALLS

- A patient with a chest radiograph abnormality may have diagnostic lung scan findings in regions where the chest radiograph is normal, but the most common result is intermediate-likelihood ratio. Thus, chest radiograph abnormalities favor pulmonary CT angiography as the initial test for pulmonary embolism.
- If the chest radiograph opacity matches the perfusion defect, the reading is usually intermediate-likelihood ratio for pulmonary embolism. If the matching chest radiograph opacity is a pleural effusion without associated atelectasis, the scan is low-likelihood ratio for pulmonary embolism (Gottschalk et al., 1993).
- Relatively normal ventilation with ^{133}Xe in the region of a perfusion abnormality matched by an infiltrate on chest radiograph should not be misinterpreted as high-likelihood ratio for pulmonary embolism. This pattern is also in the intermediate category.

Suggested Reading

Freitas JE, Sarosi MG, Nagle CC, Yeomans ME, Freitas AE, Juni JE. Modified PIOPED criteria used in clinical practice. J Nucl Med 1995;36(9):1573–1578

Gottschalk A, Sostman HD, Coleman RE, et al. Ventilation-perfusion scintigraphy in the PIOPED study, II: Evaluation of the scintigraphic criteria and interpretations. J Nucl Med 1993;34(7):1119–1126

CASE 51

Clinical Presentation

A 43-year-old woman presents with acute shortness of breath.

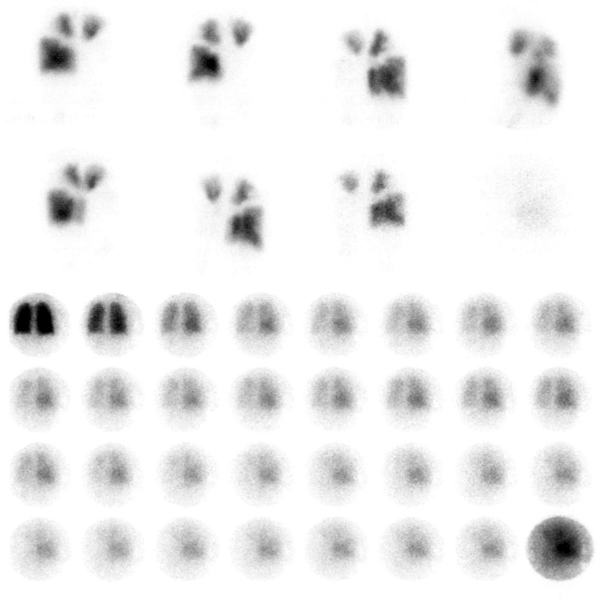

Fig. 51.1

Technique

Lung Perfusion Scan

- A 3.0 mCi dose of ^{99m}Tc-MAA is administered intravenously with the patient supine.
- The patient should cough and take several deep breaths before administration of the MAA to clear any areas of resting atelectasis.
- The patient should breathe normally during tracer injection.
- Use a low-energy, all-purpose collimator.
- Energy window 20% centered at 140 keV.
- Imaging time is 500,000 counts per view.
- Matrix size is 128 × 128.
- Views are anterior, right anterior oblique, left anterior oblique, posterior, right posterior oblique, and left posterior oblique. Lateral views can also be obtained, although it is important to remember that counts from the contralateral lung will contribute to these views.

Lung Ventilation Scan

- A 20.0 mCi dose of ^{133}Xe is breathed in via mask with the patient sitting up.
- Use a low-energy, all-purpose collimator.
- Energy window 20% centered at 80 keV.
- Matrix size is 128 × 128.
- Imaging time
  - Initial breath image: one 15-second image
  - Equilibrium phase: 15 images, 15 seconds per image
  - Washout phase: 15 images, 15 seconds per image
  - Trapping image: one 60-second image
- The view that best demonstrates the significant perfusion defects is chosen.

Image Interpretation

The lung perfusion scan (**Fig. 51.1**, upper portion) demonstrates widespread segmental and subsegmental defects throughout both lungs. Among the large defects is the entire left lower lobe, the inferior and superior segments of the lingula, and the superior segment of the right lower lobe. Both upper lobes have some preserved perfusion, although only a small portion of these lobes is perfused normally. The chest radiograph was clear. The ventilation images (**Fig. 51.1**, lower portion) are normal. Rapid washout of activity during the "equilibrium" portion of the study is likely due to leaking.

Differential Diagnosis

- Acute pulmonary thromboembolism
- Previous pulmonary thromboembolism

Diagnosis and Clinical Follow-Up

The lung scan is consistent with a high-likelihood ratio for pulmonary embolism. Furthermore, because of the extent of the pulmonary embolism, it is categorized as massive. The patient was treated for pulmonary embolism with anticoagulation and thrombolysis.

Discussion

If the segmental defects on a lung perfusion scan are moderate, large, or both, if they sum to at least two large segmental equivalents, and if they are not matched by a ventilation abnormality, the final interpretation is high-likelihood ratio for pulmonary embolism (Freitas et al., 1995). The reading will change only if a corresponding chest radiograph opacity is noted in a distribution similar to that of the perfusion defects.

In cases with widespread bilateral defects, such as this one, it is important to communicate to the referring clinician not only the likelihood ratio for pulmonary embolism but also the severity of the clot burden. Patients with a large amount of pulmonary embolus may require aggressive treatment, such as thrombolysis.

PEARLS AND PITFALLS _____

- If the widespread perfusion defects involve contiguous segments in only one lung, the possibility of another diagnosis, such as central obstructing lung cancer, should be considered. This is especially true if perfusion in the whole lung is abnormal (White et al., 1971).

- Scans demonstrating pulmonary embolism cannot reliably provide information about the age of the embolus. Elderly patients and those with poor cardiovascular function are more likely to have difficulty resolving emboli, so that ventilation-perfusion mismatch persists. Some pulmonary emboli never resolve. The differential for ventilation-perfusion mismatch therefore includes old pulmonary embolism as well as acute pulmonary embolism.

- Massive pulmonary embolism has been defined as defects including 50% of both lung fields. The case shown here, in which defects include much more than 50% of the lungs, is an extreme example of massive embolism.

- Equilibrium imaging requires rebreathing in a closed space. Leaking, which occurs more commonly when patients are severely short of breath, prevents the achievement of equilibrium.

Suggested Reading

Freitas JE, Sarosi MG, Nagle CC, Yeomans ME, Freitas AE, Juni JE. Modified PIOPED criteria used in clinical practice. J Nucl Med 1995;36(9):1573–1578

White RI Jr, James AE Jr, Wagner HN Jr. The significance of unilateral absence of pulmonary artery perfusion by lung scanning. Am J Roentgenol Radium Ther Nucl Med 1971;111(3):501–509

CASE 52

Clinical Presentation

A 63-year-old woman presents with shortness of breath, a swollen left calf, and a normal chest radiograph.

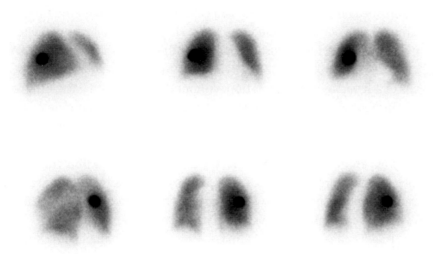

Fig. 52.1

Technique

- A 3.0 mCi dose of ^{99m}Tc-MAA is administered intravenously with the patient supine.
- The patient should cough and take several deep breaths before administration of the MAA to clear any areas of resting atelectasis.
- The patient should breathe normally during tracer injection.
- Use a low-energy, all-purpose collimator.
- Energy window 20% centered at 140 keV.
- Imaging time is 500,000 counts per view.
- Matrix size is 128 × 128.
- Views are anterior, right anterior oblique, left anterior oblique, posterior, right posterior oblique, and left posterior oblique. Lateral views can also be obtained, although it is important to remember that counts from the contralateral lung will contribute to these views.

Image Interpretation

Images in multiple projections (**Fig. 52.1**) show a focus of intensely increased tracer activity in the mid right lung field. The finding is characteristic of clumping of injected tracer.

Differential Diagnosis

- Clumping of MAA
- Small focus of normally perfused lung in a patient with massive pulmonary embolism

Diagnosis and Clinical Follow-Up

No evidence of pulmonary embolism. Shortness of breath was thought to be secondary to exacerbation of congestive heart failure.

Discussion

Clumping of MAA at the time of injection is not an uncommon problem. The MAA particles may clump together to form a large particle with intense activity. The MAA should be carefully prepared, and the syringe should be inverted several times before injection to minimize clumping.

MAA is very "sticky." It will be adsorbed onto microthrombi on a catheter tip or even on the tip of a butterfly needle. If even a small amount of blood is aspirated into the syringe during injection, microthrombi can form onto which the MAA will be avidly adsorbed. Whatever the cause, the clump of MAA will lodge in the lung, resulting in a focal "hot spot."

It is best to inject MAA by means of a separate needle insertion without drawing blood back into the radiopharmaceutical. When a well-flushed existing intravenous line has to be used, it is common to see adsorption of MAA, especially near the tip of the line. At times, the adsorption can be severe enough to render the study uninterpretable.

There are no causes of pulmonary hyperemia. Neoplasms generally derive their blood flow from the oxygen-rich bronchial blood supply; furthermore, neoplastic blood flow is much less than normal pulmonary blood flow, which is by far the greatest blood flow in the body. Arteriovenous malformations will not trap the particles, which will pass through to the systemic circulation.

True hot spots are always artifactual. Occasionally, in very massive pulmonary embolism, a small area of remaining normal lung can appear as a hot spot. However, the pattern of perfusion elsewhere in the lung usually provides a clue to the correct diagnosis.

PEARLS AND PITFALLS

- Clumping of the injected tracer can be distinguished from residual tracer in an implanted injection reservoir, such as a portacath, by noting how the focal abnormality moves in association with the lung parenchyma on the various views.
- There are no causes of pulmonary hyperemia. True hot spots are always artifactual.
- If blood is aspirated into a syringe containing MAA, that dose should be discarded and a fresh dose used.

Suggested Reading

Preston DF, Greenlaw RH. "Hot spots" in lung scans. J Nucl Med 1970;11(7):422–425

CASE 53

Clinical Presentation

An 83-year-old woman presents with shortness of breath following an airplane ride.

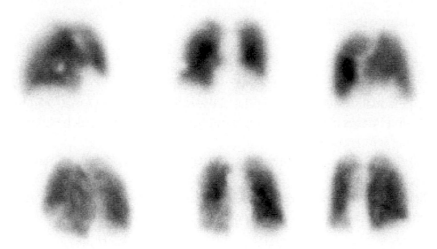

Fig. 53.1

Technique

- A 3.0 mCi dose of ^{99m}Tc-MAA is administered intravenously with the patient supine.
- The patient should cough and take several deep breaths before administration of the MAA to clear any areas of resting atelectasis.
- The patient should breathe normally during tracer injection.
- Use a low-energy, all-purpose collimator.
- Energy window 20% centered at 140 keV.
- Imaging time is 500,000 counts per view.
- Matrix size is 128 × 128.
- Views are anterior, right anterior oblique, left anterior oblique, posterior, right posterior oblique, and left posterior oblique. Lateral views can also be obtained, although it is important to remember that counts from the contralateral lung will contribute to these views.

Image Interpretation

A focal, round defect is noted over the right lung field on the right anterior oblique view (**Fig. 53.1**). It is also noted laterally on the anterior view. Patchy perfusion is noted in both lung fields.

Differential Diagnosis

(Focal, nonphysiologically shaped defect)
- Attenuation artifact
- Gamma camera defect (cracked crystal, photomultiplier tube malfunction, off-peak energy window, collimator abnormality)

Diagnosis and Clinical Follow-Up

Chest radiograph demonstrates a pacemaker over the right hemithorax.

Discussion

Pacemakers can be placed in any location on the chest, causing an attenuation artifact that may resemble a pulmonary perfusion defect. Careful analysis of the different projections of the perfusion images will demonstrate that the defect moves separately from the lung parenchyma. Of course, review of the chest radiograph will easily demonstrate the nature of the defect.

PEARLS AND PITFALLS

- Review all chest radiographs personally. Merely reading the chest radiograph report may lead to misinterpretation of the perfusion images because seemingly unimportant findings may be important for the interpretation of lung scintigraphy.
- Artifacts due to overlying high-density objects are often nonsegmental with a nonanatomic shape and sharply defined edges.
- Pacemakers can make it difficult to read defects in the underlying lung. All projections of the perfusion study should be carefully reviewed for perfusion defects in the region of the pacemaker artifact.

Suggested Reading

Busemann SE, ed. IAEA quality control atlas for scintillation camera systems 2003. http://www.pub.iaea.org/MTCD/publications/PDF/Pub11141_web.pdf

CASE 54

Clinical Presentation

A 67-year-old woman presents with worsening shortness of breath.

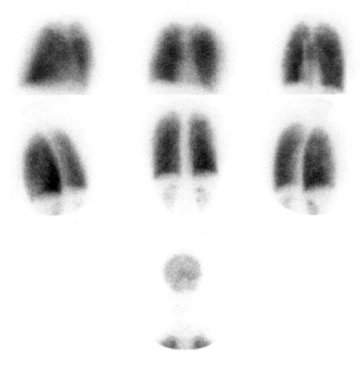

Fig. 54.1

Technique

- A 3.0 mCi dose of ^{99m}Tc-MAA is administered intravenously with the patient supine.
- The patient should cough and take several deep breaths before administration of the MAA to clear any areas of resting atelectasis.
- The patient should breathe normally during tracer injection.
- Use a low-energy, all-purpose collimator.
- Energy window 20% centered at 140 keV.
- Imaging time is 500,000 counts per view.
- Matrix size is 128 × 128.
- Views are anterior, right anterior oblique, left anterior oblique, posterior, right posterior oblique, and left posterior oblique. Lateral views can also be obtained, although it is important to remember that counts from the contralateral lung will contribute to these views.

Image Interpretation

The lung perfusion images demonstrate overall mildly heterogeneous tracer localization, without segmental defects (**Fig. 54.1**). The chest radiograph was clear. The scan was read as low-likelihood ratio for recent pulmonary embolism (Freitas et al., 1995). Tracer uptake is seen in the kidneys on the posterior views. Images of the head demonstrate tracer uptake in the brain, confirming a right-to-left shunt.

Differential Diagnosis

(For tracer uptake outside the lungs)
- Right-to-left shunt
- Particle dissolution (images obtained several hours after tracer injection)
- Radiopharmaceutical preparation problems
- Pulmonary arteriovenous malformation
- Swallowed ^{99m}Tc-DTPA aerosol

Diagnosis and Clinical Follow-Up

The patient had an atrial septal defect, which was diagnosed by echocardiography.

Discussion

Tracer uptake outside the pulmonary capillary bed can occur in several organs from a variety of causes. Uptake in segment IV, the medial segment of the left lobe of the liver (formerly the quadrate lobe), can be secondary to superior vena cava obstruction with collateral flow through the umbilical vein via a caput medusae. Uptake in the whole liver can be secondary to normal breakdown of the larger MAA particles and passage of the smaller particles through the lung with uptake in the reticuloendothelial system. Thyroid uptake is often thought to be caused by free pertechnetate. The rate of blood flow to the thyroid is quite high, however, and right-to-left shunting may also result in visualization of the thyroid. Kidney uptake can be seen with right-to-left shunts and with free pertechnetate. The most reliable way to confirm a right-to-left shunt is to image the brain.

A right-to-left shunt in adults is often caused by an atrial septal defect, although other causes include ventricular septal defect and intrapulmonic shunt. Right-to-left shunting through an atrial septal defect may be intermittent, depending on the right and left atrial pressures, or the shunting may be bidirectional.

PEARLS AND PITFALLS

- Both right-to-left shunting and free pertechnetate may be responsible for MAA tracer uptake in the kidneys. These entities may be distinguished by obtaining a view of the head. Normally, tracer should not concentrate in the brain unless there is a right-to-left shunt. Renal uptake due to free pertechnetate is not associated with tracer uptake in the brain.
- Renal uptake can also be seen following the absorption and filtration of swallowed ^{99m}Tc-DTPA aerosol.

Suggested Reading
Freitas JE, Sarosi MG, Nagle CC, Yeomans ME, Freitas AE, Juni JE. Modified PIOPED criteria used in clinical practice. J Nucl Med 1995;36(9):1573–1578

CASE 55

Clinical Presentation

A 54-year-old woman presents with hemoptysis, shortness of breath, and previous pulmonary embolism.

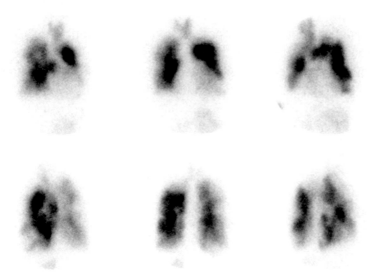

Fig. 55.1

Technique

- A 3.0 mCi dose of ^{99m}Tc-MAA is administered intravenously with the patient supine.
- The patient should cough and take several deep breaths before administration of the MAA to clear any areas of resting atelectasis.
- The patient should breathe normally during tracer injection.

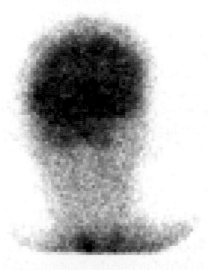

Fig. 55.2

- Use a low-energy, all-purpose collimator.
- Energy window 20% centered at 140 keV.
- Imaging time is 500,000 counts per view.
- Matrix size is 128 × 128.
- Views are anterior, right anterior oblique, left anterior oblique, posterior, right posterior oblique, and left posterior oblique. Lateral views can also be obtained, although it is important to remember that counts from the contralateral lung will contribute to these views.

Image Interpretation

The lung perfusion images (**Fig. 55.1**) demonstrate irregular perfusion throughout both lung fields, including multiple segmental and subsegmental defects that have not changed since the previous study (not shown). Anterior images (top row) show tracer uptake in the thyroid gland. A subsequent view of the head shows tracer uptake in the brain (**Fig. 55.2**). The chest radiograph was clear.

Differential Diagnosis

(For tracer uptake outside the lungs)
- Right-to-left shunt
- Particle dissolution (images obtained several hours after tracer injection)
- Radiopharmaceutical preparation problems
- Pulmonary arteriovenous malformation

Diagnosis and Clinical Follow-Up

Ventilation images in the previous study showed matched ventilation throughout both lung fields. The patient was thought to have severe chronic obstructive pulmonary disease (COPD) with pulmonary hypertension and a right-to-left shunt secondary to flow through an open atrial septal defect.

Discussion

Tracer uptake in the thyroid is often secondary to free pertechnetate. However, free pertechnetate is unusual with MAA preparation. The thyroid is an organ with a very high rate of blood flow, and it is often seen on perfusion scans when right-to-left shunting is present. Visualization of the thyroid or kidneys should raise suspicion of either free pertechnetate or right-to-left shunting (Gale et al., 1990). The blood–brain barrier excludes most radiopharmaceuticals, so a view of the head can be used as a biological assay to distinguish between poor labeling and right-to-left shunting.

Normally, the left atrial pressure is greater than the right atrial pressure, resulting either in a left-to-right shunt or in closure of the overlying flaps of a potential defect. Reversal of flow or opening of a virtual atrial septal defect can also be seen in pulmonary hypertension, including acute pulmonary hypertension due to pulmonary embolism. The acute development of right-to-left shunting is one explanation of the oxygen desaturation seen with pulmonary embolism; however, this mechanism has been shown to be unusual (Strauss et al., 1969).

PEARLS AND PITFALLS _____

- Visualization of any tracer uptake outside the lung fields should be investigated further. Special views of the area of abnormal uptake may be necessary to better define the location of the uptake.

- Views of the head are an important way to distinguish right-to-left shunt from a problem with radiopharmaceutical preparation.
- Pulmonary hypertension with a secondary elevation of right atrial pressure can be seen in both pulmonary embolism and pulmonary parenchymal disease.
- When the standard 200,000 to 400,000 particles are used in the injection of a single dose of ^{99m}Tc-MAA, approximately 1 per 1000 pulmonary capillaries are temporarily occluded. Fewer particles (60,000–100,000) may be given if the patient has a history of right-to-left shunting, pulmonary artery hypertension, or both. Care should be taken during preparation and at the time of injection to prevent clumping of the particles.

Suggested Reading

Gale B, Chen C, Chun KJ, Lan J, Cynamon J, Freeman LM. Systemic to pulmonary venous shunting in superior vena cava obstruction: unusual myocardial and thyroid visualization. Clin Nucl Med 1990;15(4):246–250

Strauss HW, Hurley PJ, Rhodes BA, Wagner HN Jr. Quantification of right-to-left transpulmonary shunts in man. J Lab Clin Med 1969;74(4):597–607

Section IV

Endocrine Scintigraphy

M. Elizabeth Oates and Rachel A. Powsner

CASE 56

Clinical Presentation

A 34-year-old woman presents with a possible right thyroid nodule palpated by the referring physician. Her thyroid function test values are normal.

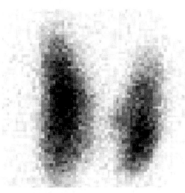 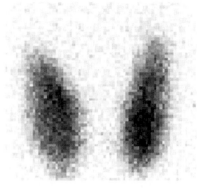 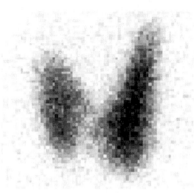

Fig. 56.1 Right anterior oblique pinhole collimator view, ^{123}I.

Fig. 56.2 Anterior pinhole collimator view, ^{123}I.

Fig. 56.3 Left anterior oblique pinhole collimator view, ^{123}I.

Technique

- 0.300 mCi of ^{123}I administered orally 4 hours before uptake and scan
- Five-minute pinhole collimator images in right anterior oblique, anterior, and left anterior oblique projections
- An appropriately shielded sodium iodide thyroid probe is positioned with the crystal surface 25 cm from the surface being measured. Obtain counts of the following for 2 minutes:
  - Thyroid bed
  - Thigh (body background)
  - Room background
  - Pill standard (in a neck phantom)
- Calculate the iodine uptake with the following formula:

$$RAIU = \frac{NeckCounts(\textbf{cpm}) - ThighCounts(\textbf{cpm})}{PillCounts(\textbf{cpm}) - BackgroundCounts(\textbf{cpm})} \times 100$$

Image Interpretation

The 24-hour uptake of radioiodine is 20%. Three views (**Figs. 56.1, 56.2,** and **56.3**) demonstrate homogeneous tracer distribution throughout the thyroid gland. The pyramid-shaped gland has smooth contours and relatively less activity at the periphery, reflecting thinner tissue there. A faint isthmus unites the right and left lobes. Each normal thyroid lobe measures approximately 5 cm in length and 2 cm in width. On physical examination, the gland feels normal in size (estimated weight, 15–30 g), configuration, and consistency. No nodule is palpated.

Differential Diagnosis

• Normal thyroid gland

Diagnosis and Clinical Follow-Up

Normal thyroid gland. Diagnosis final, no clinical follow-up.

Discussion

Thyroid scintigraphy is clinically important for the diagnosis and treatment of a variety of benign and malignant thyroid disorders, including the evaluation of goiters, differential diagnosis of hyperthyroidism, and function of thyroid nodules. Optimal thyroid scintigraphy requires an understanding of the two common imaging agents, radioactive ^{123}I and ^{99m}Tc-pertechnetate (**Table 56.1**). Normal ^{123}I scans show a variable appearance of the thyroid gland and have much less salivary activity. Thyroid scans with ^{99m}Tc look different from those with ^{123}I. With ^{99m}Tc, there is greater background activity, and the salivary glands should be clearly visible. In a euthyroid patient, the degree of normal thyroid "trapping" of ^{99m}Tc 20 minutes after injection approximates that in the salivary glands (**Figs. 56.4** and **56.5**).

The scintigraphic pattern should always be correlated with the patient history, physical examination findings, and current laboratory values.

Radioactive iodine uptake (RAIU), a measure of organification function, ranges from 5 to 15% at 4 hours to 15 to 30% at 24 hours (peak activity); these values are population-specific and laboratory-

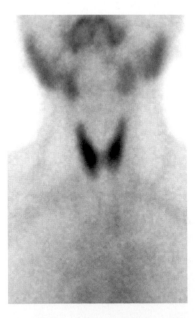

Fig. 56.4 Anterior parallel-hole collimator view, ^{99m}Tc.

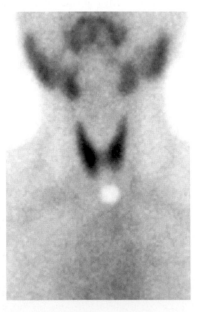

Fig. 56.5 Anterior parallel-hole collimator view with "cold" suprasternal notch marker, ^{99m}Tc.

Table 56.1   Comparison of Two Common Radiopharmaceuticals Used for Thyroid Scintigraphy

	^{123}I	^{99m}Tc-pertechnetate
Advantages	Oral administration	Inexpensive
	Tissue-specific true function (organification)	Readily available
	Uptake can be measured reliably over time	Single visit
	Higher target-to-background images	Completed in 1 h
	No blood pool activity and minimal salivary activity	Sharper images
Disadvantages	Expensive	Intravenous administration
	Special order	Pseudofunction (trapping)
	Multiple visits: (1) dosing, (2) 4-h uptake and scan, and/or (3) 24-h uptake	Activity more variable over time
	Completed in 4–24 h	Lower target-to-background images
	Less sharp images	Blood pool activity and salivary activity

specific. In most institutions, uptake values greatly influence the dose of ^{131}I prescribed to treat Graves disease and toxic nodular conditions.

For both radiotracers, patient preparation is of paramount importance. Before dosing, the patient should be questioned to ascertain the following information: no iodinated contrast for 4 to 6 weeks, no thyroid hormone for 3 to 4 weeks, no antithyroid medication for 3 to 5 days, and no iodine-containing medications such as amiodarone.

PEARLS AND PITFALLS

- The iodine administered for thyroid scintigraphy is in tracer amounts; therefore, it is safe for patients with iodine allergy or a history of reaction to previous iodinated contrast.
- As shown here, a suprasternal notch marker view provides an anatomic landmark for the position of the thyroid gland; markers can be "hot" or "cold" (**Fig. 56.5**).
- Asymmetry in lobe size, as seen here, is a common variation, with the right lobe often larger than the left.
- Oblique pinhole views allow appreciation of the posterior extent of each lobe.
- Because ^{99m}Tc is secreted by the salivary glands, salivary activity in the esophagus can mimic thyroid tissue on an anterior view (**Fig. 56.6**). On the oblique view, esophageal activity is linear and posterior in location (**Fig. 56.7**). Salivary activity should clear on repeated imaging after the ingestion of water; thus, it is prudent to ask patients to drink water before imaging.

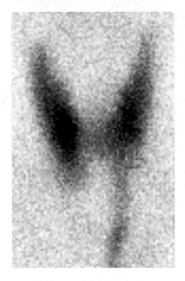

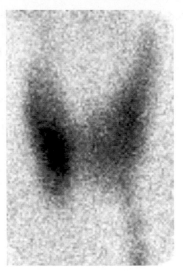

Fig. 56.6 Anterior pinhole collimator view, ^{99m}Tc.

Fig. 56.7 Left anterior oblique pinhole collimator view, ^{99m}Tc.

Suggested Reading

Sarkar SD. Benign thyroid disease: what is the role of nuclear medicine? Semin Nucl Med 2006;36(3): 185–193

Smith JR, Oates E. Radionuclide imaging of the thyroid gland: patterns, pearls, and pitfalls. Clin Nucl Med 2004;29(3):181–193

Society of Nuclear Medicine Procedure Guideline for Thyroid Scintigraphy version 2.0, approved February 7, 1999. www.snm.org. Accessed April 13, 2010

Society of Nuclear Medicine Procedure Guideline for Thyroid Uptake Measurement version 3.0, approved September 5, 2006. www.snm.org

CASE 57

Clinical Presentation

A 46-year-old woman presents with a very large palpable mass in the left thyroid lobe and markedly abnormal thyroid function test values:

- Thyrotropin (thyroid-stimulating hormone [TSH]), < 0.01 µU/mL (normal range, 0.5–6.0 µU/mL)
- Serum thyroxine (T_4), 25.4 µg/dL (normal range, 4.6–12.0 µg/dL)
- Serum triiodothyronine (T_3), 1087 ng/dL (normal range, 80–180 ng/dL)
- Thyroid peroxidase (TPO) antibodies, negative

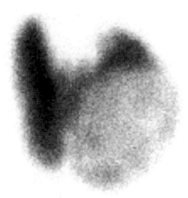 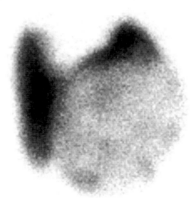 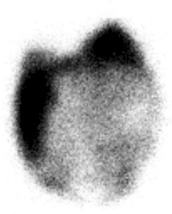

Fig. 57.1 Right anterior oblique pinhole collimator view, ^{123}I.

Fig. 57.2 Anterior pinhole collimator view, ^{123}I.

Fig. 57.3 Left anterior oblique pinhole collimator view, ^{123}I.

Technique

- 0.500 mCi of ^{123}I administered orally 24 hours before uptake and scan
- Five-minute pinhole collimator images in right anterior oblique, anterior, and left anterior oblique projections
- Appropriately shielded sodium iodide thyroid probe positioned with the crystal surface 25 cm from the surface being measured. Obtain counts of the following for 2 minutes:
  - ° Thyroid bed
  - ° Thigh (body background)
  - ° Room background
  - ° Pill standard (in a neck phantom)
- Calculate the iodine uptake with the following formula:

$$RAIU = \frac{Neck\,Counts(\text{cpm}) - Thigh\,Counts(\text{cpm})}{Pill\,Counts(\text{cpm}) - Background\,Counts(\text{cpm})} \times 100$$

Image Interpretation

The 24-hour uptake measures 85% by thyroid probe. The uptake of 85% at 24 hours is markedly increased (expected range, 15–30%). Three views (**Figs. 57.1, 57.2,** and **57.3**) demonstrate a large, well-defined "cold" nodule in the left lobe of the thyroid gland, corresponding to the palpated nodule, within an otherwise diffusely enlarged but homogeneous gland.

Differential Diagnosis

(Two coexisting thyroid conditions)
- For the right lobe and left upper lobe, Graves disease
- In the left lower lobe, primary malignant neoplasm or metastasis versus a benign condition (eg, abscess, adenoma, adenomatous hyperplasia, colloid cyst, hematoma, lymphocytic thyroiditis, parathyroid adenoma)

Diagnosis and Clinical Follow-Up

1. Graves disease (presumptive)
2. Hürthle cell lesion (follicular variant) with scant colloid (by biopsy); diagnoses final

Discussion

Graves Disease

Thyrotoxicosis and hyperthyroidism are not synonymous. The term *thyrotoxicosis* refers to the clinical condition characterized by increased systemic metabolism due to high levels of circulating T_4 and/or T_3. The term *hyperthyroidism* refers to overactivity of the thyroid gland resulting in unregulated thyroid hormone synthesis and an uncontrolled release of hormones into the circulation, leading to clinical thyrotoxicosis. Thyrotoxicosis can develop in conditions not associated with increased thyroid function, such as subacute or silent thyroiditis. The distinction is important because the management and prognosis of toxic thyroid disease depend on its etiology.

Graves disease (toxic diffuse goiter) is the most common cause of hyperthyroidism. In this disease, an immunoglobulin G autoantibody stimulates the follicular cell TSH receptor, resulting in diffuse autonomous function and concomitant thyrotoxicosis. Blood work shows elevated thyroid hormone levels and TSH levels that are low or suppressed. Radioactive iodine uptake (RAIU) is elevated, as in this case.

Scintigraphy demonstrates the functional state of the thyroid gland and thus can be used in conjunction with RAIU as the imaging modality of choice for the differential diagnosis of thyrotoxicosis. Scintigraphic patterns readily differentiate between nodular conditions and Graves disease. Whereas multinodular localization with elevated RAIU is most likely toxic nodular goiter, a diffusely "hot" gland is most likely Graves disease, as in this case.

"Cold" Nodule

Solitary thyroid nodules are common and can be found in up to half of the elderly population. Evaluation should include a careful history, physical examination, and thyroid function tests. Factors such as age, gender, size and number of nodules, and history of neck irradiation influence the likelihood of malignancy. Because the majority (90%) are benign, nonfunctioning adenomas or colloid cysts, thyroid cancer is an uncommon clinical entity. Regardless, thyroid "incidentalomas" present a vexing management problem. The major challenge remains selecting the few patients for whom surgical excision is necessary, rather than the usual conservative management.

Although its value is controversial, thyroid scintigraphy is still commonly performed in the evaluation of a palpated abnormality. Whether a solitary nodule or multiple nodules are found in the gland, the thyroid scan reliably demonstrates the function of the thyroid nodule(s). Nodules can appear hyperfunctioning ("hot"), hypofunctioning ("cold"), or relatively normally functioning ("warm") relative to the remainder of the gland. Hot nodules are generally benign and do not require fine-needle aspiration biopsy (FNAB), whereas cold nodules are potentially (10%) malignant and warrant FNAB with cytologic examination. FNAB is readily performed in an outpatient setting and is used routinely today to assess for malignancy in palpated thyroid nodules. It is considered a safe and cost-effective approach to patient management. When FNAB results are equivocal, thyroid scintigraphy can be particularly useful in risk stratification; for example, it is reassuring when the nodule in question appears autonomously functioning (hot) on the scan.

Ultrasonography can provide correlative information about the internal architecture of thyroid nodules, but the anatomic findings are nonspecific and less definitive than histologic examination.

PEARLS AND PITFALLS

- The scintigraphic pattern of Graves disease is typically diffuse and uniform, but it may be heterogeneous.
- A pyramidal lobe, which represents the caudal remnant of the thyroglossal duct, extends cephalad from the medial portion of one of the lobes, coursing anteriorly and superiorly. The pyramidal lobe is commonly prominent in Graves disease (**Figs. 57.4** and **57.5**).
- A dominant cold nodule in a multinodular gland may be benign or malignant. The cancer risk when more than three nodules are present is significantly lower than that for a solitary nodule in an otherwise normal gland. However, because malignancy remains a concern in patients with one or two nodules larger than 1 cm, those patients should undergo FNAB.
- It is important to obtain the TSH level in a patient with thyrotoxicosis because early Hashimoto thyroiditis may be associated with increased RAIU, mimicking Graves disease. However, in Hashimoto thyroiditis, hormone synthesis is inefficient, resulting in hypothyroidism with a concomitantly increased TSH level. A similar pattern is seen in the early phase of subacute thyroiditis.
- Rarely, a malignant nodule may retain its trapping function, but not organification functions, and appear warm on ^{99m}Tc imaging and cold on ^{123}I imaging. A nodule that is warm on ^{99m}Tc but cold on

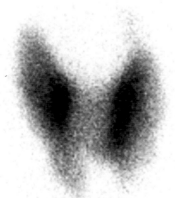

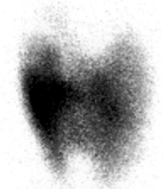

Fig. 57.4 Anterior pinhole collimator view, ^{123}I.

Fig. 57.5 Left anterior oblique pinhole collimator view, ^{123}I.

[123]I imaging is referred to as a *discordant nodule* and warrants FNAB for further evaluation. However, nodules demonstrating the much less common *reverse discordance* pattern (ie, cold on ^{99m}Tc and warm or hot on ^{123}I) are almost always benign, so that no biopsy is needed.

- Cold nodules can occur in the isthmus or at the periphery of the gland. They may be difficult to appreciate or may cause little distortion of the normal gland contour. Look for a thin rim of thyroid tissue outlining an exophytic cold nodule. If palpated, the nodule should be marked and should correlate with scan findings.

Suggested Reading

Barroeta JE, Wang H, Shiina N, Gupta PK, Livolsi VA, Baloch ZW. Is fine-needle aspiration (FNA) of multiple thyroid nodules justified? Endocr Pathol 2006;17(1):61–65

Delbridge L. Solitary thyroid nodule: current management. ANZ J Surg 2006;76(5):381–386

dell'Erba L, Gerundini P, Caputo M, Bagnasco M. Association of hyperfunctioning thyroid adenoma with thyroid cancer presenting as "trapping only" nodule at [99m]TcO4- scintigraphy. J Endocrinol Invest 2003;26(11):1124–1127

Intenzo CM, dePapp AE, Jabbour S, Miller JL, Kim SM, Capuzzi DM. Scintigraphic manifestations of thyrotoxicosis. Radiographics 2003;23(4):857–869

Lansford CD, Teknos TN. Evaluation of the thyroid nodule. Cancer Control 2006;13(2):89–98

CASE 58

Clinical Presentation

A 55-year-old woman presents with a large mediastinal mass on CT of the thorax. Thyroid function tests show normal values: thyroid-stimulating hormone (TSH), 0.1 µU/mL;, thyroxine (T_4), 10.5 µg/dL.

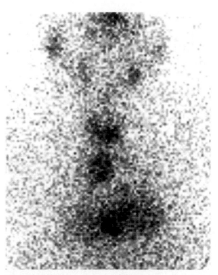

Fig. 58.1 Anterior parallel-hole collimator view of neck and thorax, [123]I.

Technique

- 0.500 mCi of ^{123}I administered orally 4 hours before scan
- Five-minute anterior parallel-hole collimator view (**Fig. 58.1**); SPECT with low-energy, high-resolution collimators on dual-detector gamma camera
- Acquisition parameters
    - 64 × 64 matrix
    - 180 degrees
    - 64 views
    - 30 seconds per view per detector
- Processing parameters
    - Gaussian iterative reconstruction, filter 10.0 (**Fig. 58.2**)
    - Thoracic CT (**Fig. 58.3**)
    - Fused SPECT/CT (**Fig. 58.4**) with commercial software

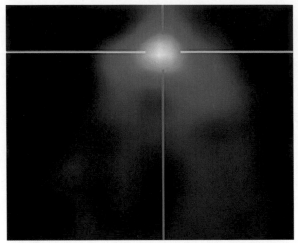

Fig. 58.2 Selected transaxial SPECT image of thorax, ^{123}I.

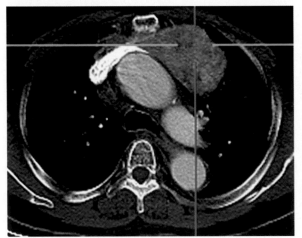

Fig. 58.3 Selected transaxial CT image of thorax, same level as **Fig. 58.2**.

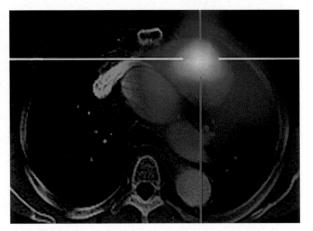

Fig. 58.4 SPECT/CT fusion (**Figs. 58.2** and **58.3**).

Image Interpretation

A large region of heterogeneous ^{123}I localization extending from the neck into the thorax characterizes the mediastinal mass as thyroid tissue, consistent with a large substernal goiter. SPECT/CT image fusion confirms the functional/anatomic relationship.

Differential Diagnosis

Based on CT scan alone, the differential diagnosis of mediastinal masses includes the following:

- Lymphoma
- Metastasis
- Thymoma
- Teratoma
- Thyroid tissue

Diagnosis and Clinical Follow-Up

Substernal goiter. Diagnosis final, no clinical follow-up.

Discussion

Multinodular goiter may result from goitrogens, iodine deficiency (endemic goiter), or thyroiditis. Goitrogens inhibit hormone synthesis, leading to increased TSH levels that result in goiter formation. Goitrogens include large doses of iodine, lithium, and some foods in their raw form (eg, cabbage, peanuts, walnuts, mustard, cassava, and soybeans). Biochemically, multinodular goiter may be euthyroid or toxic. Patients with Hashimoto thyroiditis may acquire a multinodular goiter if some portions of the gland grow in response to the increased TSH level.

Substernal goiter accounts for approximately 5 to 10% of mediastinal masses and is the most common cause of a superior mediastinal mass. Diagnostically, it needs to be differentiated from primary and metastatic tumors. ^{123}I is the preferred agent for characterizing substernal goiters because of its higher target-to-background images, greater tissue specificity, and decreased blood pool activity in comparison with ^{99m}Tc-pertechnetate.

Clinically, a large substernal goiter can be significant because as it grows between the sternum anteriorly and vertebral bodies posteriorly, it may impinge on adjacent vital structures and cause compressive symptoms; some require surgical removal.

PEARLS AND PITFALLS

- Goiter often demonstrates calcifications, high density, and contrast enhancement on CT.
- Most intrathoracic goiters are contiguous with the cervical thyroid gland, but they may appear as separate ^{123}I imagery because of a lack of functional intervening tissue.
- If a patient receives iodinated contrast during CT, then radionuclide imaging must be postponed for at least 4 weeks.
- ^{123}I is the preferred agent for confirming a substernal goiter, but uptake of ^{123}I may be poor because of impaired function of the goitrous tissue.
- Hyperextension of the head during thyroid scintigraphy can greatly affect the apparent location of the thyroid tissue in relation to other anatomic structures because it is "pulled up." Because the patient's head is usually in a neutral position for the CT scan, correlation between the imaging modalities may be misleading unless positioning is the same for all the studies.

Suggested Reading

Infante JR, Serrano J, Rayo JI, et al. Primary intrathoracic goiter on scintigraphy. Clin Nucl Med 2005;30(7):523–524

Shah PJ, Bright T, Singh SS, et al. Large retrosternal goitre: a diagnostic and management dilemma. Heart Lung Circ 2006;15(2):151–152

CASE 59

Clinical Presentation

A 35-year-old man presents with an asymptomatic right thyroid nodule noted on routine physical examination. Thyroid function test values are normal.

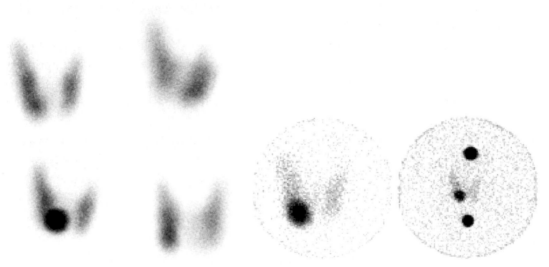

Fig. 59.1 Multiple pinhole collimator views: anterior, right anterior oblique, left anterior oblique, and anterior with "hot" ^{57}Co marker over palpated nodule, ^{123}I.

Fig. 59.2 Two pinhole collimator views: anterior without and with anatomic markers (superior marker at chin, inferior marker at sternal notch), ^{123}I after suppression with thyroid hormone.

Technique

- 0.400 mCi of ^{123}I at 24 hours before scan
- Five-minute pinhole collimator views in anterior, right anterior oblique, and left anterior oblique projections, and anterior projection with a "hot" ^{57}Co marker placed over the palpated nodule (**Fig. 59.1**; look at the images clockwise, beginning with the ^{57}Co marker image in the lower left-hand corner).
- After suppression with oral thyroid hormone, repeated anterior pinhole views without and with anatomic markers on the chin (superior marker) and sternal notch (inferior marker) (**Fig. 59.2**)

Image Interpretation

Figure 59.1 shows a normal-appearing thyroid gland except for minimal asymmetry in tracer uptake. The right lobe appears larger than the left, but this can be a normal variant. The "hot spot" represents the ^{57}Co marker placed on the palpated nodule. **Figure 59.2** demonstrates imaging of the same patient after administration of a suppressive dose of thyroid hormone, which "turns off" thyroid-stimulating hormone (TSH) and thus suppresses normally responsive thyroid tissue. The palpated nodule continues to function despite TSH suppression and so is termed *autonomous*. It is unlikely for a single autonomously functioning nodule to be cancerous, and therefore no further management is required.

Differential Diagnosis

- Thyroid adenoma
- Autonomous adenoma (common) versus thyroid carcinoma (uncommon)

Diagnosis and Clinical Follow-Up

Autonomous adenoma with incomplete suppression of the remainder of the thyroid gland, consistent with a euthyroid state. Diagnosis final, no clinical follow-up.

Discussion

Solitary thyroid nodules are common; the majority of them are benign. Radionuclide imaging can characterize toxic or autonomous hot nodules, which are frequently functioning adenomas and rarely malignant. Not all functioning adenomas cause clinical toxicity, although the likelihood of toxicity increases with nodule size (> 2.5 cm). Suppression of the remainder of the gland implies autonomy of the nodule; this pattern may be associated with overt or subclinical thyrotoxicosis. Thus, correlation with thyroid function test values is essential because a low or suppressed TSH level may be the first clinical indicator of toxicity.

When a palpated nodule does not clearly correspond to focally decreased or increased tracer uptake on the scan, several causes should be considered (eg, "cold" nodule hidden by surrounding functioning tissue, weakly functioning hot nodule, extrathyroidal mass). If the nodule is functioning, it may be autonomously functioning but not hyperfunctioning to the extent that it suppresses the surrounding normal thyroid tissue, so that it is difficult to appreciate. To distinguish an autonomously functioning nodule from a cold nodule, a suppression scan may be helpful, as shown here. A suppression scan is simply repeated ^{123}I imaging following the oral administration of a suppressive dose of thyroid hormone (**Fig. 59.2**). The thyroid hormone should suppress iodine uptake in all tissue normally responsive to TSH, but not in the autonomous nodule. This is an important clinical distinction because if the nodule is functioning and autonomous, it is very unlikely to be cancer. Conversely, if the nodule is cold (or not seen on the suppression scan), then it is potentially malignant and requires further investigation.

Physical examination is very important in the interpretation of the thyroid scan. Palpated nodules should be indicated with radioactive markers to document how they correspond to the scintigraphic appearance. However, caution is in order when a pinhole collimator is used for imaging. The pinhole collimator provides magnification and the highest spatial resolution, but it results in spatial distortion, which can interfere with proper coregistration of a palpated nodule and the scintigraphic abnormality (**Fig. 59.3**). The pinhole should be centered over the nodule to avoid parallax distortion.

Simple observation and thyroid hormone suppressive therapy are acceptable management options for patients with presumably benign thyroid nodules. Radioiodine therapy may be used for the management of patients with hyperfunctioning (hot) thyroid nodules.

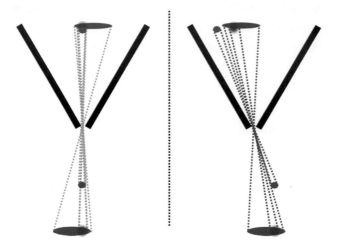

Fig. 59.3 Diagram of relationship of marker to nodule and parallax effect.

PEARLS AND PITFALLS

- Images should be viewed on a computer monitor so that image intensity and contrast can be manipulated to look for subtly increased or decreased uptake in the thyroid gland.

- An adenoma usually appears homogeneous, but a large adenoma may have central necrosis or hemorrhage or undergo cystic degeneration, leading to central photopenia (cold center) with a hot rim of surrounding activity.

- More than one hot nodule may be identified in an otherwise normal gland. *Plummer disease* originally described a single toxic adenoma in a multinodular gland, but the eponym now implies multiple toxic foci, usually in a multinodular gland.

- Not all functioning nodules are autonomous; therefore, the lack of uptake in a nodule on a suppression scan does not necessarily mean that it is a cold nodule.

- When properly done, marker views can establish that the palpated nodule does or does not correspond to the visualized hyperfunctioning nodule. However, it is important technically to position the palpated nodule in the center of the pinhole collimator field of view. Given that the marker is not in the same plane as the thyroid gland (ie, the marker is on the skin surface, whereas the thyroid gland is deeper), the parallax effect may artifactually misregister the nodule in relation to the marker (**Fig. 59.3**).

Suggested Reading

Britto-Fioretti AM, Furlanetto RP, Paiva ER, Kunii IS, Silva MR, Maciel RM. Thyroid suppression test with a single oral dose of levothyroxine in the diagnosis of functional thyroid autonomy. Endocr Pract 1999;5(6):330–336

Niepomniszcze H, Suárez H, Pitoia F, et al. Follicular carcinoma presenting as autonomous functioning thyroid nodule and containing an activating mutation of the TSH receptor (T620I) and a mutation of the Ki-RAS (G12C) genes. Thyroid 2006;16(5):497–503

Sakorafas GH, Peros G. Thyroid nodule: a potentially malignant lesion; optimal management from a surgical perspective. Cancer Treat Rev 2006;32(3):191–202

CASE 60

Clinical Presentation

A 33–year-old woman presents with palpitations and heat intolerance. Laboratory values confirm thyrotoxicosis with suppressed thyroid-simulating hormone (TSH) and elevated thyroxine (T$_4$) levels. She is 3 months postpartum.

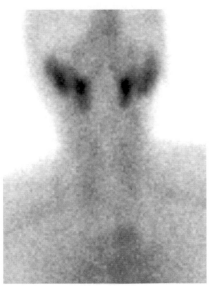

Fig. 60.1 Anterior parallel-hole collimator view, ^{99m}Tc.

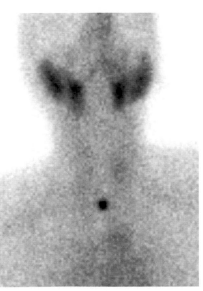

Fig. 60.2 Anterior parallel-hole collimator view with "hot" suprasternal notch marker, ^{99m}Tc.

Technique

- 12 mCi of ^{99m}Tc-pertechnetate administered intravenously at 10 minutes before scan
- Five-minute anterior parallel-hole collimator images without (**Fig. 60.1**) and with (**Fig. 60.2**) "hot" sternal notch marker

Image Interpretation

Absence of ^{99m}Tc localization and nonvisualization of the thyroid gland. Note prominent, symmetric salivary glands.

Differential Diagnosis

See **Table 60.1** for a comparative analysis of poorly visualized or nonvisualized thyroid glands.

Table 60.1 Differential Diagnosis of a Poorly Visualized or Nonvisualized Thyroid Gland

Hypothyroid	Euthyroid	Hyperthyroid
After ^{131}I ablation, surgery, radiation therapy	Diet rich in iodine	Subacute (granulomatous), silent (lymphocytic), postpartum thyroiditis
End-stage goiter	Recent iodinated contrast media	Factitious thyrotoxicosis
Hashimoto thyroiditis	Concomitant medications: amiodarone (high iodine), antithyroid medications, thyroid hormone	Concomitant medication: amiodarone (high iodine)
Amyloidosis	Incomplete dose	Ectopic thyroid tissue: struma ovarii, hyperfunctioning thyroid, cancer metastases

Diagnosis and Clinical Follow-Up

Postpartum thyroiditis. Diagnosis final, no clinical follow-up.

Discussion

Radionuclide evaluation of the thyroid gland helps considerably in the differential diagnosis of thyrotoxicosis. As in this clinical setting, nonvisualization of the thyroid gland suggests a destructive thyroiditis, which is a self-limited disorder, whereas normal or elevated ^{99m}Tc trapping (or ^{123}I uptake) would indicate toxic nodular goiter or Graves disease. Because the management of these disorders is quite different, a specific diagnosis is very important.

A common cause of primary thyrotoxicosis is subacute (granulomatous) thyroiditis, usually secondary to viral illness. A painful, tender thyroid gland, sore throat, and systemic symptoms characterize subacute thyroiditis (**Figs. 60.3** and **60.4**). The associated inflammatory process is self-limited; it begins with a thyrotoxic phase, manifested by low radioactive iodine uptake (RAIU) and poor visualization/

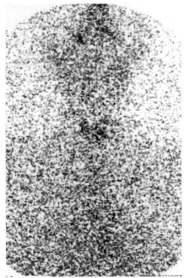

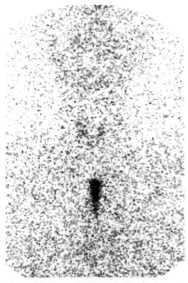

Fig. 60.3 Anterior parallel-hole collimator view, ^{123}I.

Fig. 60.4 Anterior parallel-hole collimator view with "hot" suprasternal notch marker, ^{123}I.

nonvisualization of the thyroid gland on scintigraphy, which is followed by short euthyroid and hypothyroid phases before complete recovery. During the hypothyroid stage, "uptake" may actually be mildly increased, although the thyroid gland has not yet regained efficient hormonogenesis. A similar triphasic response of thyroid dysfunction/function can be seen with silent (lymphocytic) thyroiditis and postpartum thyroiditis. Postpartum thyroiditis is considered a subtype of silent thyroiditis and occurs in 5 to 10% of pregnancies, as shown here.

The term *autoimmune thyroiditis* encompasses multiple inflammatory conditions of the thyroid gland, each with variable clinical manifestations. The more acute forms, silent (painless) thyroiditis and postpartum thyroiditis, are associated with transient thyrotoxicosis and sometimes mistaken for Graves disease clinically. The chronic form, Hashimoto thyroiditis (chronic autoimmune thyroiditis), results in a goiter and eventual hypothyroidism.

As shown in **Table 60.1**, low RAIU and poor visualization/nonvisualization may be associated with other variables (eg, Hashimoto thyroiditis, excess dietary iodine, recent administration of iodinated contrast, ingestion of thyroid hormone or other medications, notably amiodarone). Thyroiditis with these causes can easily be distinguished from subacute or silent thyroiditis because the patients are biochemically hypothyroid or euthyroid, not thyrotoxic.

Amiodarone can have significant effects on the thyroid gland. Amiodarone contains 75 mg of iodine per 200-mg tablet (500 times the Recommended Daily Allowance of iodine). Although amiodarone induced hypothyroidism is more common, amiodarone can cause hyperthyroidism in patients with normal glands or preexisting thyroiditis. It can also lead to thyrotoxicosis, which is caused by excess thyroid hormone synthesis resulting from the high iodine levels, or be associated with the destructive release of hormone, as in subacute thyroiditis. RAIU will be low in all cases because of the high iodine content.

PEARLS AND PITFALLS

- ^{99m}Tc can quickly establish a diagnosis of subacute or silent thyroiditis in patients with thyrotoxicosis.
- Salivary gland activity and the sternal notch marker provide anatomic landmarks because the thyroid gland is not well visualized.
- Careful questioning about medications, dietary sources of iodine (eg, kelp), and recent administration of iodinated contrast is important. Before dosing, speak with the patient yourself and be aware of factors that may suppress iodine uptake.
- Hypertrapping of ^{99m}Tc can be seen in the hypothyroid phase of subacute thyroiditis before recovery of organification function; this occurs only when TSH levels are no longer suppressed and have rebounded. Because that scintigraphic pattern alone could be misinterpreted as Graves disease, it is important to correlate temporally the scan findings with the thyroid function test values. In some cases, ^{123}I can be used for a more accurate assessment of organification function.

Suggested Reading

Intenzo CM, Capuzzi DM, Jabbour S, Kim SM, dePapp AE. Scintigraphic features of autoimmune thyroiditis. Radiographics 2001;21(4):957–964

Ross DS. Syndromes of thyrotoxicosis with low radioactive iodine uptake. Endocrinol Metab Clin North Am 1998;27(1):169–185

CASE 61

Clinical Presentation

A 48-year-old woman with a history of thyroid cancer has undergone thyroidectomy and requires evaluation for thyroid remnant tissue and possible metastases.

Fig. 61.1 Emission parallel-hole collimator view, ^{131}I.

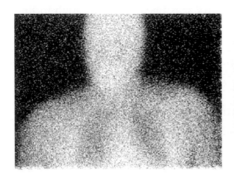

Fig. 61.2 Transmission parallel-hole collimator view, ^{57}Co.

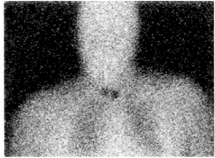

Fig. 61.3 Composite image: ^{131}I + ^{57}Co.

Technique

- 5.0 mCi of ^{131}I administered orally at 72 hours before scan
- Use of a high-energy collimator for parallel-hole collimator imaging of the neck and thorax without (**Fig. 61.1**) and with (**Fig. 61.2**) cobalt 57 flood source behind patient (ie, patient between flood source and detector)
- Emission image on ^{131}I photopeak (364 keV); transmission image on ^{57}Co photopeak (122 keV) without moving patient; superimposition of the two images (^{131}I and ^{57}Co) for composite image (**Fig. 61.3**)

Image Interpretation

Figures 61.1, 61.2, and **61.3** all show a silhouette of the head, torso, and lungs, with two discrete foci in the thyroid bed. No other abnormal ^{131}I-avid sites.

Differential Diagnosis

- Residual functioning thyroid tissue in the thyroid bed
- Surface contamination

Diagnosis and Clinical Follow-Up

Remnants in thyroid bed only. No regional or distant metastases. Diagnosis final, no clinical follow-up.

Discussion

Physiologic biodistribution of radioiodine occurs to the following: salivary glands, nose, stomach (and gastrointestinal tract from gastric emptying), bowel, kidneys, thyroid, choroid plexus, and bladder (renal excretion). The detection of pathologic ^{131}I-avid foci is the first step in evaluating a patient with thyroid cancer. However, localization can be difficult without anatomic landmarks. If there are no landmarks, a transmission image with use of a ^{57}Co flood source behind the patient to outline the lungs and the body can aid in localization (**Fig. 61.2**). The lungs are visualized with ^{57}Co because air in the lungs attenuates the ^{57}Co photons less than surrounding tissues do. **Figures 61.1** and **61.2** also demonstrate how the ^{131}I and ^{57}Co images look before they are combined to form the final composite image (**Fig. 61.3**). Although a flood source may increase radiation exposure to the patient, the additional exposure is minimal and the benefits far outweigh the theoretical risks, particularly in a patient receiving radioiodine therapy. Another localization method is to use a "hot" point source to manually outline the patient's body during image acquisition. More recently, SPECT/CT imaging has also been used for localization.

Traditionally, ^{131}I has been the radiopharmaceutical used for the diagnostic imaging of patients with differentiated thyroid cancer. Recently, ^{123}I has become more widely available and has become well accepted in many practices. ^{123}I is a pure gamma emitter with a 159-keV photopeak that has excellent imaging characteristics. Thus, superior image quality is obtained without sacrificing diagnostic accuracy. Also, ^{123}I avoids the "stunning" effect that can be associated with diagnostic scan doses of ^{131}I before high-dose ablative therapy.

The management of patients with differentiated thyroid cancer has changed significantly during the last few decades. Mortality has decreased as the result of earlier detection, refined surgical approaches, the standardization of radioiodine ablation, and the development of more sensitive methods of detecting and monitoring disease recurrence. Follow-up has been facilitated by serum thyroglobulin measurements, the use of recombinant human thyrotropin, in combination with ^{131}I and/or serum thyroglobulin measurements and the availability of ^{18}F-FDG-PET in selected patients in whom radioiodine imaging fails to locate suspected recurrence or metastases.

PEARLS AND PITFALLS

- Patients must be properly prepared for imaging and therapy (e.g., no iodinated contrast within 4 to 6 weeks and an elevated thyroid-stimulating hormone [TSH] level, either naturally through withdrawal of thyroid hormone or after administration of exogenous TSH).

- A low-iodine diet for one to two week depletes "cold" iodine stores before dosing with radioactive iodine, enhancing sensitivity.
- Scintigraphy is advantageous in that it provides a sensitive and specific approach to whole-body surveillance.
- Women of child-bearing potential should have a negative quantitative serum BHCG pregnancy test result within 24 hours before receiving [131]I.
- By first reviewing standard emission images to identify sites of ^{131}I uptake, faint abnormal tracer concentration in lung metastases will not be masked by the transmission flood source.

Suggested Reading

Intenzo CM, Jabbour S, Dam HQ, Capuzzi DM. Changing concepts in the management of differentiated thyroid cancer. Semin Nucl Med 2005;35(4):257–265

Lind P, Kohlfürst S. Respective roles of thyroglobulin, radioiodine imaging, and positron emission tomography in the assessment of thyroid cancer. Semin Nucl Med 2006;36(3):194–205

Mandel SJ, Shankar LK, Benard F, Yamamoto A, Alavi A. Superiority of iodine-123 compared with iodine-131 scanning for thyroid remnants in patients with differentiated thyroid cancer. Clin Nucl Med 2001;26(1):6–9

Morris LF, Waxman AD, Braunstein GD. The nonimpact of thyroid stunning: remnant ablation rates in 131I-scanned and nonscanned individuals. J Clin Endocrinol Metab 2001;86(8):3507–3511

Society of Nuclear Medicine Procedure Guideline for Scintigraphy for Differentiated Papillary and Follicular Thyroid Cancer, approved September 5, 2006. http://interactive.snm.org/docs/scintigraphy%20for%20Differentiated%20Thyroid%20Cancer%20v3%200%20(9-2s-06).pdf

CASE 62

Clinical Presentation

A 42-year-old woman with stage I papillary thyroid cancer presents for pre-therapy whole-body scan, ^{131}I ablation therapy, and post-therapy whole-body scan. Her serum thyroglobulin level is markedly elevated at 300 ng/mL (normal, < 0.5 ng/mL).

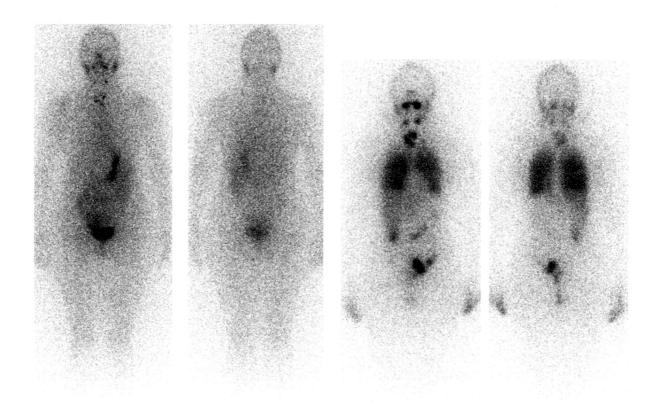

Fig. 62.1 Whole-body parallel-hole collimator views, anterior and posterior projections, ^{123}I (pre-therapy, diagnostic dose).

Fig. 62.2 Whole-body parallel-hole collimator views, anterior and posterior projections, ^{131}I (post-therapy dose).

Technique

- Pre-therapy scan: 2 mCi of oral ^{123}I 24 hours before scan
- Post-therapy scan: 200 mCi of oral ^{131}I one week before scan
- Whole-body diagnostic (pre-therapy) imaging (**Fig. 62.1**)
- Whole-body post-therapy imaging (**Fig. 62.2**)

Image Interpretation

On the diagnostic (pre-therapy) [123]I scan, multiple small, scattered foci in the neck suggest remnant tissue and possibly regional nodal metastases. On the post-therapy scan, marked diffuse activity throughout the lungs and liver is new; the neck activity is much more intense and extensive.

Differential Diagnosis

- Metastatic thyroid carcinoma
- Salivary or urinary contamination

Diagnosis and Clinical Follow-Up

Thyroid remnant tissue, regional lymph node metastases, and diffuse pulmonary metastases; physiologic uptake of tracer in the liver on post-therapy scan. Diagnosis final.

Discussion

Following thyroidectomy, radioiodine therapy is the most effective treatment option and is indicated for differentiated thyroid carcinomas (papillary and follicular). The withdrawal of thyroid hormone replacement causes the thyroid-stimulating hormone (TSH) level to rise, which in turn stimulates functional tissue to concentrate radioiodine. This avidity for radioiodine allows the effective treatment of metastatic sites with high doses of locally delivered radiation following ^{131}I administration. Despite such targeted therapy, distant metastases carry a poorer prognosis than disease confined to the thyroid bed.

Proper patient preparation is critical for optimal scan and therapy results. To achieve an appropriate hypothyroid state, patients are withdrawn from thyroxine (T_4) replacement 6 weeks before testing. Some practitioners transition the patient by converting to triiodothyronine (T_3) at this time, then stopping the T_3 2 weeks before testing. The TSH level is measured a few days before planned testing; if the TSH level is above 30 μU/mL, imaging and subsequent therapy can proceed. Patients are also put on a low-iodine diet to maximize tracer uptake. All women of child-bearing age must have a negative serum quantitative BHCG level within 24 hours of dosing with [131]I.

One criterion for treatment with radioactive iodine is tumor avidity, which can be assessed on a low-dose whole-body scan with 2 to 5 mCi of radioactive iodine (^{123}I or ^{131}I). Although controversial, it is believed there is no pre-therapy "stunning" of thyroid tissue after [123]I. For this reason ^{123}I whole-body scanning is preferred by some practitioners. Because of the relatively low level of tumor avidity (compared with normal thyroid tissue) and relatively higher background counts, metastases may not be visualized on the low-dose diagnostic scan.

Post-therapy scanning provides important information, even in patients whose pre-therapy scan is positive for metastases. After administration of a therapeutic dose of [131]I (100–200 mCi), it is not uncommon to visualize additional sites of metastatic disease. Reasons include the much higher ^{131}I dose and delayed imaging at 7 to 10 days, which allow clearance of background activity. Visualization of the liver is a common finding, occurring in approximately half the post-therapy scans; the intensity in the liver is roughly proportional to the amount of ^{131}I-avid functional thyroid tissue seen elsewhere.

PEARLS AND PITFALLS

- Even though distant disease may not be seen with a low-dose whole-body scan, a post-therapy whole-body scan should always be obtained to search for additional sites and complete scintigraphic staging of ^{131}I-avid disease.

- Pinhole collimator views of the thyroid bed can resolve separate foci and therefore may be helpful to assess the efficacy of therapy relative to individual sites.
- Diagnostic imaging doses of ^{131}I following thyroidectomy can "stun" thyrocytes and diminish the uptake of subsequent therapeutic doses of radioiodine.
- Normal physiologic ^{131}I activity in the esophagus, mediastinum, liver, bowel, and urinary collecting system may be misinterpreted as metastatic disease.

Suggested Reading

Dam HQ, Kim SM, Lin HC, Intenzo CM. 131 I therapeutic efficacy is not influenced by stunning after diagnostic whole-body scanning.

Donohoe KP, Shah NP, Lee S, Oates ME. Initial staging of differentiated thyroid carcinoma: the continued utility of post-therapy 1–131 whole body scintigraphy. Radiology 2008;246:887–894

Gerard SK, Cavalieri RR. I-123 diagnostic thyroid tumor whole-body scanning with imaging at 6, 24, and 48 hours. Clin Nucl Med 2002;27(1):1–8

Rosenbaum RC, Johnston GS, Valente WA. Frequency of hepatic visualization during I-131 imaging for metastatic thyroid carcinoma. Clin Nucl Med 1988;13(9):657–660

Souza Rosário PW, Barroso AL, Rezende LL, et al. Post I-131 therapy scanning in patients with thyroid carcinoma metastases: an unnecessary cost or a relevant contribution? Clin Nucl Med 2004;29(12):795–798

Thyroid. In: American Joint Committee on Cancer. AJCC Cancer Staging Manual. 6th ed. New York, NY: Springer; 2002:77–87

CASE 63

Clinical Presentation

A 34-year-old man with papillary thyroid cancer has undergone thyroidectomy and presents for imaging after radioiodine ablation.

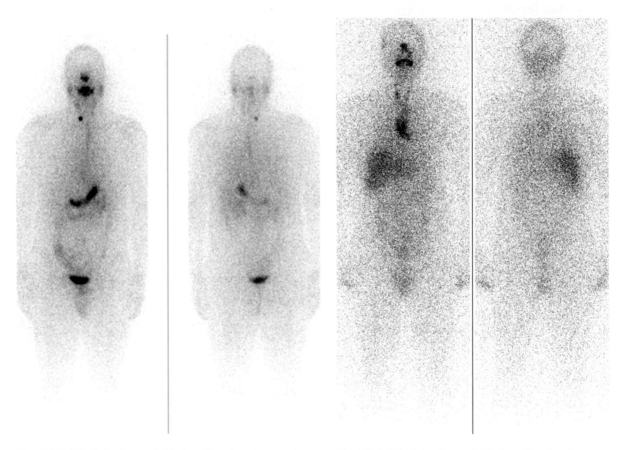

Fig. 63.1 Whole-body parallel-hole collimator views, anterior and posterior projections, ^{123}I (pre-therapy).

Fig. 63.2 Whole-body parallel-hole collimator views, anterior and posterior projections, ^{131}I (therapeutic dose).

Technique

- Pre-therapy scan: 2 mCi of ^{123}I administered orally for diagnostic scan 2 days before ^{131}I therapy
- Post-therapy scan: 100 mCi of therapeutic ^{131}I administered orally 1 week before scan
- Whole-body ^{123}I imaging in anterior and posterior projections with a dual-detector gamma camera equipped with low-energy collimators (**Fig. 63.1**)
- Whole-body ^{131}I imaging in anterior and posterior projections with a dual-detector gamma camera equipped with high-energy collimators (**Fig. 63.2**)

Image Interpretation

Physiologic distribution and a focus of thyroid tissue in the right side of the neck are seen on pre-therapy diagnostic ^{123}I imaging (**Fig. 63.1**). On post-therapy images, an additional intense site of uptake is noted in the region of the thymus (**Fig. 63.2**).

Differential Diagnosis

- Metastatic thyroid cancer
- Thymus uptake
- Contamination artifact

Diagnosis and Clinical Follow-Up

Physiologic variant: thymus on post-therapy scan only. Diagnosis final.

Discussion

Unusual biodistribution can be seen on post-therapy scans. The gallbladder is occasionally visualized (**Fig. 63.3**); this pattern suggests an abnormal gallbladder (eg, gallstones), and correlative evaluation with ultrasound or hepatobiliary scan can be diagnostic. Known or unsuspected renal cysts can accumulate radioiodine and be dramatic on post-therapy scans (**Fig. 63.4**); again, correlative imaging will confirm the cause.

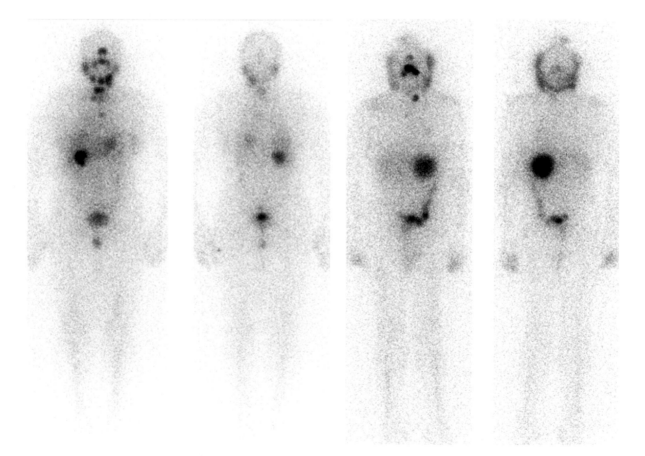

Fig. 63.3 Whole-body parallel-hole collimator views, anterior and posterior projections, ^{131}I (therapeutic dose).

Fig. 63.4 Whole-body parallel-hole collimator views, anterior and posterior projections, ^{131}I (therapeutic dose).

- Take advantage of a therapeutic (high) dose of ^{131}I by obtaining whole-body imaging a week after treatment; additional clinically relevant metastases, not apparent on pre-therapy diagnostic images, can be detected in a significant minority of patients.
- Delayed images can verify persistent activity in unexpected structures and can help differentiate physiologic (often clears with time) from pathologic (often persists over time) localization.
- Normal physiologic ^{131}I uptake in the salivary glands, esophagus, stomach, bowel, liver, and urinary collecting system may be misinterpreted as metastatic disease.
- Contamination of clothing, skin, and hair (**Fig. 63.4**) can yield false-positive results.

Suggested Reading

Thymus

Muratet JP, Giraud P. Thymus accumulation of I-131 after therapeutic dose for thyroid carcinoma. Clin Nucl Med 1996;21(9):736–737

Biliary System and Gallbladder

Achong DM, Oates E, Lee SL, Doherty FJ. Gallbladder visualization during post-therapy iodine-131 imaging of thyroid carcinoma. J Nucl Med 1991;32(12):2275–2277

Carlisle M, Cortés A, McDougall IR. Uptake of I-131 in the biliary tract: a potential cause of a false-positive result of scintiscan. Clin Nucl Med 1998;23(8):524–527

McEwan LM, Fong W. Unusual extrathyroidal iodine accumulation in a post-ablative I-131 scan. Australas Radiol 2001;45(4):512–513

Seok JW, Kim SJ, Kim IJ, Kim YS, Kim YK. Normal gallbladder visualization during post-ablative iodine-131 scan of thyroid cancer. J Korean Med Sci 2005;20(3):521–523

Renal Cyst

Letaief B, Boughattas S, Guezguez M, Hassine H, Essabbah H. Abdominal uptake of I-131 revealing a renal cyst. Clin Nucl Med 2001;26(3):255–256

Wen C, Iuanow E, Oates E, Lee SL, Perrone R. Post-therapy iodine-131 localization in unsuspected large renal cyst: possible mechanisms. J Nucl Med 1998;39(12):2158–2161

CASE 64

Clinical Presentation

A 43-year-old woman presents with a recent diagnosis of renal stones. The patient has elevated calcium and parathyroid hormone levels.

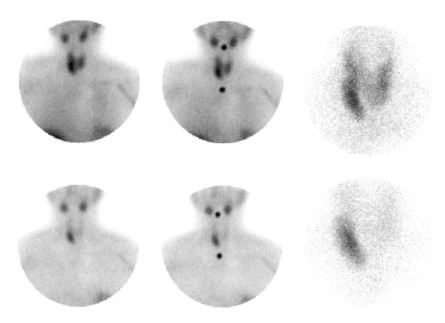

Fig. 64.1 Top row: 20-minute images; bottom row: 2-hour images.

Technique

- Approximately 20 mCi of ^{99m}Tc-sestamibi injected intravenously
- High-resolution collimator
- Anterior view of the neck and chest done at 20 minutes and 2 hours after injection
- Pinhole view of the thyroid bed done at 20 minutes and 2 hours after injection

Image interpretation

Initial images at 20 minutes (**Fig. 64.1**, top row) show relatively diffuse uptake in the thyroid and a focus of increased tracer uptake in the right lower pole. Two-hour–delayed images (**Fig. 64.1**, bottom row) show washout of tracer from the thyroid and residual tracer concentration in the region of the right lower pole.

Differential Diagnosis

- Parathyroid adenoma
- Parathyroid hyperplasia
- Thyroid adenoma (less common)
- Thyroid carcinoma
- Parathyroid carcinoma

Diagnosis and Clinical Follow-Up

Ultrasound demonstrated a possible nodule on the left side, but no abnormality on the right side. Surgical exploration revealed a 3 × 2-cm right inferior parathyroid adenoma. Parathyroid hormone levels returned to normal after resection of the adenoma.

Discussion

Parathyroid imaging with ^{99m}Tc-sestamibi can provide important information about the location of parathyroid adenomas and to a lesser extent multiple hyperplastic glands. There is disagreement about its clinical utility in the initial workup of hyperparathyroidism. Many surgeons feel it is important to do a full exploration of the thyroid bed and to locate, palpate, and often biopsy all four parathyroid glands; for these surgeons, there is often no added benefit to be derived from scanning. For those surgeons who are interested in performing minimally invasive surgery, the scan, in combination with the use of an intraoperative probe, can help direct the surgical incision and localization of the abnormal gland. Additionally, in cases in which an initial surgical procedure has failed to cure the hyperparathyroidism and the anatomy of the surgical bed is distorted and/or scarred, the scan can aid in directing surgical exploration.

[99m]Tc-sestamibi localizes in mitochondria, and mitochondria-rich oxyphil cells are often, although not always, found in abundance in parathyroid adenomas. In general, larger adenomas demonstrate greater uptake of nuclide. The scan is most accurate for the diagnosis of abnormal parathyroid tissue when one or more focal areas of abnormality on the initial images demonstrate prolonged retention of nuclide on the delayed images relative to the surrounding thyroid tissue. Some abnormal parathyroid glands demonstrate increased uptake on initial images only, however, and some thyroid nodules show retention on delayed images. These factors must be taken into consideration when the scan is interpreted. Additional imaging studies, such as thyroid scan, ultrasound, and CT, should be correlated with the results of the parathyroid scan.

PEARLS AND PITFALLS

- The field of view should include the entire thyroid bed and as much of the mediastinum as possible. The identification of an ectopic hyperfunctioning gland is one of the strengths of the scintigraphic study.
- The classic pattern is an initial increase of uptake by a parathyroid adenoma followed by prolonged retention of nuclide in the adenoma compared with uptake in normal thyroid tissue. Some parathyroid adenomas, however, demonstrate rapid washout of nuclide and are not well visualized on delayed imaging.
- When anatomic imaging studies are available, they should be correlated with the findings on the scintigraphic study.
- The utility of imaging in the initial surgical workup of patients with hyperparathyroidism is controversial in those who are scheduled for extensive exploratory surgery. Presurgical localization with additional intraoperative probe does aid, however, in the performance of minimally invasive surgery.

Suggested Reading

Bénard F, Lefebvre B, Beuvon F, Langlois MF, Bisson G. Rapid washout of [99m]TC-MIBI from a large parathyroid adenoma. J Nucl Med 1995;36(2):241–243

Johnson NA, Tublin ME, Ogilvie JB. Parathyroid imaging: technique and role in the preoperative evaluation of primary hyperparathyroidism. AJR Am J Roentgenol 2007;188(6):1706–1715

Kettle AG, O'Doherty MJ. Parathyroid imaging: how good is it and how should it be done? Semin Nucl Med 2006;36(3):206–211

Mariani G, Gulec SA, Rubello D, et al. Preoperative localization and radioguided parathyroid surgery. J Nucl Med 2003;44(9):1443–1458

Melloul M, Paz A, Koren R, Cytron S, Feinmesser R, Gal R. 99mTc-MIBI scintigraphy of parathyroid adenomas and its relation to tumour size and oxyphil cell abundance. Eur J Nucl Med 2001;28(2):209–213

Palestro CJ, Tomas MB, Tronco GG. Radionuclide imaging of the parathyroid glands. Semin Nucl Med 2005;35(4):266–276

CASE 65

Clinical Presentation

A 34-year-old woman presents with a ureteral stone. Subsequent workup reveals elevated calcium and parathyroid hormone levels.

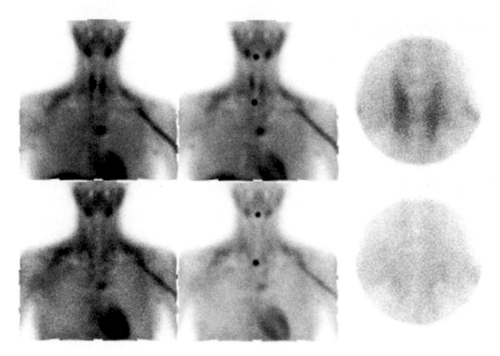

Fig. 65.1 Top row: 20-minute images; bottom row: 2-hour images. The middle column shows marker views.

Technique

- Approximately 20 mCi of ^{99m}Tc-sestamibi injected intravenously
- High-resolution collimator
- Anterior view of the neck and chest done at 20 minutes and 2 hours after injection
- Pinhole view of the thyroid bed done at 20 minutes and 2 hours after injection

Image Interpretation

Normal uptake and washout are noted in the region of the thyroid bed (**Fig. 65.1**). A focus of tracer concentration is noted just to the left of midline in the mediastinum, just superior to the heart.

Differential Diagnosis

- Parathyroid adenoma
- Other malignancy that can be seen in the mediastinum or lung

Diagnosis and Clinical Follow-Up

CT scan demonstrated a nodule in the aortopulmonic window. Resection resulted in normalization of the parathyroid hormone levels. Histologic examination revealed a parathyroid adenoma. The patient recovered uneventfully.

Discussion

Parathyroid adenomas are usually found in the region of the thyroid bed but can be seen in the anterior mediastinum in approximately 5% of patients. Nuclear medicine parathyroid scintigraphy is particularly helpful in these patients because many have undergone an earlier surgical procedure in the region of the thyroid bed that failed to identify the abnormality. This study demonstrates the importance of using a camera with a large field of view.

PEARLS AND PITFALLS

- Views of the mediastinum should always be obtained in parathyroid scintigraphy.
- Focal sestamibi uptake is not specific for parathyroid adenomas. Other tumors should be included in the differential diagnosis, particularly when the uptake is in an unusual location.

Suggested Reading

Palestro CJ, Tomas MB, Tronco GG. Radionuclide imaging of the parathyroid glands. Semin Nucl Med 2005;35(4):266–276

Phitayakorn R, McHenry CR. Incidence and location of ectopic abnormal parathyroid glands. Am J Surg 2006;191(3):418–423

Smith JR, Oates ME. Radionuclide imaging of the parathyroid glands: patterns, pearls, and pitfalls. Radiographics 2004;24(4):1101–1115

CASE 66

Clinical Presentation

A 34-year-old man presents with a long history of hyperparathyroidism. A sestamibi study is obtained for parathyroid localization.

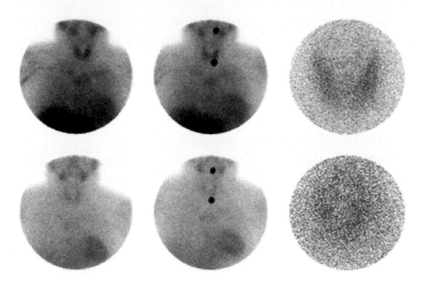

Fig. 66.1 Top row: 20-minute images; bottom row: 2-hour images. The middle column shows marker views.

Technique

- Approximately 20 mCi of ^{99m}Tc-sestamibi injected intravenously
- High-resolution collimator
- Anterior view of the neck and chest done at 20 minutes and 2 hours after injection
- Pinhole view of the thyroid bed done at 20 minutes and 2 hours after injection

Image Interpretation

Normal uptake is seen in the region of the thyroid bed (**Fig. 66.1**). A vague blush in the region of the mediastinum is also noted but not seen clearly enough to be diagnostic. Retention of nuclide in this area is unchanged on the delayed images, which is consistent with delayed washout.

Differential Diagnosis

(For mediastinal uptake)
- Normal blood pool structure
- Parathyroid adenoma
- Other malignancy

Diagnosis and Clinical Follow-Up

Angiography showed a blush of vascularity in the mediastinum at the site of the blush noted on the sestamibi images. MRI and CT showed equivocal soft tissue density in that region. Thoracoscopy re-

202

vealed a parathyroid adenoma at that location. Thoracoscopic resection of mediastinal parathyroid adenoma was performed, after which the patient became hypoparathyroid.

Discussion

The tracer uptake in the neck was normal. The mediastinal scintigraphic findings were reported as equivocal. This patient demonstrated other equivocal findings in the same location on several studies. This case, a "real world" case of an equivocal study, illustrates the importance of correlating borderline findings on scintigraphic imaging with the findings on other imaging modalities. The uptake of sestamibi generally depends on the size of an adenoma and the prevalence of mitochondria-rich oxyphil cells in the adenoma. The deeper the location of the adenoma in the mediastinum, the more likely the adenoma will be poorly visualized because of soft tissue attenuation. SPECT, SPECT/CT, and/or image fusion with CT can aid in the identification of mediastinal parathyroid adenomas.

PEARLS AND PITFALLS

- Before nondiagnostic findings are dismissed as unimportant, the findings of the scintigraphic study should be correlated with other test results.
- Reading any study with other test results in hand may bias the reading of the current study. The scintigraphic study is best read initially without additional information, then rechecked after all other available test results have been reviewed.

Suggested Reading

Melloul M, Paz A, Koren R, Cytron S, Feinmesser R, Gal R. 99mTc-MIBI scintigraphy of parathyroid adenomas and its relation to tumour size and oxyphil cell abundance. Eur J Nucl Med 2001;28(2):209–213

Phitayakorn R, McHenry CR. Incidence and location of ectopic abnormal parathyroid glands. Am J Surg 2006;191(3):418–423

Rubello D, Casara D, Fiore D, Muzzio P, Zonzin G, Shapiro B. An ectopic mediastinal parathyroid adenoma accurately located by a single-day imaging protocol of 99mTc pertechnetate-MIBI subtraction scintigraphy and MIBI-SPECT-computed tomographic image fusion. Clin Nucl Med 2002;27(3):186–190

Smith JR, Oates ME. Radionuclide imaging of the parathyroid glands: patterns, pearls, and pitfalls. Radiographics 2004;24(4):1101–1115

CASE 67

Clinical Presentation

A 37-year-old woman with a history of hypertensive renal failure and a renal transplant now presents with hyperparathyroidism. A surgical exploration of the neck shows four benign-appearing parathyroid glands. Three are removed, and a portion of the fourth is left behind. The patient remains hyperparathyroid, with parathyroid hormone (PTH) levels above 700 ng/L following surgery. A sestamibi study is done to search for additional parathyroid tissue.

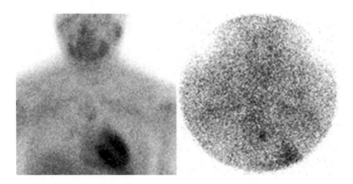

Fig. 67.1

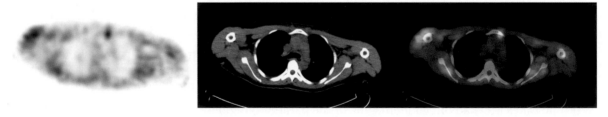

Fig. 67.2

Technique

- Approximately 20 mCi of ^{99m}Tc-sestamibi injected intravenously
- High-resolution collimator
- Anterior view of the neck and chest done at 20 minutes and 2 hours after injection
- Pinhole view of the thyroid bed done at 20 minutes and 2 hours after injection
- SPECT/CT of the thyroid bed and mediastinum

Image Interpretation

Anterior planar and pinhole images at 2 hours (**Fig. 67.1**) show faint focal tracer uptake between the thyroid bed and the heart.

SPECT/CT images (**Fig. 67.2**) show a substernal focus of tracer uptake, consistent with a fifth parathyroid gland.

Differential Diagnosis

- Parathyroid adenoma
- Other malignancy

Diagnosis and Clinical Follow-Up

Because the PTH levels remained elevated (> 700 ng/L following surgery, it was felt that the substernal lesion was likely a fifth parathyroid gland. The patient's comorbidities dictated that she be treated medically.

Discussion

Because the initial surgery failed to alleviate the hyperparathyroidism, a sestamibi study to search for additional parathyroid tissue was performed. The planar images showed a faint area of uptake but did a poor job of localizing the site of uptake. SPECT imaging alone can help to localize tracer uptake, but localization, particularly in the axial direction, can remain difficult. SPECT/CT is very helpful for providing a more precise localization of parathyroid tissue, which allows a more accurate assessment of the feasibility of surgery. Once surgery is determined to be possible, SPECT/CT provides important information for surgical planning.

PEARLS AND PITFALLS

- SPECT alone may not provide enough information beyond planar imaging to assist the surgeon in localizing a parathyroid adenoma.
- The differential diagnosis of focal sestamibi uptake can be aided by the addition of fused anatomic imaging, such as with SPECT/CT.

Suggested Reading

Lavely WC, Goetze S, Friedman KP, et al. Comparison of SPECT/CT, SPECT, and planar imaging with single- and dual-phase ^{99m}Tc-sestamibi parathyroid scintigraphy. J Nucl Med 2007;48(7):1084–1089

Martin P, Alcan I, Fuss M, et al. Preoperative localization of parathyroid adenoma: a comparison between the information provided by traditional SPECT-radiological CT fusion and direct hybrid SPECT-CT fusion. Eur J Nucl Med Mol Imaging 2006;33:S143

Núñez R, Namwongprom S, Kim EE, et al. Added value of parathyroid scintigraphy with a hybrid SPECT/multislice CT scanner in patients with primary hyperparathyroidism. Eur J Nucl Med Mol Imaging 2006;33:S111

Serra A, Bolasco P, Satta L, Nicolosi A, Uccheddu A, Piga M. Role of SPECT/CT in the preoperative assessment of hyperparathyroid patients. Radiol Med (Torino) 2006;111(7):999–1008

Section V

Scintigraphy of Neoplastic Disease
Part A PET/CT

Steven C. Burrell, Niall P. Sheehy, Victor H. Gerbaudo,
Francine L. Jacobson, and Annick D. Van den Abbeele

CASE 68

Clinical Presentation

A 35-year-old woman is referred for PET with 2-deoxy-2-[18F-FDG].

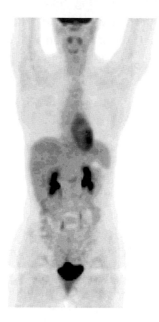

Fig. 68.1 PET scan with 18F-FDG.

Technique

- The patient is instructed to avoid vigorous exercise for 24 hours prior to the scan, fast for at least 4 hours before the study, drink water during the fasting and uptake periods, and void prior to the scan
- A venous serum glucose sample is obtained prior to the injection of 18F-FDG (reference range is < 120 mg/dl for non-diabetic patients and < 200 mg/dl for diabetic patients), and the patient's height and weight are recorded
- A 10–20 mCi dose of 18F-FDG is injected intravenously (in a dimly lit quiet room for brain PET scans), and the patient is asked to rest comfortably in a room that is kept warm
- Most PET scans are now acquired on a hybrid PET/CT scanner, and a low dose spiral CT is acquired for attenuation correction of the PET images and for anatomic localization. Some centers may choose to perform oral and/or intravenous contrast-enhanced diagnostic CT as part of the PET/CT examination
- Sixty minutes following the 18F-FDG injection, the spiral CT is performed using a weight-based algorithm from the skull base to the upper thighs (for most oncologic indications), or from the vertex to the feet, or centered over the brain depending on the tumor being evaluated

- A 2D or 3D PET acquisition (depending on the manufacturer) is then performed over the same region(s), and all PET images are corrected for attenuation, detector efficiency, scatter, decay, and random coincidences
- Consistency in ^{18}F-FDG injected dose, scan acquisition time relative to the injection time, and acquisition and reconstruction protocols is important when performing serial scanning on the same patient

Image Interpretation

Anterior view from the three-dimensional maximum-intensity pixel (MIP) image (**Fig. 68.1**) demonstrates intense ^{18}F-FDG uptake in the brain, heart, renal collecting systems, ureters, and bladder. There is more moderate uptake in the liver, spleen, colon, and various mucosal structures of the head and neck, as well as mild uptake in the thyroid, mediastinal blood pool, bone marrow, and skeletal muscles.

Differential Diagnosis

Normal ^{18}F-FDG-PET scan.

Diagnosis and Clinical Follow-Up

Normal ^{18}F-FDG-PET scan. Diagnosis final, no clinical follow-up.

Discussion

This case reflects the typical normal findings in an ^{18}F-FDG-PET scan. However, there are several normal variants that nuclear medicine physicians must be aware of when interpreting PET scans. A gallery of normal variants follows; **Fig. 68.2** demonstrates some generalized variants that are not uncommonly encountered, whereas **Fig. 68.3** depicts several focal variants, some common and some rare.

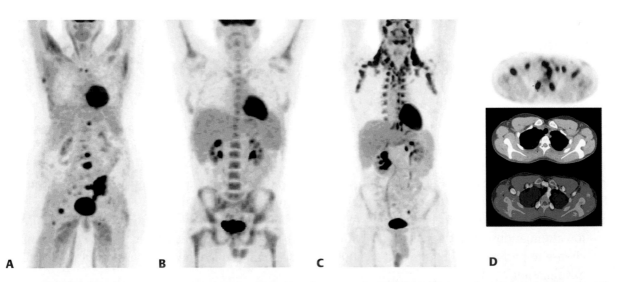

A   **B**   **C**   **D**

Fig. 68.2 **(A)** Increased skeletal muscle uptake in a hyperinsulinemic patient (along with several metastases). **(B)** Increased generalized bone marrow and splenic uptake in a patient receiving granulocyte colony–stimulating factor (G-CSF). **(C,D)** Increased uptake in brown fat of the neck and thorax. **(D)** Axial slices from the coregistered PET (top), CT (middle), and fused PET/CT (bottom) images clearly demonstrate that these areas of intense uptake are indeed within fat (dark areas on CT).

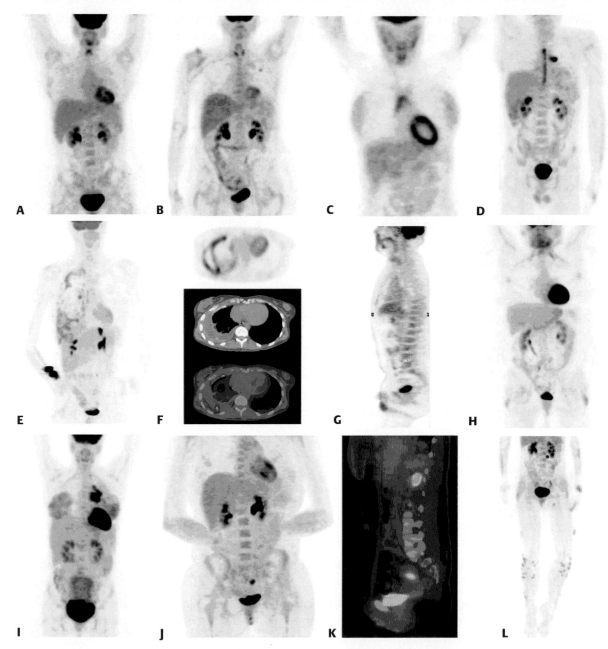

Fig. 68.3 **(A)** Prominent uptake in the laryngeal muscles, a common finding. Several different configurations are possible. **(B)** Diffuse uptake in the thyroid, which is occasionally encountered. There is moderate joint-based uptake, particularly in the shoulders and hips, not uncommon in patients with arthritis. There is moderate uptake in the colon, also a common physiologic finding. Uptake at the left lung apex is pathologic. **(C)** Diffuse uptake in the thymus, which can be seen in children and young adults, particularly following therapy ("thymic rebound"). **(D)** Uptake along the site of a sternotomy is often seen after surgery. Mild–moderate uptake in the testicles is a normal finding. Uptake in the left hilum is pathologic. **(E)** MIP image and **(F)** axial PET, CT, and fused PET/CT images showing fairly intense pleura-based uptake resulting from prior talc pleurodesis that can mimic mesothelioma, pleural metastases, or pleural infection. **(G)** Decreased uptake in the bone marrow of the cervical and upper thoracic spine secondary to radiation therapy. **(H)** Moderate uptake at the greater trochanter of each hip due to trochanteric bursitis. Note also normal mild–moderate uptake throughout the stomach. **(I)** Prominent uptake in the breasts and enlarged uterus in a postpartum woman. Mild–moderate symmetric uptake in the breasts is commonly seen. Focal uptake in a breast raises the possibility of a malignancy. Uptake in the left lung and hilum in this patient is pathologic. **(J,K)** A focus of intense uptake in the pelvis on the anterior MIP image is demonstrated on the lateral fused PET/CT image to be within the uterus in this menstruating patient. **(L)** Scattered foci of superficial uptake over the lower legs are due to varicose veins.

Given the wide acceptance of ^{18}F-FDG-PET scanning in oncology, standardization of imaging protocols and consistency in scanning methodologies in the follow-up of patients with cancer are important factors to consider. Shankar et al. provide useful recommendations for the use of ^{18}F-FDG-PET in patients with cancer.

PEARLS AND PITFALLS

- Although ^{18}F-FDG-PET scans are generally excellent at distinguishing neoplastic from normal tissue, several benign pitfalls and variants can hinder evaluation of the scan by either simulating or masking malignancy.
- Generalized increased uptake can be seen in the skeletal muscles of hyperglycemic patients as a result of elevated insulin levels, which may decrease the sensitivity of the study. To avoid this, patients undergoing an oncology ^{18}F-FDG-PET scan should fast for at least 4 hours before injection. If the patient has diabetes, the glucose levels may be controlled with insulin no less than 4 hours before the scan.
- Hyperinsulinemia also causes increased ^{18}F-FDG uptake in the myocardium. However, cardiac uptake on oncologic PET scans can be extremely variable, even when patients have been appropriately fasting.
- Uptake in the brown fat of the neck and upper thorax may be mistaken for disease or may obscure disease. Brown fat uptake can be reduced by keeping the patient warm during the injection and uptake period. If necessary, benzodiazepines may be used to reduce brown fat uptake.
- When an unexplained abnormality is encountered, a directed patient history is very helpful.

Suggested Reading

Bakheet SM, Powe J. Benign causes of 18-FDG uptake on whole body imaging. Semin Nucl Med 1998;28(4):352–358

Burrell SC, Van den Abbeele AD. 2-Deoxy-2-[F-18]fluoro-D-glucose-positron emission tomography of the head and neck: an atlas of normal uptake and variants. Mol Imaging Biol 2005;7(3):244–256

Cohade C, Osman M, Pannu HK, Wahl RL. Uptake in supraclavicular area fat ("USA-Fat"): description on ^{18}F-FDG PET/CT. J Nucl Med 2003;44(2):170–176

Cook GJ, Fogelman I, Maisey MN. Normal physiological and benign pathological variants of 18-fluoro-2-deoxyglucose positron-emission tomography scanning: potential for error in interpretation. Semin Nucl Med 1996;26(4):308–314

Delbeke D, Coleman RE, Guiberteau MJ, et al. Procedure guideline for tumor imaging with ^{18}F-FDG PET/CT 1.0. J Nucl Med 2006;47(5):885–895

Hollinger EF, Alibazoglu H, Ali A, Green A, Lamonica G. Hematopoietic cytokine-mediated FDG uptake simulates the appearance of diffuse metastatic disease on whole-body PET imaging. Clin Nucl Med 1998;23(2):93–98

Kwek BH, Aquino SL, Fischman AJ. Fluorodeoxyglucose positron emission tomography and CT after talc pleurodesis. Chest 2004;125(6):2356–2360

Shankar LK, Hoffman JM, Bacharach S, et al. Consensus recommendations for the use of F-18-FDG PET as an indicator of therapeutic response in patients in national cancer institute trials. J Nucl Med 2006;47(6):1059–1066

Shreve PD, Anzai Y, Wahl RL. Pitfalls in oncologic diagnosis with FDG PET imaging: physiologic and benign variants. Radiographics 1999;19(1):61–77, quiz 150–151

CASE 69

Clinical Presentation

A 55-year-old man with a 6-year history of grade 1 follicular lymphoma presents for assessment today (**Fig. 69.2**) and six-months earlier (**Fig. 69.1**). The patient's lactate dehydrogenase level is elevated.

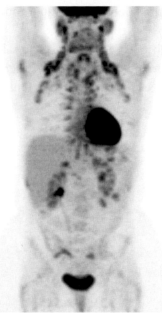
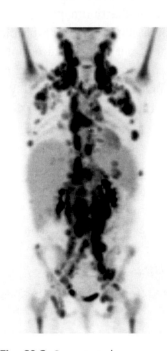

Fig. 69.1 Six months earlier.   **Fig. 69.2** Current study.

Technique

- The patient is instructed to avoid vigorous exercise for 24 hours prior to the scan, fast for at least 4 hours before the study, drink water during the fasting and uptake periods, and void prior to the scan
- A venous serum glucose sample is obtained prior to the injection of ^{18}F-FDG (reference range is < 120 mg/dl for non-diabetic patients and < 200 mg/dl for diabetic patients), and the patient's height and weight are recorded
- A 10–20 mCi dose of ^{18}F-FDG is injected intravenously (in a dimly lit quiet room for brain PET scans), and the patient is asked to rest comfortably in a room that is kept warm
- Most PET scans are now acquired on a hybrid PET/CT scanner, and a low dose spiral CT is acquired for attenuation correction of the PET images and for anatomic localization. Some centers may choose to perform oral and/or intravenous contrast-enhanced diagnostic CT as part of the PET/CT examination
- Sixty minutes following the ^{18}F-FDG injection, the spiral CT is performed using a weight-based algorithm from the skull base to the upper thighs (for most oncologic indications), or from the vertex to the feet, or centered over the brain depending on the tumor being evaluated

- A 2D or 3D PET acquisition (depending on the manufacturer) is then performed over the same region(s), and all PET images are corrected for attenuation, detector efficiency, scatter, decay, and random coincidences
- Consistency in ^{18}F-FDG injected dose, scan acquisition time relative to the injection time, and acquisition and reconstruction protocols is important when performing serial scanning on the same patient

Image Interpretation

When the patient underwent scintigraphy 6 months earlier (**Fig. 69.1**), symmetric tracer uptake was noted in the neck, supraclavicular fossae, mediastinum, paraspinal regions, and perinephric fat. These regions of uptake corresponded to brown adipose tissue. Multiple minimally enlarged lymph nodes were seen on the corresponding CT images, but without tracer uptake.

At this presentation (**Fig. 69.2**), the picture is very different. Although there is still tracer uptake in brown adipose tissue, interval development of ^{18}F-FDG–avid lymphadenopathy is seen in the neck, chest, abdomen, and pelvis. In addition, the bone marrow also demonstrates multiple focal regions of increased tracer uptake.

Differential Diagnosis

- Transformation from low-grade to aggressive lymphoma
- Interval development of sarcoidosis
- Interval development of new ^{18}F-FDG–avid disseminated malignancy

Diagnosis and Clinical Follow-Up

The patient's lymphoma had transformed from a low-grade to an aggressive lymphoma.

Discussion

Non-Hodgkin lymphomas can be divided into slow-growing types (marginal zone, small-cell lymphocytic lymphoma, lymphoplasmacytic lymphoma, and follicular lymphoma), more aggressive types (diffuse large B-cell lymphoma and mantle cell lymphoma), and fast-growing types (Burkitt lymphoma and lymphoblastic lymphoma). The last two are considered aggressive lymphomas.

Several studies have attempted to assess tumor grade by ^{18}F-FDG-PET. In general, the more aggressive types of lymphoma have higher standardized uptake values (SUVs). However, tracer uptake varies widely, and it is not possible to accurately assess grade by PET. Illustrating this fact, a study of 97 patients (Schöder et al., 2005) correlated biopsy findings with the highest SUV in PET scans obtained from untreated patients or patients with relapsed or persistent disease who had not been treated within 6 months of undergoing PET. All indolent lymphomas had an SUV of less than 13, but 35% of the 63 patients with aggressive disease also had tumors with an SUV of less than 13. The study concluded that ^{18}F-FDG uptake is higher in aggressive disease than in indolent lymphomas, and the authors suggested that an SUV of more than 10 confers a higher likelihood of aggressive disease.

In this case, the dramatic change in the ^{18}F-FDG uptake suggests transformation of the lymphoma from an indolent form to an aggressive form, but this must be confirmed by biopsy. ^{18}F-FDG-PET can be used in this instance to guide biopsy because lower- and higher-grade lymphomas often coexist within the same patient.

PEARLS AND PITFALLS

- In general, aggressive lymphomas show intense ^{18}F-FDG uptake and low-grade, indolent lymphomas show low-level uptake, but overlaps in appearance may occur.
- Both aggressive and low-grade lymphomas may coexist in the same patient.
- ^{18}F-FDG-PET may be used to guide biopsy to prevent the incorrect classification of an aggressive lymphoma.

Suggested Reading

Jhanwar YS, Straus DJ. The role of PET in lymphoma. J Nucl Med 2006;47(8):1326–1334

Rodriguez M, Rehn S, Ahlström H, Sundström C, Glimelius B. Predicting malignancy grade with PET in non-Hodgkin's lymphoma. J Nucl Med 1995;36(10):1790–1796

Schöder H, Noy A, Gönen M, Weng L, Green D, Erdi YE, Larson SM, Yeung HW. Intensity of 18fluorodeoxyglucose uptake in positron emission tomography distinguishes between indolent and aggressive non-Hodgkin's lymphoma. J Clin Oncol 2005;23(21):4643–4651

CASE 70

Clinical Presentation

A 25-year-old woman presents with bulky anterior mediastinal lymphadenopathy. Biopsy confirms the diagnosis of Hodgkin lymphoma. The patient is scheduled for six cycles of ABVD (adriamycin [doxorubicin], bleomycin, vinblastine, dacarbazine) chemotherapy, and PET/CT is performed at baseline and after three cycles of chemotherapy to assess the response to chemotherapy.

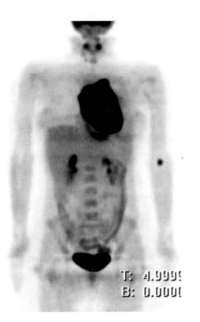

Fig. 70.1

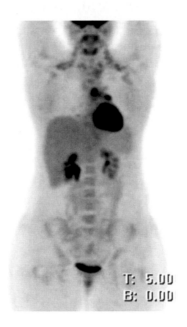

Fig. 70.2

Technique

- The patient is instructed to avoid vigorous exercise for 24 hours prior to the scan, fast for at least 4 hours before the study, drink water during the fasting and uptake periods, and void prior to the scan
- A venous serum glucose sample is obtained prior to the injection of ¹⁸F-FDG (reference range is < 120 mg/dl for non-diabetic patients and < 200 mg/dl for diabetic patients), and the patient's height and weight are recorded
- A 10–20 mCi dose of ¹⁸F-FDG is injected intravenously (in a dimly lit quiet room for brain PET scans), and the patient is asked to rest comfortably in a room that is kept warm
- Most PET scans are now acquired on a hybrid PET/CT scanner, and a low dose spiral CT is acquired for attenuation correction of the PET images and for anatomic localization. Some centers may choose to perform oral and/or intravenous contrast-enhanced diagnostic CT as part of the PET/CT examination
- Sixty minutes following the ¹⁸F-FDG injection, the spiral CT is performed using a weight-based algorithm from the skull base to the upper thighs (for most oncologic indications), or from the vertex to the feet, or centered over the brain depending on the tumor being evaluated

- A 2D or 3D PET acquisition (depending on the manufacturer) is then performed over the same region(s), and all PET images are corrected for attenuation, detector efficiency, scatter, decay, and random coincidences
- Consistency in ^{18}F-FDG injected dose, scan acquisition time relative to the injection time, and acquisition and reconstruction protocols is important when performing serial scanning on the same patient

Image Interpretation

Anterior maximum-intensity pixel (MIP) views of the ^{18}F-FDG-PET scan are obtained at baseline (**Fig. 70.1**) and after three cycles of chemotherapy (**Fig. 70.2**). On the baseline images, there is a large focus of intense tracer uptake in the mediastinum that represents the patient's Hodgkin lymphoma. There is no abnormal ^{18}F-FDG uptake outside the chest.

After three cycles of chemotherapy, there has been a marked reduction in both the size and the intensity of tracer uptake in the mediastinal lymphoma, but there is residual ^{18}F-FDG–avid disease. There is also tracer uptake in brown adipose tissue in the supraclavicular regions and intense uptake in the left ventricle, which are normal variants.

Differential Diagnosis

- Partial response to therapy with residual disease
- Complete response to therapy with a new ^{18}F-FDG–avid process in the mediastinum

Diagnosis and Clinical Follow-Up

Partial response to therapy with residual ^{18}F-FDG–avid lymphoma. The patient received three further courses of chemotherapy. A whole-body ^{18}F-FDG-PET scan was then performed after six cycles of chemotherapy (**Fig. 70.3**). The size and tracer uptake of the Hodgkin lymphoma, which showed an incomplete

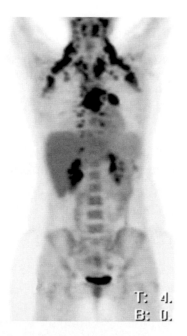

Fig. 70.3

response after three cycles, have increased between cycle 3 and cycle 6 of therapy, indicating that it has grown through three cycles of chemotherapy.

Discussion

^{18}F-FDG-PET is increasingly being used to assess the response of various tumors to chemotherapy and radiotherapy. When reading scans performed to assess response to therapy, the nuclear medicine physician needs to be aware of the expected responses of the individual tumors in given situations. For example, in a recent study of non–small-cell lung cancer, a decrease of 20% in the standardized uptake value (SUV) 3 weeks after the initiation of chemotherapy predicted which patients would respond to therapy (metabolic responders). In most solid tumors, a decrease of 30 to 50% in the SUV seems to predict a metabolic response.

In patients with Hodgkin and aggressive non-Hodgkin lymphomas, a substantial response to chemotherapy may be evident within 24 hours of the initiation of therapy. Several studies have examined the use of midtherapy scans to assess the chemosensitivity of aggressive lymphomas. An absence of abnormal tracer uptake, which can be visually assessed by comparing the site of the lymphoma with the mediastinal blood pool activity, is called a *complete metabolic response (CMR)*. Multiple studies have shown that a CMR in a midcycle ^{18}F-FDG-PET study is the most powerful predictor of disease-free survival. In fact, patients without a CMR in a midcycle study should be considered for more aggressive therapy, a point dramatically indicated in this patient, whose lymphoma actually grew through three additional cycles of the same chemotherapy regimen.

PEARLS AND PITFALLS

- ^{18}F-FDG-PET is a powerful tool for assessing the chemosensitivity of Hodgkin and aggressive non-Hodgkin lymphomas.
- Hodgkin and aggressive non-Hodgkin lymphomas have the best prognosis when they show a complete response on midtherapy restaging scans.

Suggested Reading

Hutchings M, Loft A, Hansen M, Pedersen LM, Buhl T, Jurlander J, Buus S, Keiding S, D'Amore F, Boesen AM, Berthelsen AK, Specht L. FDG-PET after two cycles of chemotherapy predicts treatment failure and progression-free survival in Hodgkin lymphoma. Blood 2006;107(1):52–59

MacManus MP, Seymour JF, Hicks RJ. Overview of early response assessment in lymphoma with FDG-PET. Cancer Imaging 2007;7:10–18

Mikhaeel NG, Hutchings M, Fields PA, O'Doherty MJ, Timothy AR. FDG-PET after two to three cycles of chemotherapy predicts progression-free and overall survival in high-grade non-Hodgkin lymphoma. Ann Oncol 2005;16(9):1514–1523

CASE 71

Clinical Presentation

Approximately 15 months after receiving an autologous bone marrow transplant, a 43-year-old man with a history of Hodgkin lymphoma feels well and, in particular, does not have any respiratory distress. A re-staging examination is performed three months (**Fig. 71.2**) following the last follow-up (**Fig. 71.1**).

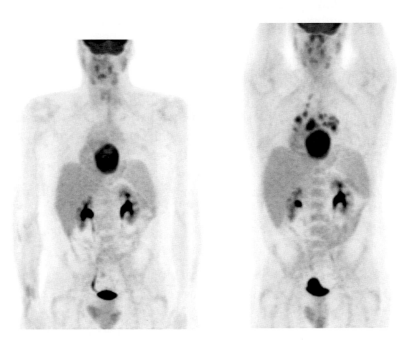

Fig. 71.1   **Fig. 71.2**

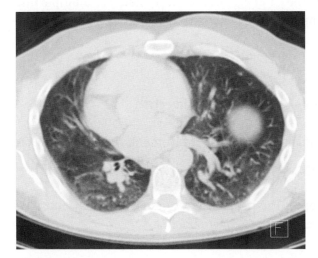

Fig. 71.3

219

Technique

- The patient is instructed to avoid vigorous exercise for 24 hours prior to the scan, fast for at least 4 hours before the study, drink water during the fasting and uptake periods, and void prior to the scan
- A venous serum glucose sample is obtained prior to the injection of ^{18}F-FDG (reference range is < 120 mg/dl for non-diabetic patients and < 200 mg/dl for diabetic patients), and the patient's height and weight are recorded
- A 10–20 mCi dose of ^{18}F-FDG is injected intravenously (in a dimly lit quiet room for brain PET scans), and the patient is asked to rest comfortably in a room that is kept warm
- Most PET scans are now acquired on a hybrid PET/CT scanner, and a low dose spiral CT is acquired for attenuation correction of the PET images and for anatomic localization. Some centers may choose to perform oral and/or intravenous contrast-enhanced diagnostic CT as part of the PET/CT examination
- Sixty minutes following the ^{18}F-FDG injection, the spiral CT is performed using a weight-based algorithm from the skull base to the upper thighs (for most oncologic indications), or from the vertex to the feet, or centered over the brain depending on the tumor being evaluated
- A 2D or 3D PET acquisition (depending on the manufacturer) is then performed over the same region(s), and all PET images are corrected for attenuation, detector efficiency, scatter, decay, and random coincidences
- Consistency in ^{18}F-FDG injected dose, scan acquisition time relative to the injection time, and acquisition and reconstruction protocols is important when performing serial scanning on the same patient

Image Interpretation

Anterior maximum-intensity pixel (MIP) views of ^{18}F-FDG-PET scans obtained 3 months earlier (**Fig. 71.1**) and at this presentation (**Fig. 71.2**). Selected current CT image of the chest on lung windows (**Fig. 71.3**).

On the current study, multiple ^{18}F-FDG–avid lymph nodes are seen in the mediastinum. These are present in both pulmonary hila and in the paratracheal and subcarinal stations. They were not present on the PET scan performed 3 months earlier. On the CT images of the chest, there are multiple tiny pulmonary nodules. These appear to have a predominantly perilymphatic distribution.

Differential Diagnosis

- Recurrent Hodgkin lymphoma
- Unusual pulmonary infective process, such as atypical mycobacterial infection
- Metastatic carcinoma in the chest
- Generalized inflammatory disease with predominantly pulmonary involvement, such as sarcoidosis

Diagnosis and Clinical Follow-Up

The patient underwent a mediastinoscopy and biopsy. The pathologic results favored a diagnosis of sarcoidosis. There was no histologic evidence of recurrent Hodgkin lymphoma.

Discussion

Sarcoidosis is a systemic granulomatous disorder of unknown etiology. It is a frequent cause of diagnostic difficulty in ^{18}F-FDG-PET examinations because regions of sarcoidosis demonstrate intense tracer uptake. It has been demonstrated that ^{18}F-FDG-PET provides a more accurate delineation of extrapulmonary disease than do ^{67}Ga whole-body examinations.

Sarcoidosis frequently demonstrates symmetric ^{18}F-FDG–avid lymph nodes, most commonly in the mediastinal and hilar regions. In this patient, in whom the major diagnostic consideration was recurrent Hodgkin lymphoma, the perilymphatic pulmonary nodules strongly suggested sarcoidosis rather than recurrent lymphoma. However, the overall appearance is similar, and a biopsy is mandatory to discriminate between them.

PEARLS AND PITFALLS

- Sarcoidosis, a systemic granulomatous disease, may demonstrate intense tracer uptake and is frequently misdiagnosed as malignancy.
- The combination of symmetric mediastinal lymphadenopathy and pulmonary parenchymal nodules is suggestive of sarcoidosis. However, this pattern of disease may also be seen with metastatic malignancy and with certain infectious processes. Therefore, in most cases, histologic examination is recommended to confirm the diagnosis of sarcoidosis when it is suggested by a PET scan.

Suggested Reading

Braun JJ, Kessler R, Constantinesco A, Imperiale A. ^{18}F-FDG PET/CT in sarcoidosis management: review and report of 20 cases. Eur J Nucl Med Mol Imaging 2008;35(8):1537–1543

Nishiyama Y, Yamamoto Y, Fukunaga K, Takinami H, Iwado Y, Satoh K, Ohkawa M. Comparative evaluation of ^{18}F-FDG PET and ^{67}Ga scintigraphy in patients with sarcoidosis. J Nucl Med 2006;47(10):1571–1576

Teirstein AS, Machac J, Almeida O, Lu P, Padilla ML, Iannuzzi MC. Results of 188 whole-body fluorodeoxyglucose positron emission tomography scans in 137 patients with sarcoidosis. Chest 2007;132(6):1949–1953

CASE 72

Clinical Presentation

An 82-year-old man with a diagnosis of pneumonia is treated with antibiotics. Follow-up chest radiograph reveals a 16-mm lesion in the right upper lobe.

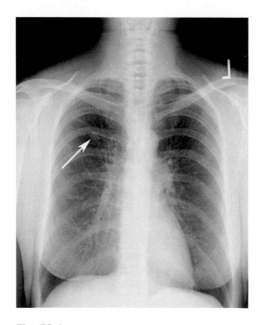

Fig. 72.1

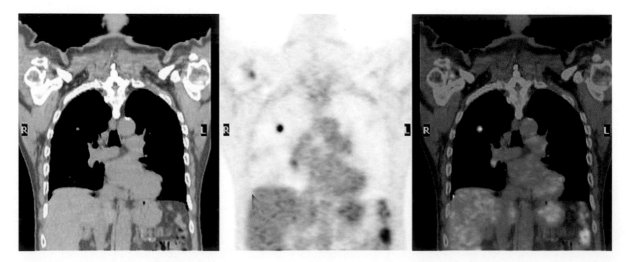

Fig. 72.2

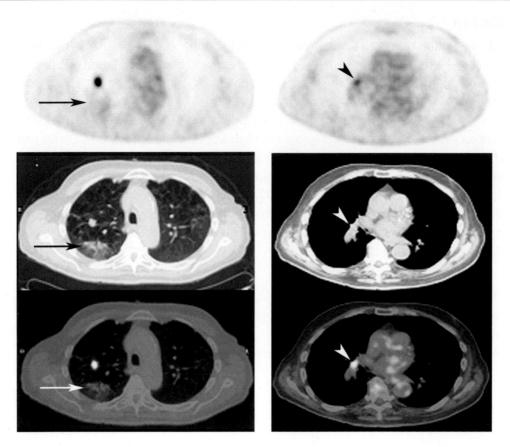

Fig. 72.3   **Fig. 72.4**

Technique

- The patient is instructed to avoid vigorous exercise for 24 hours prior to the scan, fast for at least 4 hours before the study, drink water during the fasting and uptake periods, and void prior to the scan
- A venous serum glucose sample is obtained prior to the injection of ^{18}F-FDG (reference range is < 120 mg/dl for non-diabetic patients and < 200 mg/dl for diabetic patients), and the patient's height and weight are recorded
- A 10–20 mCi dose of ^{18}F-FDG is injected intravenously (in a dimly lit quiet room for brain PET scans), and the patient is asked to rest comfortably in a room that is kept warm
- Most PET scans are now acquired on a hybrid PET/CT scanner, and a low dose spiral CT is acquired for attenuation correction of the PET images and for anatomic localization. Some centers may choose to perform oral and/or intravenous contrast-enhanced diagnostic CT as part of the PET/CT examination
- Sixty minutes following the ^{18}F-FDG injection, the spiral CT is performed using a weight-based algorithm from the skull base to the upper thighs (for most oncologic indications), or from the vertex to the feet, or centered over the brain depending on the tumor being evaluated
- A 2D or 3D PET acquisition (depending on the manufacturer) is then performed over the same region(s), and all PET images are corrected for attenuation, detector efficiency, scatter, decay, and random coincidences
- Consistency in ^{18}F-FDG injected dose, scan acquisition time relative to the injection time, and acquisition and reconstruction protocols is important when performing serial scanning on the same patient

Image Interpretation

Posteroanterior chest radiograph (**Fig. 72.1**) demonstrates an indistinct nodular opacity (*arrow*) projecting over the right second anterior rib. Elsewhere, the lungs are clear. There is no pleural effusion or evidence of central lymph node enlargement. The heart size is normal.

Coronal (**Fig. 72.2**) and axial (**Fig. 72.3**) images reveal a 1.4 × 1.1 cm right upper lobe nodule with intense focal uptake of ^{18}F-FDG greater than mediastinal blood pool activity, suggestive of malignancy. Posterior to the nodule on the axial views, there is an area of ill-defined patchy opacity on CT with just mild ^{18}F-FDG uptake (*arrows*), consistent with incomplete resolution of the known pneumonia.

Axial images more inferiorly (**Fig. 72.4**) reveal mild–moderate uptake focally in the right hilar region (*arrowheads*), also appreciated on the coronal images (**Fig. 72.2**). This finding represents small nodes of indeterminate significance on CT, but malignancy cannot be excluded. There is no pleural or pericardial effusion. No pathologically enlarged axillary or supraclavicular lymph nodes are seen. Physiologic biodistribution of ^{18}F-FDG is present in the abdomen.

Differential Diagnosis

- Primary lung cancer
- Metastatic tumor to the lung
- Inflammation (coccidioidomycosis, histoplasmosis, tuberculosis, sarcoidosis, anthracosilicosis, subacute abscess, focal pneumonia)
- Hamartoma

Diagnosis and Clinical Follow-Up

Flexible bronchoscopy followed by right upper lobectomy revealed a moderately differentiated adenocarcinoma (1.1 cm). The tumor did not involve the visceral pleura, and there was no evidence of lymphovascular invasion. The paratracheal, peribronchial, and right hilar lymph nodes were found to be negative for tumor.

Discussion

The morphologic evaluation of solitary pulmonary nodules (SPNs) helps differentiate benign from malignant lesions when typical benign or malignant features are present; however, considerable overlap occurs in many cases. PET has proved to be an accurate, noninvasive diagnostic test, with an average sensitivity and specificity of 93.9% and 85.3%, respectively, for detecting malignancy in SPNs and a negative predictive value of 95%. Increased blood flow, a high steady-state metabolic rate with overexpression of active GLUT transporters, and a high hexokinase-to-phosphatase ratio in viable tumor cells are responsible for the high net ^{18}F-FDG uptake in neoplastic conditions, enhancing the ability of ^{18}F-FDG-PET imaging to discriminate between benign and malignant lesions.

Hybrid imaging technology such as PET/CT has gained rapid clinical acceptance. The superior anatomic detail provided by CT scans is evaluated in the context of its biological significance when fused with the metabolic information provided by PET images. In these images, where structure and function meet, the PET findings are presented in a clear, defined anatomic context. Thus, the main advantage of hybrid imaging is its ability not only to accurately correlate metabolic with anatomic features of malignancy but also to clarify the significance of high ^{18}F-FDG uptake in otherwise normal structures. Thus, in this context, integrated PET/CT imaging provides a more detailed and complete characterization of lung lesions than does PET or CT alone. PET/CT imaging also serves as a promising tool to guide biopsy to the area of highest metabolic rate in the lesion, thus minimizing sampling errors.

Although ^{18}F-FDG can be considered a probe of a specific altered process in cancer cells, it is by no means a marker of a tumor-specific process. Inflammatory cells also have upregulated glucose transporters. ^{18}F-FDG uptake has been demonstrated in granulation tissue, and in both activated macrophages and neutrophils. In inflammatory processes, the low hexokinase-to-phosphatase ratio favors dephosphorylation, with the final outcome "generally" a relatively low but noticeable rate of ^{18}F-FDG uptake compared with that in tumor. However, it is not uncommon to observe high levels of ^{18}F-FDG avidity in the acute phase of infection/inflammation, which can be mistaken for malignancy. Low-moderate uptake in nodes that are negative for tumor, such as in this case, is certainly not common. It may represent ^{18}F-FDG uptake in nodes reactive to the chronic inflammation associated with occupational lung disease, a generalized inflammatory response to infection (in this case, pneumonia), or lymphoid follicular hyperplasia in patients with long histories of smoking, chronic airway disease, or tuberculosis.

PEARLS AND PITFALLS

- Morphologic characteristics of a malignant nodule are the following: an ill-defined and/or spicular solitary upper lobe lesion with endobronchial extension, pleural retraction, and ground-glass opacity or solid, eccentric calcification that enhances more than 25 Hounsfield units (HU) following contrast administration.
- However, 25 to 39% of malignant nodules are incorrectly classified as benign based on their morphologic characteristics alone.
- ^{18}F-FDG-PET imaging interrogates the biological behavior of the lesion, so that it is a better noninvasive predictor of malignancy in indeterminate SPNs than are conventional imaging modalities.
- ^{18}F-FDG-PET imaging is a cost-effective procedure in the setting of an SPN because it reduces the number of unnecessary invasive procedures.
- False-positive results in PET are often due to inflammation or infection; thus a positive finding always requires biopsy.
- False-negative findings in PET may be due to the small size of nodules (< 7 mm) and/or to the low rate of metabolic activity in tumors such as bronchioloalveolar carcinomas, carcinoids, and other mucinous malignancies. Patients who have negative findings on PET should be followed up clinically and with conventional imaging at 6- to 12-month intervals.

Suggested Reading

Chung JH, Cho KJ, Lee SS, Baek HJ, Park JH, Cheon GJ, Choi CW, Lim SM. Overexpression of Glut1 in lymphoid follicles correlates with false-positive ^{18}F-FDG PET results in lung cancer staging. J Nucl Med 2004;45(6):999–1003

Erasmus JJ, Connolly JE, McAdams HP, Roggli VL. Solitary pulmonary nodules, I: Morphologic evaluation for differentiation of benign and malignant lesions. Radiographics 2000;20(1):43–58

Erasmus JJ, McAdams HP, Connolly JE. Solitary pulmonary nodules, II: Evaluation of the indeterminate nodule. Radiographics 2000;20(1):59–66

Goerres GW, von Schulthess GK, Steinert HC. Why most PET of lung and head-and-neck cancer will be PET/CT. J Nucl Med 2004;45(Suppl 1):66S–71S

Gould MK, Maclean CC, Kuschner WG, Rydzak CE, Owens DK. Accuracy of positron emission tomography for diagnosis of pulmonary nodules and mass lesions: a meta-analysis. JAMA 2001;285(7):914–924

Jones HA, Clark RJ, Rhodes CG, Schofield JB, Krausz T, Haslett C. Positron emission tomography of 18FDG uptake in localized pulmonary inflammation. Acta Radiol Suppl 1991;376:148

Lardinois D, Weder W, Hany TF, Kamel EM, Korom S, Seifert B, von Schulthess GK, Steinert HC. Staging of non-small-cell lung cancer with integrated positron-emission tomography and computed tomography. N Engl J Med 2003;348(25):2500–2507

Siegelman SS, Khouri NF, Leo FP, Fishman EK, Braverman RM, Zerhouni EA. Solitary pulmonary nodules: CT assessment. Radiology 1986;160(2):307–312

Yamada S, Kubota K, Kubota R, Ido T, Tamahashi N. High accumulation of ^{18}F-1D6 in turpentine-induced inflammatory tissue. J Nucl Med 1995;36(7):1301–1306

CASE 73

Clinical Presentation

A 47-year-old man presents with a left lower lobe solitary pulmonary nodule (SPN). PET/CT is obtained for initial staging.

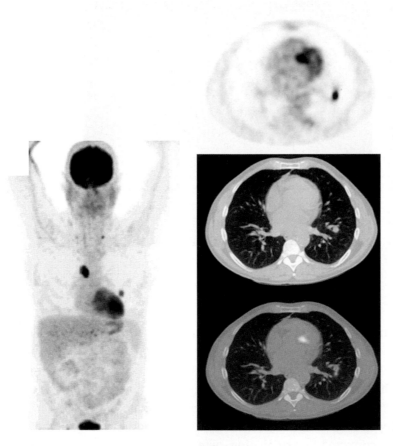

Fig. 73.1   **Fig. 73.2**

Technique

- The patient is instructed to avoid vigorous exercise for 24 hours prior to the scan, fast for at least 4 hours before the study, drink water during the fasting and uptake periods, and void prior to the scan
- A venous serum glucose sample is obtained prior to the injection of ^{18}F-FDG (reference range is < 120 mg/dl for non-diabetic patients and < 200 mg/dl for diabetic patients), and the patient's height and weight are recorded
- A 10-20 mCi dose of ^{18}F-FDG is injected intravenously (in a dimly lit quiet room for brain PET scans), and the patient is asked to rest comfortably in a room that is kept warm
- Most PET scans are now acquired on a hybrid PET/CT scanner, and a low dose spiral CT is acquired for attenuation correction of the PET images and for anatomic localization. Some centers may

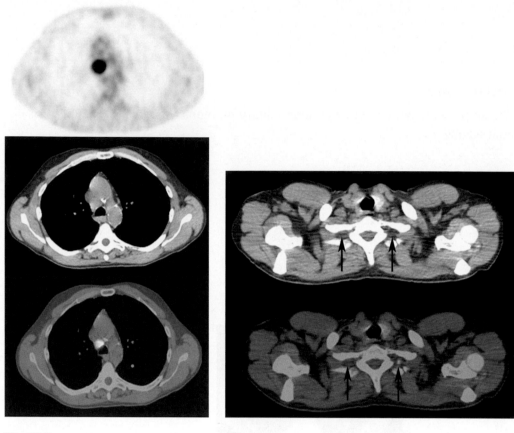

Fig. 73.3   **Fig. 73.4**

choose to perform oral and/or intravenous contrast-enhanced diagnostic CT as part of the PET/CT examination

- Sixty minutes following the ^{18}F-FDG injection, the spiral CT is performed using a weight-based algorithm from the skull base to the upper thighs (for most oncologic indications), or from the vertex to the feet, or centered over the brain depending on the tumor being evaluated

- A 2D or 3D PET acquisition (depending on the manufacturer) is then performed over the same region(s), and all PET images are corrected for attenuation, detector efficiency, scatter, decay, and random coincidences

- Consistency in ^{18}F-FDG injected dose, scan acquisition time relative to the injection time, and acquisition and reconstruction protocols is important when performing serial scanning on the same patient

Image Interpretation

An anterior maximum-intensity pixel (MIP) image (**Fig. 73.1**) demonstrates asymmetric foci of increased ^{18}F-FDG uptake in the posterior cervical regions bilaterally, a focus of increased uptake at the midlevel of the chest just to the right of midline, and a focus in the left lung. Axial images (**Fig. 73.2**) confirm a round, 1.1-cm nodule in the left lower lobe that is highly ^{18}F-FDG–avid. Images more superiorly (**Fig. 73.3**) reveal an enlarged right paratracheal lymph node of approximately 2.1 cm with high ^{18}F-FDG metabolism. Images through the neck (**Fig. 73.4**) indicate that the bilateral cervical uptake corresponds to brown fat (*arrows*).

Differential Diagnosis

- Stage IIIb lung cancer
- Stage I lung cancer with indeterminate contralateral reactive lymphadenitis
- Granulomatous disease
- Other inflammatory disease
- Metastatic disease

Diagnosis and Clinical Follow-Up

Biopsy of the left lower lobe lesion showed a poorly differentiated squamous cell carcinoma. A 4R node biopsy confirmed the presence of nodal metastasis.

Discussion

PET/CT imaging characterized the solitary pulmonary lesion as worrisome for malignancy and confirmed the presence of contralateral disease, correctly upstaging an SPN to unresectable stage IIIb disease.

Nodal status is a major determinant of the resectability of lung tumors. Metastases to the contralateral and/or supraclavicular nodes (N3 disease) deny the possibility of curative resection. ^{18}F-FDG-PET imaging has been shown to be more accurate than CT for the detection of lymph node metastases in patients with non–small-cell lung cancer. The use of integrated PET/CT imaging further improves determination of the N stage compared with PET alone or with PET and CT evaluated side by side.

PEARLS AND PITFALLS

- Unlike mediastinoscopy, ^{18}F-FDG-PET/CT imaging is an accurate tool for the noninvasive anatomic-metabolic characterization of the entire mediastinum. Moreover, the ^{18}F-FDG-PET information is useful to guide mediastinoscopy to metabolically active lymph nodes.
- Unlike anatomic imaging modalities, ^{18}F-FDG-PET accurately characterizes nodal disease in small nodes and excludes malignancy in enlarged nodes.
- However, ^{18}F-FDG-PET may yield false-positive results in inflammatory reactive lymph nodes and false-negative results in nodes harboring micrometastases.
- The synergistic information derived from the PET/CT images provides a more detailed and complete characterization of nodal status than does PET or CT alone, increasing the level of confidence in image interpretation.
- By CT criteria, the right paratracheal region is divided into 2R and 4R nodal stations by the top of the aortic arch, to reflect the poorer prognosis of nodal metastases above the aortic arch.

Suggested Reading

Dwamena BA, Sonnad SS, Angobaldo JO, Wahl RL. Metastases from non-small cell lung cancer: mediastinal staging in the 1990s–meta-analytic comparison of PET and CT. Radiology 1999;213(2):530–536

Lardinois D, Weder W, Hany TF, Kamel EM, Korom S, Seifert B, von Schulthess GK, Steinert HC. Staging of non-small-cell lung cancer with integrated positron-emission tomography and computed tomography. N Engl J Med 2003;348(25):2500–2507

CASE 74

Clinical Presentation

A 71-year-old man has biopsy-proven adenocarcinoma of the lung. PET/CT is obtained for initial staging.

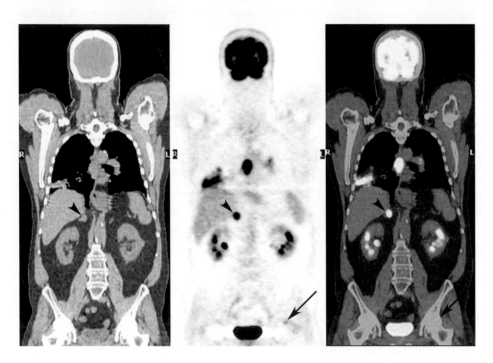

Fig. 74.1

Technique

- The patient is instructed to avoid vigorous exercise for 24 hours prior to the scan, fast for at least 4 hours before the study, drink water during the fasting and uptake periods, and void prior to the scan
- A venous serum glucose sample is obtained prior to the injection of ^{18}F-FDG (reference range is < 120 mg/dl for non-diabetic patients and < 200 mg/dl for diabetic patients), and the patient's height and weight are recorded
- A 10–20 mCi dose of ^{18}F-FDG is injected intravenously (in a dimly lit quiet room for brain PET scans), and the patient is asked to rest comfortably in a room that is kept warm
- Most PET scans are now acquired on a hybrid PET/CT scanner, and a low dose spiral CT is acquired for attenuation correction of the PET images and for anatomic localization. Some centers may choose to perform oral and/or intravenous contrast-enhanced diagnostic CT as part of the PET/CT examination
- Sixty minutes following the ^{18}F-FDG injection, the spiral CT is performed using a weight-based algorithm from the skull base to the upper thighs (for most oncologic indications), or from the vertex to the feet, or centered over the brain depending on the tumor being evaluated

- A 2D or 3D PET acquisition (depending on the manufacturer) is then performed over the same region(s), and all PET images are corrected for attenuation, detector efficiency, scatter, decay, and random coincidences
- Consistency in ^{18}F-FDG injected dose, scan acquisition time relative to the injection time, and acquisition and reconstruction protocols is important when performing serial scanning on the same patient

Image Interpretation

Unenhanced coronal CT, PET, and fused PET/CT slices (**Fig. 74.1**) show a dominant mass in the right lower lung that has a broad base of contact with the posterolateral pleural surface and a heterogeneous pattern of high ^{18}F-FDG activity. In addition, highly ^{18}F-FDG–avid mediastinal and right hilar lymphadenopathy is present. There is also a left paramediastinal parenchymal lesion with moderate-high ^{18}F-FDG uptake (not shown).

In the upper abdomen, a 1.4-cm right adrenal nodule (*arrowheads*) is highly ^{18}F-FDG–avid and most likely metastatic. A lytic, 1.6-cm lesion in the left superior acetabulum (*arrows*) is moderately ^{18}F-FDG–avid and suspected to be a metastasis. The unenhanced liver, spleen, kidneys, and left adrenal gland are unremarkable.

Differential Diagnosis

Stage IV lung cancer.

Diagnosis and Clinical Follow-Up

Fine-needle aspiration biopsy of the right adrenal gland was positive for malignant cells, consistent with a metastasis from the patient's known lung adenocarcinoma.

Discussion

In patients with lung cancer, an important advantage of ^{18}F-FDG-PET over anatomic imaging modalities is its greater accuracy for the detection of unsuspected systemic metastases. ^{18}F-FDG-PET correctly defines the presence or absence of contralateral and extrathoracic involvement in one whole-body scan.

The advantage of PET/CT in this setting is that it enables the precise localization of extrathoracic lesions. It allows a determination of the clinical significance of metabolically active foci by localizing them to specific morphologic structures, in this case the right adrenal gland and left superior acetabulum.

The adrenal gland is a common site of extrathoracic metastases in patients with lung cancer. When the uptake in adrenal lesions is greater than that in the liver, ^{18}F-FDG-PET has been shown to have a sensitivity of 100% and a specificity ranging from 80 to 94% for the detection of metastases to the adrenal glands. The less-than-perfect specificity is due to ^{18}F-FDG uptake in some benign adrenal adenomas. A recently published report demonstrated that when contrast-enhanced PET/CT and delayed imaging are used, the specificity may reach 100%.

The skeleton is also a common site for lung cancer metastases. ^{18}F-FDG-PET is a very accurate technique to evaluate for the presence of bone metastases. ^{18}F-FDG-PET has sensitivity similar to that of bone scintigraphy, but higher specificity, for the detection and characterization of osseous metastases from lung cancer.

- ^{18}F-FDG-PET interrogates the biological behavior of a lesion and thus is a better noninvasive predictor of malignancy in indeterminate extrathoracic lesions than are conventional imaging modalities.
- ^{18}F-FDG-PET imaging is a cost-effective test because patients in whom unresectable disease is diagnosed will be excluded from additional invasive procedures, such as unnecessary surgery.
- Some benign adrenal masses are ^{18}F-FDG–avid. Moreover, false-positive results of PET are expected in inflammation or infection, so that a positive finding always requires biopsy.
- False-negative findings in PET may occur in small lesions (< 7 mm) and in micrometastatic disease. Some tumors with a low rate of metabolic activity, such as bronchioloalveolar carcinomas, carcinoids, and other mucinous malignancies, may also be ^{18}F-FDG–negative.

Suggested Reading

Blake MA, Slattery JM, Kalra MK, Halpern EF, Fischman AJ, Mueller PR, Boland GW. Adrenal lesions: characterization with fused PET/CT image in patients with proved or suspected malignancy—initial experience. Radiology 2006;238(3):970–977

Erasmus JJ, Patz EF Jr, McAdams HP, Murray JG, Herndon J, Coleman RE, Goodman PC. Evaluation of adrenal masses in patients with bronchogenic carcinoma using 18F-fluorodeoxyglucose positron emission tomography. AJR Am J Roentgenol 1997;168(5):1361–1362

Fogelman I, Cook G, Israel O, Van der Wall H. Positron emission tomography and bone metastases. Semin Nucl Med 2005;35(2):135–142

Yun M, Kim W, Alnafisi N, Lacorte L, Jang S, Alavi A. 18F-FDG PET in characterizing adrenal lesions detected on CT or MRI. J Nucl Med 2001;42(12):1795–1799

CASE 75

Clinical Presentation

A 62-year-old man had follicular lymphoma. The patient is in clinical remission, having completed chemotherapy 3 years earlier. PET is requested for routine follow-up.

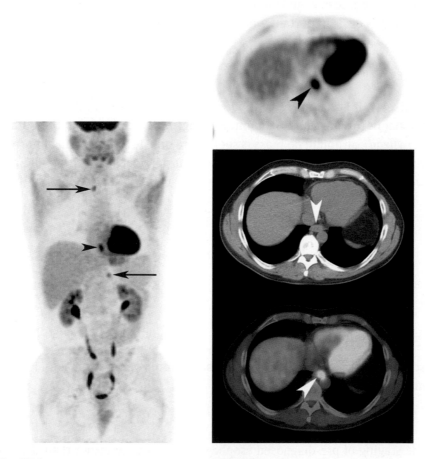

Fig. 75.1   Fig. 75.2

Technique

- The patient is instructed to avoid vigorous exercise for 24 hours prior to the scan, fast for at least 4 hours before the study, drink water during the fasting and uptake periods, and void prior to the scan
- A venous serum glucose sample is obtained prior to the injection of ¹⁸F-FDG (reference range is < 120 mg/dl for non-diabetic patients and < 200 mg/dl for diabetic patients), and the patient's height and weight are recorded
- A 10–20 mCi dose of ¹⁸F-FDG is injected intravenously (in a dimly lit quiet room for brain PET scans), and the patient is asked to rest comfortably in a room that is kept warm

- Most PET scans are now acquired on a hybrid PET/CT scanner, and a low dose spiral CT is acquired for attenuation correction of the PET images and for anatomic localization. Some centers may choose to perform oral and/or intravenous contrast-enhanced diagnostic CT as part of the PET/CT examination
- Sixty minutes following the ^{18}F-FDG injection, the spiral CT is performed using a weight-based algorithm from the skull base to the upper thighs (for most oncologic indications), or from the vertex to the feet, or centered over the brain depending on the tumor being evaluated
- A 2D or 3D PET acquisition (depending on the manufacturer) is then performed over the same region(s), and all PET images are corrected for attenuation, detector efficiency, scatter, decay, and random coincidences
- Consistency in ^{18}F-FDG injected dose, scan acquisition time relative to the injection time, and acquisition and reconstruction protocols is important when performing serial scanning on the same patient

Image Interpretation

Anterior maximum-intensity pixel (MIP) image (**Fig. 75.1**) demonstrates a focus of intense ^{18}F-FDG accumulation in the distal esophagus (*arrowhead*). Axial images (**Fig. 75.2**) confirm that the uptake is in the distal esophagus (*arrowhead*), although no mass is seen there on CT. There is also abnormal uptake in two small lymph nodes (**Fig. 75.1**, *arrows*), one in the right paratracheal station and one in the celiac axis. There is normal physiologic uptake in the stomach at the gastroesophageal junction.

Differential Diagnosis

- Esophageal cancer
- Focal inflammatory disease related to gastric reflux
- Lymphoma

Diagnosis and Clinical Follow-Up

The patient underwent endoscopy and was found to have an adenocarcinoma of the esophagus. He was treated with surgery and chemoradiotherapy.

Discussion

PET/CT is typically used for the staging of pre-diagnosed esophageal malignancy rather than the initial diagnosis. However, esophageal cancer may be an incidental finding, and focal esophageal uptake should always be reported. Focal tracer accumulation in the distal esophagus is a relatively common finding on ^{18}F-FDG-PET examinations. It is most commonly due to low-level esophagitis, and the typical picture is one of low-level, linear tracer accumulation. Focal esophagitis is usually due to gastric reflux and therefore is most commonly present at the gastroesophageal junction. Focal esophagitis can also be caused by radiotherapy, and in these cases it will be within the treated region and can show very intense tracer uptake. Less common causes of focal esophagitis include viral or fungal infection, which typically shows linear or diffuse moderate-high tracer uptake.

In this patient, the finding is more focal and intense than is usual for an inflammatory condition. Esophageal cancer may have an associated esophageal mass or proximal esophageal dilatation on CT; however, in some cases the CT scan may not show any abnormality. The incidental esophageal malignancy discovered in this patient showed intense tracer uptake. The lymph node uptake in this patient would not be expected in simple esophagitis and likely represented nodal involvement by the esophageal cancer; it would less likely be related to the patient's lymphoma.

PEARLS AND PITFALLS_____

- Inflammatory esophagitis is typically linear, low-grade, and located at the gastroesophageal junction. However, early esophageal cancer can also have this appearance, and a clinical correlation should always be sought.
- Early esophageal cancer in the esophageal lumen may not appear abnormal on coregistered CT images. Therefore, normal CT findings do not exclude malignancy.

Suggested Reading

Bruzzi JF, Munden RF, Truong MT, Marom EM, Sabloff BS, Gladish GW, Iyer RB, Pan TS, Macapiniac HA, Erasmus JJ. PET/CT of esophageal cancer: its role in clinical management. Radiographics 2007;27(6):1635–1652

Flanagan FL, Dehdashti F, Siegel BA, Trask DD, Sundaresan SR, Patterson GA, Cooper JD. Staging of esophageal cancer with ^{18}F-fluorodeoxyglucose positron emission tomography. AJR Am J Roentgenol 1997;168(2):417–424

Yasuda S, Raja S, Hubner KF. Application of whole-body positron emission tomography in the imaging of esophageal cancer: report of a case. Surg Today 1995;25(3):261–264

CASE 76

Clinical Presentation

A 50-year-old woman with a history of metastatic colon cancer completed chemotherapy 1 year ago. During the last 3 months, she has started to experience fleeting abdominal pains and has lost about 6 to 8 lb. Furthermore, her carcinoembryonic antigen (CEA) level has risen from 1.1 to 2.7 ng/mL (the upper limit of normal is 2.5 ng/mL).

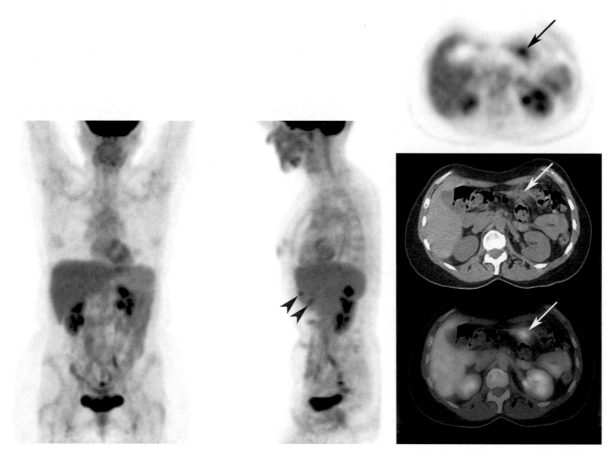

Fig. 76.1   Fig. 76.2

Technique

- The patient is instructed to avoid vigorous exercise for 24 hours prior to the scan, fast for at least 4 hours before the study, drink water during the fasting and uptake periods, and void prior to the scan
- A venous serum glucose sample is obtained prior to the injection of ¹⁸F-FDG (reference range is < 120 mg/dl for non-diabetic patients and < 200 mg/dl for diabetic patients), and the patient's height and weight are recorded
- A 10–20 mCi dose of ¹⁸F-FDG is injected intravenously (in a dimly lit quiet room for brain PET scans), and the patient is asked to rest comfortably in a room that is kept warm

236

- Most PET scans are now acquired on a hybrid PET/CT scanner, and a low dose spiral CT is acquired for attenuation correction of the PET images and for anatomic localization. Some centers may choose to perform oral and/or intravenous contrast-enhanced diagnostic CT as part of the PET/CT examination
- Sixty minutes following the ^{18}F-FDG injection, the spiral CT is performed using a weight-based algorithm from the skull base to the upper thighs (for most oncologic indications), or from the vertex to the feet, or centered over the brain depending on the tumor being evaluated
- A 2D or 3D PET acquisition (depending on the manufacturer) is then performed over the same region(s), and all PET images are corrected for attenuation, detector efficiency, scatter, decay, and random coincidences
- Consistency in ^{18}F-FDG injected dose, scan acquisition time relative to the injection time, and acquisition and reconstruction protocols is important when performing serial scanning on the same patient

Image Interpretation

Anterior (**Fig. 76.1A**) and sagittal (**Fig. 76.1B**) three-dimensional maximum-intensity pixel (MIP) views from the ^{18}F-FDG-PET scan show two ^{18}F-FDG–avid mesenteric deposits. They are best appreciated on the sagittal view (*arrowheads*), as they are obscured by renal activity on the anterior view. The more prominent one is in the mesentery adjacent to the site of resection in the transverse colon and is demonstrated on the axial slices (**Fig. 76.2**, *arrows*).

Differential Diagnosis

- Peritoneal metastatic disease
- Physiologic tracer uptake in bowel
- Abcess or other inflammatory lesion

Diagnosis and Clinical Follow-Up

The ^{18}F-FDG–avid soft-tissue mass adjacent to the transverse colon was biopsied under CT guidance. Recurrent adenocarcinoma was confirmed. The patient went on to receive salvage chemotherapy.

Discussion

The most established use of PET/CT for colorectal carcinoma in clinical practice has been to detect tumor recurrence in patients with rising levels of CEA and otherwise normal radiologic studies. Many reports have shown that ^{18}F-FDG-PET is more accurate than conventional radiologic imaging for the detection of intra-abdominal metastases.

One important pitfall to be aware of is that tracer uptake is lower in tumors with a mucinous histology than in those with other histologies because of the large amount of acellular mucin within the former.

PEARLS AND PITFALLS_____

- PET/CT is an important tool in the investigation of patients with a history of colorectal cancer and a rising CEA level.
- In the setting of a rising CEA level, particular care should be taken to assess the mesenteric fat for ^{18}F-FDG–avid soft tissue masses, which may represent peritoneal metastases.
- Mucinous colorectal carcinoma tumor deposits may demonstrate minimal ^{18}F-FDG uptake.

Suggested Reading

Choi MY, Lee KM, Chung JK, Lee DS, Jeong JM, Park JG, Kim JH, Lee MC. Correlation between serum CEA level and metabolic volume as determined by FDG PET in postoperative patients with recurrent colorectal cancer. Ann Nucl Med 2005;19(2):123–129

Delbeke D, Martin WH. PET and PET-CT for evaluation of colorectal carcinoma. Semin Nucl Med 2004;34(3):209–223

Flanagan FL, Dehdashti F, Ogunbiyi OA, Kodner IJ, Siegel BA. Utility of FDG-PET for investigating unexplained plasma CEA elevation in patients with colorectal cancer. Ann Surg 1998;227(3):319–323

CASE 77

Clinical Presentation

A 63-year-old man has a history of large-cell lymphoma. The patient has returned for a routine restaging examination.

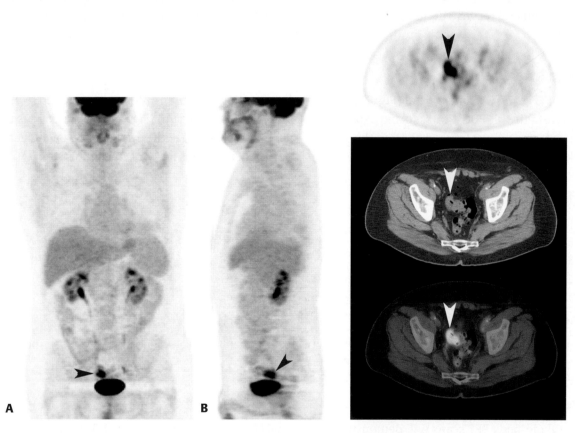

Fig. 77.1

Fig. 77.2

Technique

- The patient is instructed to avoid vigorous exercise for 24 hours prior to the scan, fast for at least 4 hours before the study, drink water during the fasting and uptake periods, and void prior to the scan
- A venous serum glucose sample is obtained prior to the injection of ^{18}F-FDG (reference range is < 120 mg/dl for non-diabetic patients and < 200 mg/dl for diabetic patients), and the patient's height and weight are recorded
- A 10–20 mCi dose of 18F-FDG is injected intravenously (in a dimly lit quiet room for brain PET scans), and the patient is asked to rest comfortably in a room that is kept warm
- Most PET scans are now acquired on a hybrid PET/CT scanner, and a low dose spiral CT is acquired for attenuation correction of the PET images and for anatomic localization. Some centers may

choose to perform oral and/or intravenous contrast-enhanced diagnostic CT as part of the PET/CT examination

- Sixty minutes following the ^{18}F-FDG injection, the spiral CT is performed using a weight-based algorithm from the skull base to the upper thighs (for most oncologic indications), or from the vertex to the feet, or centered over the brain depending on the tumor being evaluated

- A 2D or 3D PET acquisition (depending on the manufacturer) is then performed over the same region(s), and all PET images are corrected for attenuation, detector efficiency, scatter, decay, and random coincidences

- Consistency in ^{18}F-FDG injected dose, scan acquisition time relative to the injection time, and acquisition and reconstruction protocols is important when performing serial scanning on the same patient

Image Interpretation

Anterior (**Fig. 77.1A**) and sagittal (**Fig. 77.1B**) three-dimensional maximum-intensity projection (MIP) views from the ^{18}F-FDG-PET scan and axial images at the level of the sacrum (**Fig. 77.2**) show a focus of intense tracer uptake (*arrowheads*) in the sigmoid colon. On the CT images, the sigmoid colon appears thickened, and there is diverticular disease. There is no other suspicious focus of tracer uptake.

Differential Diagnosis

- Physiologic tracer uptake
- Diverticulitis
- Sigmoid carcinoma
- Other pre-cancerous neoplastic disease, such as adenoma

Diagnosis and Clinical Follow-Up

The patient underwent a sigmoidoscopy and biopsy, which resulted in a diagnosis of adenocarcinoma. The patient subsequently underwent surgery.

Discussion

Most whole-body PET scans will demonstrate physiologic tracer uptake in the bowel. This is most frequently seen in the terminal ileum and cecum. The source of tracer uptake is uncertain, but it may be extraluminal, perhaps in smooth muscle or lymphoid tissue. Alternatively, ^{18}F-FDG may be secreted into the bowel lumen or taken up by bowel microorganisms. Antibiotics, laxatives, and glucagon have all been used in an effort to reduce the tracer uptake, but with minimal success.

It can be very difficult to differentiate pathologic from physiologic tracer uptake. Knowledge of the normal patterns of tracer uptake is essential to differentiate uptake in a patient with colon cancer from that seen in a normal bowel. PET/CT is more accurate than PET alone because it allows the reader to correlate tracer uptake with anatomic abnormalities. In this instance, an abnormality on the CT portion of the examination, the thickened bowel wall, led the reporting nuclear medicine physician to recommend a sigmoidoscopy. Physiologic tracer uptake in the bowel normally varies between examinations in the same patient, and another finding that should be considered suggestive of a neoplasm is a persistent focus of tracer uptake in the same location on two separate examinations.

Bowel uptake of ^{18}F-FDG can also be seen in inflammatory or infectious/inflammatory conditions such as ulcerative colitis and diverticulitis. Correlation with the patient's history can be useful to help differentiate this uptake from normal tracer uptake. Diffuse small and large bowel uptake is also seen in diabetic patients treated with the oral hypoglycemic agent metformin.

PEARLS AND PITFALLS

- Physiologic tracer uptake in the bowel is common and most frequently seen in the terminal ileum and cecum.
- A persistent focus of tracer uptake in one location in the bowel in the same patient on multiple scans is a very suspicious finding and merits further investigation.
- Abnormalities such as a soft tissue mass or thickened bowel wall on CT images that correspond to a focus of ^{18}F-FDG tracer uptake should also prompt concern.

Suggested Reading

Gutman F, Alberini JL, Wartski M, Vilain D, Le Stanc E, Sarandi F, Corone C, Tainturier C, Pecking AP. Incidental colonic focal lesions detected by FDG PET/CT. AJR Am J Roentgenol 2005;185(2):495–500

Hannah A, Scott AM, Akhurst T, Berlangieri S, Bishop J, McKay WJ. Abnormal colonic accumulation of fluorine-18-FDG in pseudomembranous colitis. J Nucl Med 1996;37(10):1683–1685

Yasuda S, Takahashi W, Takagi S, Fujii H, Ide M, Shohtsu A. Factors influencing physiological FDG uptake in the intestine. Tokai J Exp Clin Med 1998;23(5):241–244

CASE 78

Clinical Presentation

A 55-year-old man has been shown to have a mass in the head of the pancreas. PET is requested for staging.

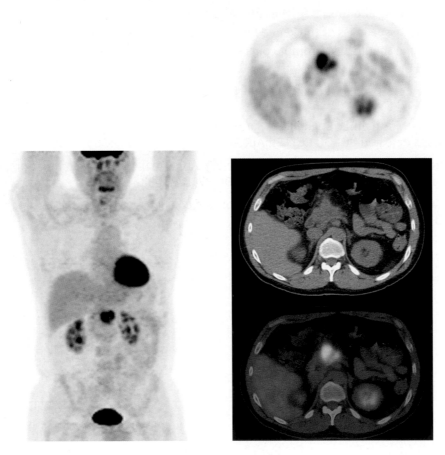

Fig. 78.1   Fig. 78.2

Technique

- The patient is instructed to avoid vigorous exercise for 24 hours prior to the scan, fast for at least 4 hours before the study, drink water during the fasting and uptake periods, and void prior to the scan
- A venous serum glucose sample is obtained prior to the injection of ^{18}F-FDG (reference range is < 120 mg/dl for non-diabetic patients and < 200 mg/dl for diabetic patients), and the patient's height and weight are recorded
- A 10–20 mCi dose of ^{18}F-FDG is injected intravenously (in a dimly lit quiet room for brain PET scans), and the patient is asked to rest comfortably in a room that is kept warm
- Most PET scans are now acquired on a hybrid PET/CT scanner, and a low dose spiral CT is acquired for attenuation correction of the PET images and for anatomic localization. Some centers may choose to perform oral and/or intravenous contrast-enhanced diagnostic CT as part of the PET/CT examination

- Sixty minutes following the ¹⁸F-FDG injection, the spiral CT is performed using a weight-based algorithm from the skull base to the upper thighs (for most oncologic indications), or from the vertex to the feet, or centered over the brain depending on the tumor being evaluated
- A 2D or 3D PET acquisition (depending on the manufacturer) is then performed over the same region(s), and all PET images are corrected for attenuation, detector efficiency, scatter, decay, and random coincidences
- Consistency in ¹⁸F-FDG injected dose, scan acquisition time relative to the injection time, and acquisition and reconstruction protocols is important when performing serial scanning on the same patient

Image Interpretation

The anterior maximum-intensity pixel (MIP) image from the PET scan (**Fig. 78.1**) demonstrates increased ¹⁸F-FDG uptake in the midline of the upper abdomen. There is otherwise normal physiologic uptake, with no pathologic uptake in the local lymph nodes and no distant metastases. Axial PET, CT, and fused PET/CT (**Fig. 78.2**) confirm ¹⁸F-FDG uptake in a pancreatic mass.

Differential Diagnosis

- Pancreatic adenocarcinoma
- Other pancreatic malignancy
- Pancreatitis

Diagnosis and Clinical Follow-Up

Pancreatic adenocarcinoma. Diagnosis final, no clinical follow-up.

Discussion

Cancer of the pancreas is the second most common gastrointestinal malignancy, after colorectal cancer. It is the fourth leading cause of cancer death. The incidence of pancreatic cancer increases steadily with age. Adenocarcinomas account for 95% of primary malignancies of the exocrine pancreas. Pancreatic cancer usually presents late, resulting in a poor outcome. Only 10 to 20% of patients are candidates for resection surgery, and the overall 5-year survival is 5%. Symptoms are nonspecific and include jaundice, weight loss, and pain. Glucose intolerance or frank diabetes is present in as many as 70% of patients as the consequence of pancreatic duct obstruction and resultant atrophy.

In the diagnosis of pancreatic cancer, the primary imaging modality is CT. However, PET can play an important complementary role—for example, when pancreatic cancer is suspected but CT fails to identify a mass or when fine-needle aspiration is nondiagnostic. Normal pancreatic tissue does not take up ¹⁸F-FDG, whereas pancreatic cancers selectively overexpress GLUT1 receptors, resulting in significantly increased ¹⁸F-FDG uptake. However, the normal pancreas is visualized when imaged with ¹¹C-methionine or ¹¹C-acetate. Unfortunately, active pancreatitis also exhibits increased ¹⁸F-FDG uptake and is the most common cause of a false-positive study. Uptake in pancreatitis tends to be more diffuse, with lower intensity and standardized uptake value (SUV), than uptake in pancreatic cancer, but there is overlap. Correlation with enzymatic and C-reactive protein levels is recommended to differentiate pancreatitis from cancer. Tissue diagnosis may be required.

Figures 78.3 (MIP) and **78.4** (axial PET, CT, fused PET/CT) are from the ¹⁸F-FDG-PET scan of a 58-year-old man with non-Hodgkin lymphoma. In addition to several foci of uptake in lymph nodes in the head, neck, and thorax, there is moderate uptake throughout the body and tail of the pancreas (partially

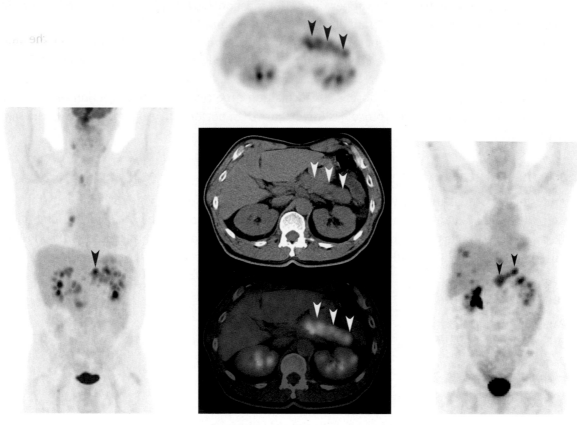

Fig. 78.3   **Fig. 78.4**   **Fig. 78.5**

overlapping left renal uptake on the MIP image, *arrowhead*) as a result of pancreatitis. Other causes of false-positive studies have included placement of a nasobiliary probe, portal vein thrombosis, hemorrhagic pseudocyst, and microcystic cystadenoma.

A common cause of a false-negative study is hyperglycemia, which results in decreased ^{18}F-FDG uptake in the tumor through competitive inhibition. As noted, as many as 70% of patients with pancreatic cancer are hyperglycemic. In one study, 10 of 11 false-negative examinations were in patients with hyperglycemia. The sensitivity was 98% in euglycemic patients versus 63% in hyperglycemic patients with pancreatic cancer. A summary of 305 cases from five studies yielded an overall sensitivity of 92%, specificity of 79%, and accuracy of 87% in the diagnosis of pancreatic cancer.

The accurate staging of pancreatic cancer is difficult. In up to 40% of patients with presumed resectable cancer, the cancer has been found to be unresectable at surgery. Both PET and CT are limited in N (node) staging because of the small size of the local nodes and their close proximity to the primary tumor. The major staging impact of PET is in M (metastasis) staging, with the identification of metastases in the liver in particular, but also in the lungs, bone marrow, and peritoneum. **Figure 78.5** is from a 67-year-old man with ^{18}F-FDG uptake in a primary pancreatic cancer (*arrowheads*) as well as in several small liver metastases.

PET may be useful in the follow-up of patients with pancreatic cancer, particularly in distinguishing fibrosis from recurrence when CT is not definitive, in evaluating new liver lesions that are too small to biopsy, and in the setting of a rising tumor marker (cancer antigen [CA] 19-9) and negative or equivocal results of conventional imaging.

- The most common cause of a false-positive study is active pancreatitis. This should be excluded on clinical and biochemical grounds, including a measurement of C-reactive protein.
- A common cause of a false-negative examination is hyperglycemia, which is prevalent in this patient population. Other causes of a false-negative study include small tumor size and neuroendocrine tumors.
- PET is of limited utility in staging lymph nodes adjacent to the primary tumor. However, PET is helpful in staging more distant nodes, such as the Virchow node, and in identifying metastases.
- PET can be useful in the surveillance of patients with pancreatic cancer, particularly when the results of anatomic imaging are equivocal or negative in the setting of a rising tumor marker.

Suggested Reading

Delbeke D, Rose DM, Chapman WC, Pinson CW, Wright JK, Beauchamp RD, Shyr Y, Leach SD. Optimal interpretation of FDG PET in the diagnosis, staging and management of pancreatic carcinoma. J Nucl Med 1999;40(11):1784–1791

Delbeke D, Pinson CW. Pancreatic tumors: role of imaging in the diagnosis, staging, and treatment. J Hepatobiliary Pancreat Surg 2004;11(1):4–10

Maemura K, Takao S, Shinchi H, Noma H, Mataki Y, Kurahara H, Jinnouchi S, Aikou T. Role of positron emission tomography in decisions on treatment strategies for pancreatic cancer. J Hepatobiliary Pancreat Surg 2006;13(5):435–441

Pakzad F, Groves AM, Ell PJ. The role of positron emission tomography in the management of pancreatic cancer. Semin Nucl Med 2006;36(3):248–256

Redlich PN, Ahrendt SA, Pitt HA. Tumors of the pancreas, gallbladder, and bile ducts. In: Lenhard RE Jr, Osteen RT, Gansler T, eds. The American Cancer Society's Clinical Oncology. Atlanta, GA: American Cancer Society; 2001:373–394

Zimny M, Fass J, Bares R, Cremerius U, Sabri O, Buechin P, Schumpelick V, Buell U. Fluorodeoxyglucose positron emission tomography and the prognosis of pancreatic carcinoma. Scand Gastroenterol 2000;35(8):883–888

CASE 79

Clinical Presentation

A 57-year-old woman has a 4-month history of a right breast lump. An ultrasound-guided biopsy of the breast mass demonstrates invasive ductal carcinoma.

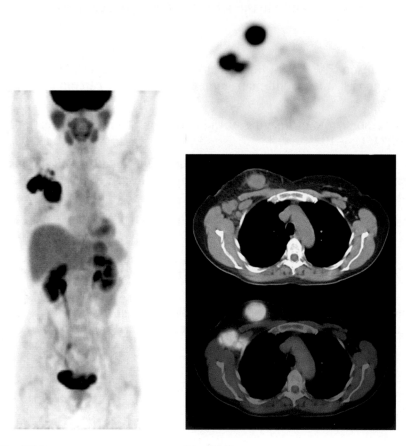

Fig. 79.1   **Fig. 79.2**

Technique

- The patient is instructed to avoid vigorous exercise for 24 hours prior to the scan, fast for at least 4 hours before the study, drink water during the fasting and uptake periods, and void prior to the scan
- A venous serum glucose sample is obtained prior to the injection of ^{18}F-FDG (reference range is < 120 mg/dl for non-diabetic patients and < 200 mg/dl for diabetic patients), and the patient's height and weight are recorded
- A 10–20 mCi dose of ^{18}F-FDG is injected intravenously (in a dimly lit quiet room for brain PET scans), and the patient is asked to rest comfortably in a room that is kept warm
- Most PET scans are now acquired on a hybrid PET/CT scanner, and a low dose spiral CT is acquired for attenuation correction of the PET images and for anatomic localization. Some centers may

choose to perform oral and/or intravenous contrast-enhanced diagnostic CT as part of the PET/CT examination

- Sixty minutes following the ^{18}F-FDG injection, the spiral CT is performed using a weight-based algorithm from the skull base to the upper thighs (for most oncologic indications), or from the vertex to the feet, or centered over the brain depending on the tumor being evaluated

- A 2D or 3D PET acquisition (depending on the manufacturer) is then performed over the same region(s), and all PET images are corrected for attenuation, detector efficiency, scatter, decay, and random coincidences

- Consistency in ^{18}F-FDG injected dose, scan acquisition time relative to the injection time, and acquisition and reconstruction protocols is important when performing serial scanning on the same patient

Image Interpretation

Anterior maximum-intensity projection (MIP) image (**Fig. 79.1**) and axial images through the thorax (**Fig. 79.2**). The mass in the right breast is clearly seen on both the PET and CT data sets. It demonstrates intense ^{18}F-FDG uptake. There are also several ^{18}F-FDG–avid masses in the right axilla.

Differential Diagnosis

- Breast cancer avid for ^{18}F-FDG and ispilateral axillary nodal metastases
- Breast cancer avid for ^{18}F-FDG with inflammatory tracer uptake in the axilla related to the recent biopsy

Diagnosis and Clinical Follow-Up

The patient went on to mastectomy and axillary dissection, which confirmed metastatic involvement of the axillary lymph nodes with invasive ductal breast cancer. Because the primary tumor was bulky, the clinicians were concerned about the possibility of internal thoracic lymph node metastases. However, the ^{18}F-FDG-PET/CT results did not support this.

Discussion

The accuracy of PET/CT in the detection of primary breast cancers varies depending on the histologic type and size of the tumor. Uptake of ^{18}F-FDG is lower in pure lobular carcinoma, tubular carcinoma, and small in situ carcinomas than in other types of breast cancer. The sensitivity of ^{18}F-FDG-PET for tumors smaller than 1 cm is limited, as is its sensitivity in detecting axillary nodal metastases. One large trial demonstrated a sensitivity of 61% and a specificity of 80% for axillary metastases. Therefore, ^{18}F-FDG-PET is not recommended as an accurate tool for the initial staging of breast cancer.

Nonetheless, in certain circumstances ^{18}F-FDG-PET may have a role in the initial staging of breast cancer. These include planning neoadjuvant therapy in patients with bulky tumors and assessing internal thoracic lymph node involvement in patients with bulky medial primary breast tumors. Metastatic involvement of the axillary nodes can be confirmed by sentinel node biopsy. However, internal thoracic lymph node metastases may occur in up to 25% of patients. These metastatic nodes may not be included in the radiation field, and recurrence in them is common. **Figure 79.3** demonstrates an ^{18}F-FDG–avid internal thoracic lymph node (*arrowheads*) in a different patient with recurrent breast cancer.

Low-level tracer uptake in axillary nodes may be present after biopsy, so caution is advised when studies are interpreted under these circumstances.

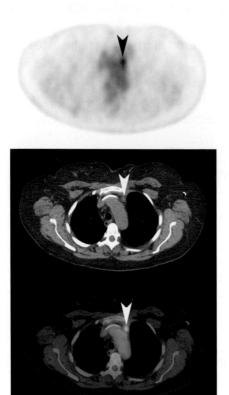

Fig. 79.3

PEARLS AND PITFALLS _____

- ^{18}F-FDG-PET/CT is not currently indicated for the routine staging of breast cancer, but is useful in the evaluation of therapeutic response.
- ^{18}F-FDG uptake in primary tumors may be low, especially if the tumor is smaller than 1 cm and/or of pure lobular etiology.
- ^{18}F -FDG uptake in axillary lymph nodes after biopsy may be inflammatory.

Suggested Reading

Avril N, Dose J, Jänicke F, Ziegler S, Römer W, Weber W, Herz M, Nathrath W, Graeff H, Schwaiger M. Assessment of axillary lymph node involvement in breast cancer patients with positron emission tomography using radiolabeled 2-(fluorine-18)-fluoro-2-deoxy-D-glucose. J Natl Cancer Inst 1996;88(17):1204–1209

Bos R, van Der Hoeven JJ, van Der Wall E, van Der Groep P, van Diest PJ, Comans EF, Joshi U, Semenza GL, Hoekstra OS, Lammertsma AA, Molthoff CF. Biologic correlates of (18)fluorodeoxyglucose uptake in human breast cancer measured by positron emission tomography. J Clin Oncol 2002;20(2):379–387

Eubank WB, Mankoff DA. Current and future uses of positron emission tomography in breast cancer imaging. Semin Nucl Med 2004;34(3):224–240

CASE 80

Clinical Presentation

A 56-year-old woman presents with a palpable mass in the right breast and nipple inversion. Ultrasound-guided biopsy reveals a poorly differentiated invasive ductal carcinoma. After radical mastectomy, 13 of 15 axillary lymph nodes are involved by tumor. PET/CT with ^{18}F-FDG is performed postoperatively for further staging.

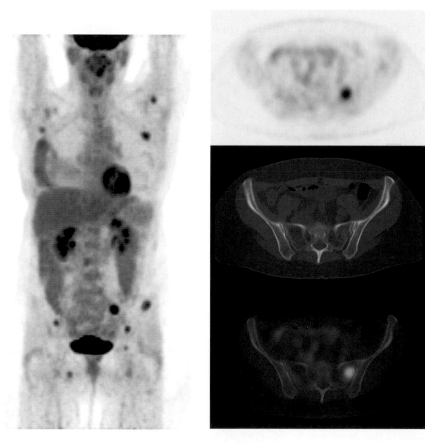

Fig. 80.1　　　　　　　　Fig. 80.2

Technique

- The patient is instructed to avoid vigorous exercise for 24 hours prior to the scan, fast for at least 4 hours before the study, drink water during the fasting and uptake periods, and void prior to the scan
- A venous serum glucose sample is obtained prior to the injection of ^{18}F-FDG (reference range is < 120 mg/dl for non-diabetic patients and < 200 mg/dl for diabetic patients), and the patient's height and weight are recorded

- A 10-20 mCi dose of ^{18}F-FDG is injected intravenously (in a dimly lit quiet room for brain PET scans), and the patient is asked to rest comfortably in a room that is kept warm
- Most PET scans are now acquired on a hybrid PET/CT scanner, and a low dose spiral CT is acquired for attenuation correction of the PET images and for anatomic localization. Some centers may choose to perform oral and/or intravenous contrast-enhanced diagnostic CT as part of the PET/CT examination
- Sixty minutes following the ^{18}F-FDG injection, the spiral CT is performed using a weight-based algorithm from the skull base to the upper thighs (for most oncologic indications), or from the vertex to the feet, or centered over the brain depending on the tumor being evaluated
- A 2D or 3D PET acquisition (depending on the manufacturer) is then performed over the same region(s), and all PET images are corrected for attenuation, detector efficiency, scatter, decay, and random coincidences
- Consistency in ^{18}F-FDG injected dose, scan acquisition time relative to the injection time, and acquisition and reconstruction protocols is important when performing serial scanning on the same patient

Image Interpretation

Anterior maximum-intensity pixel (MIP) image (**Fig. 80.1**) and axial images (**Fig. 80.2**) at the level of the sacrum show multiple foci of tracer uptake throughout the skeleton. There is also a linear focus of low-grade tracer uptake in the right anterior chest wall, the site of the recent surgery. On the co-registered images, no focal abnormalities are seen in the bones on the CT scan in the regions of tracer uptake on the PET scan.

Differential Diagnosis

- Multiple metastases, based primarily in the bone marrow
- Residual tumor in the right anterior chest wall

Diagnosis and Clinical Follow-Up

Multiple osseous metastases in a patient who presented with advanced breast cancer.

Discussion

Chest radiography, liver ultrasound, bone scintigraphy, CT, and MRI are currently used to stage breast cancer after the initial diagnosis has been made. ^{18}F-FDG-PET/CT allows whole-body staging with a single examination. The reported sensitivity and specificity are 86% and 90%, respectively. Cancers that are advanced at diagnosis are more likely to have distant metastases, and ^{18}F-FDG-PET may be more appropriate in these cases.

When compared with bone scintigraphy, ^{18}F-FDG-PET has a higher sensitivity for osseous metastases. Bone metastases may be characterized by their appearance on CT as either osteoblastic or osteolytic. A third pattern of bone metastasis detected on ^{18}F-FDG-PET/CT has no CT abnormality and is localized within the bone marrow. Osteolytic and bone marrow–based metastases are particularly ^{18}F-FDG–avid, and ^{18}F-FDG-PET/CT is more sensitive for these lesions. Some osteoblastic metastases may not be ^{18}F-FDG–avid, and a careful review of the CT images on bone windows is advised. When a patient has been treated previously, ^{18}F-FDG–avid lytic or marrow based–metastases may become sclerotic on CT while losing their avidity for ^{18}F-FDG. This pattern is typical of treated disease.

PEARLS AND PITFALLS

- ^{18}F-FDG-PET is most sensitive for osteolytic and bone marrow–based metastases.
- Lytic ^{18}F-FDG–avid metastases typically become sclerotic and lose their avidity for ^{18}F-FDG with treatment.
- ^{18}F-FDG negative sclerotic/osteoblastic skeletal metastases may not be falsely negative but represent treated lesions.

Suggested Reading

Cook GJ, Houston S, Rubens R, Maisey MN, Fogelman I. Detection of bone metastases in breast cancer by [18]FDG PET: differing metabolic activity in osteoblastic and osteolytic lesions. J Clin Oncol 1998;16(10):3375–3379

Du Y, Cullum I, Illidge TM, Ell PJ. Fusion of metabolic function and morphology: sequential ^{18}F-FDG/CT studies yield new insights into the natural history of bone metastases in breast cancer. J Clin Oncol 2007;25(23):3440–3447

CASE 81

Clinical Presentation

A 65-year-old woman has breast cancer. The patient was previously shown to have metastatic disease in the chest (**Figs. 81.1** and **81.2**). A re-staging examination after a course of chemotherapy was performed (**Fig. 81.3**).

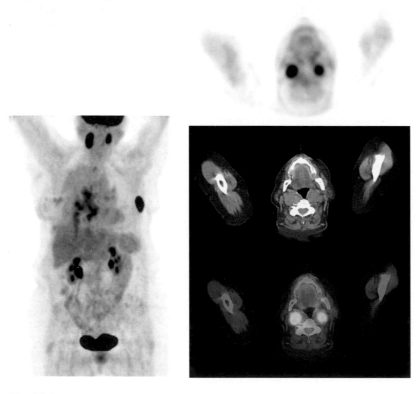

Fig. 81.1　　　　　**Fig. 81.2**

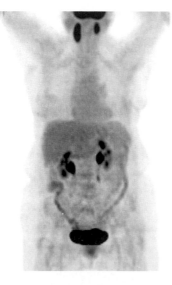

Fig. 81.3

Technique

- The patient is instructed to avoid vigorous exercise for 24 hours prior to the scan, fast for at least 4 hours before the study, drink water during the fasting and uptake periods, and void prior to the scan
- A venous serum glucose sample is obtained prior to the injection of ^{18}F-FDG (reference range is < 120 mg/dl for non-diabetic patients and < 200 mg/dl for diabetic patients), and the patient's height and weight are recorded
- A 10–20 mCi dose of ^{18}F-FDG is injected intravenously (in a dimly lit quiet room for brain PET scans), and the patient is asked to rest comfortably in a room that is kept warm
- Most PET scans are now acquired on a hybrid PET/CT scanner, and a low dose spiral CT is acquired for attenuation correction of the PET images and for anatomic localization. Some centers may choose to perform oral and/or intravenous contrast-enhanced diagnostic CT as part of the PET/CT examination
- Sixty minutes following the ^{18}F-FDG injection, the spiral CT is performed using a weight-based algorithm from the skull base to the upper thighs (for most oncologic indications), or from the vertex to the feet, or centered over the brain depending on the tumor being evaluated
- A 2D or 3D PET acquisition (depending on the manufacturer) is then performed over the same region(s), and all PET images are corrected for attenuation, detector efficiency, scatter, decay, and random coincidences
- Consistency in ^{18}F-FDG injected dose, scan acquisition time relative to the injection time, and acquisition and reconstruction protocols is important when performing serial scanning on the same patient

Image Interpretation

Anterior maximum-intensity pixel (MIP) image (**Fig. 81.1**) and axial images (**Fig. 81.2**) at the level of the carotid bulbs from the initial PET scan before chemotherapy show intense tracer uptake in the chest, which was proven to be metastatic disease. There is also tracer uptake in the left axilla and in bilateral neck masses. **Figure 81.3** is from the re-staging examination following chemotherapy.

Differential Diagnosis

- Mixed response to treatment with resistant disease in the neck
- Different ^{18}F-FDG–avid process in the neck
- Bilateral internal jugular vein thromboses

Diagnosis and Clinical Follow-Up

The bilateral ^{18}F-FDG–avid process in the neck had originally been felt to represent metastatic breast cancer. However, after failure of the response to therapy while excellent response was seen elsewhere in the chest and axilla, further diagnostic studies were performed. These demonstrated that the neck lesions were in fact bilateral carotid body tumors.

Discussion

Monitoring of response to chemotherapy is a common indication for PET/CT in patients with breast cancer. Metabolic changes will precede anatomic changes, and the greater the reduction in tracer uptake, the better the response to treatment and the better the outcome. Restaging PET/CT is usually performed after one to three cycles of chemotherapy. In this patient, the true metastatic disease demonstrated a complete metabolic response to therapy. A mixed response to treatment may indicate that a clone of resistant cells is present within certain anatomic locations. Another cause of a mixed response is the use of radiotherapy for some metastatic lesions and not others. In the current case, the apparent lack of response to therapy of the ^{18}F-FDG–avid disease in the neck prompted a search for a separate ^{18}F-FDG–avid process that might explain the apparent failure to respond to chemotherapy.

Carotid body tumors are paragangliomas. Paragangliomas usually demonstrate intense ^{18}F-FDG tracer uptake. Bilateral carotid body tumors may be seen in 30% of cases and may be familial.

PEARLS AND PITFALLS

- Mixed responses to therapy most commonly occur when radiotherapy has been used in one anatomic site of disease and not another.
- Mixed responses to therapy can indicate resistant disease at one anatomic site.
- A marked difference between responses to therapy at two disease sites may also suggest the possibility of a second ^{18}F-FDG–avid process.

Suggested Reading

Jansson T, Westlin JE, Ahlström H, Lilja A, Långström B, Bergh J. Positron emission tomography studies in patients with locally advanced and/or metastatic breast cancer: a method for early therapy evaluation? J Clin Oncol 1995;13(6):1470–1477

Macfarlane DJ, Shulkin BL, Murphy K, Wolf GT. FDG PET imaging of paragangliomas of the neck: comparison with MIBG SPET. Eur J Nucl Med 1995;22(11):1347–1350

Rousseau C, Devillers A, Sagan C, Ferrer L, Bridji B, Campion L, Ricauld M, Bourbouloux E, Doutriax I, Clovet M, Benton-Rigaud D, Bouriel C, Delecroix V, Garin E, Rouquette S, Resche I, Kerbrat P, Chatal JF, Campone M. Monitoring of early response to neoadjuvant chemotherapy in stage II and III breast cancer by [18F]fluorodeoxyglucose positron emission tomography. J Clin Oncol 2006;24(34):5366–5372

CASE 82

Clinical Presentation

A 58-year-old man has a recently identified mass in the right piriform sinus, confirmed by biopsy to be squamous cell carcinoma. PET is ordered for purposes of staging.

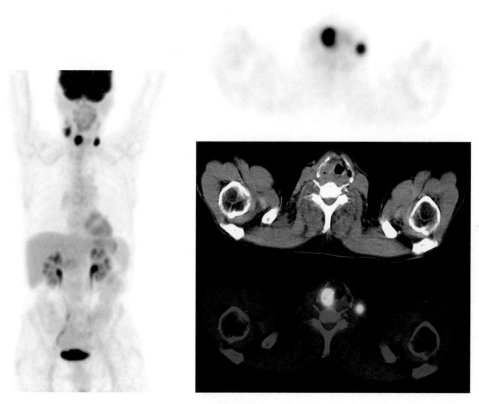

Fig. 82.1   **Fig. 82.2**

Technique

- The patient is instructed to avoid vigorous exercise for 24 hours prior to the scan, fast for at least 4 hours before the study, drink water during the fasting and uptake periods, and void prior to the scan
- A venous serum glucose sample is obtained prior to the injection of ^{18}F-FDG (reference range is < 120 mg/dl for non-diabetic patients and < 200 mg/dl for diabetic patients), and the patient's height and weight are recorded
- A 10–20 mCi dose of ^{18}F-FDG is injected intravenously (in a dimly lit quiet room for brain PET scans), and the patient is asked to rest comfortably in a room that is kept warm
- Most PET scans are now acquired on a hybrid PET/CT scanner, and a low dose spiral CT is acquired for attenuation correction of the PET images and for anatomic localization. Some centers may choose to perform oral and/or intravenous contrast-enhanced diagnostic CT as part of the PET/CT examination

- Sixty minutes following the ^{18}F-FDG injection, the spiral CT is performed using a weight-based algorithm from the skull base to the upper thighs (for most oncologic indications), or from the vertex to the feet, or centered over the brain depending on the tumor being evaluated
- A 2D or 3D PET acquisition (depending on the manufacturer) is then performed over the same region(s), and all PET images are corrected for attenuation, detector efficiency, scatter, decay, and random coincidences
- Consistency in ^{18}F-FDG injected dose, scan acquisition time relative to the injection time, and acquisition and reconstruction protocols is important when performing serial scanning on the same patient

Image Interpretation

A maximum-intensity pixel (MIP) image (**Fig. 82.1**) from the ^{18}F-FDG-PET scan demonstrates three foci of intense ^{18}F-FDG uptake in the neck. Axial images (**Fig. 82.2**) from PET, CT, and fused PET/CT localize two of the foci of abnormal uptake to the primary tumor in the right piriform sinus and a contralateral lymph node. The third focus was in an ipsilateral lymph node not included at this axial level.

Differential Diagnosis

- Squamous cell carcinoma of the larynx with nodal metastases
- Three sites of metastatic disease from an unknown primary

Diagnosis and Clinical Follow-Up

Squamous cell carcinoma of the larynx with bilateral neck nodal metastases but no distal metastases. The disease is stage IVa. Diagnosis final, no clinical follow-up.

Discussion

Head and neck carcinomas account for approximately 5% of all cancers in Western society. The incidence is highest in men in their fifth and sixth decades. There is a strong association with tobacco and alcohol use. Because the upper aerodigestive tract is lined by squamous epithelium, the vast majority of cancers in this region are squamous cell cancers. Squamous cell cancers tend to be highly ^{18}F-FDG–avid, making ^{18}F-FDG-PET an excellent tool for evaluating head and neck cancers.

Knowledge of the normal ^{18}F-FDG uptake patterns, which can be quite variable, is essential for the accurate evaluation of any PET scan. The head and neck region presents some unique challenges for several reasons, including the large number of anatomic structures in this region, their small size, and the prominent yet variable physiologic ^{18}F-FDG uptake seen within some of these normal structures. ^{18}F-FDG is taken up and retained to varying degrees within the mucosal structures of the oropharynx, including the tongue and soft palate, as well as the sublingual glands and lingual tonsil. There can be prominent uptake as well throughout the remainder of the salivary glands, particularly in the post-therapy setting. A high level of uptake can be seen in the palatine and pharyngeal tonsils, particularly in young patients. In the laryngeal region, uptake can be seen within several of the small muscles of phonation. Although the laryngeal muscles involved, and the resultant pattern on ^{18}F-FDG-PET can be quite variable, asymmetry can be an important clue to an abnormality, particularly in the pre-therapy setting, or a sign of recurrent laryngeal nerve paralysis. Diffuse uptake is occasionally seen throughout the thyroid. More focal uptake in the thyroid should raise the possibility of thyroid cancer, although this finding is not specific, as benign thyroid adenomas can also demonstrate increased ^{18}F-FDG uptake. Diffuse uptake is occasionally seen in the thymus, typically in pediatric and young adult patients.

PET is effectively used in several scenarios in head and neck cancer, including staging. Most clinically detected head and neck cancers have already spread to lymph nodes. Correct establishment of the lymph node status is important for planning therapy and for prognosis. Survival decreases by 50% when nodal involvement is present. The lymph node status has been traditionally assessed through physical examination and anatomic imaging, including CT, MRI, and ultrasound. Assessment with these modalities is based on structural parameters, most notably lymph node size. Metabolic imaging with ^{18}F-FDG-PET has been shown to be significantly more sensitive and more specific than anatomic imaging in establishing lymph node status. Because PET cannot identify microscopic disease, some advocate proceeding to a sentinel node biopsy following a node-negative PET scan in an algorithm that exploits the high specificity of PET in this setting and the high sensitivity of sentinel node biopsy. As in many other cancers, the whole-body nature of PET scanning allows staging for distal metastases. Furthermore, patients with head and neck cancers are at significantly increased risk for having a synchronous primary tumor, usually in the upper aerodigestive tract, often the result of the common risk factors of tobacco and alcohol use. PET has been shown to identify previously unknown metastases and synchronous primaries in patients with head and neck cancer.

PEARLS AND PITFALLS

- The uptake of ^{18}F-FDG-PET in the head and neck region can be complex, with normal and variant uptake in several structures. Knowledge of these potential variants is essential for proper image interpretation. The reader is referred to the references for further review.
- Traditional staging in head and neck cancers has relied on clinical examination and anatomic imaging, including CT and MRI. These modalities rely primarily on size criteria and as such are less sensitive and specific than PET in the loco-regional staging of lymph nodes.
- PET assessment of the head and neck is significantly improved with combined PET/CT, which improves anatomic localization and decreases the number of equivocal lesions.
- Because of the nearly whole-body nature of PET imaging, PET can identify previously unsuspected distant metastases and second primaries.

Suggested Reading

Burrell SC, Van den Abbeele AD. [18]FDG-PET of the head and neck: an atlas of normal uptake and variants. Mol Imaging Biol 2005;7(3):244–256

Menda Y, Graham MM. Update on ^{18}F-fluorodeoxyglucose/positron emission tomography and positron emission tomography/computed tomography imaging of squamous head and neck cancers. Semin Nucl Med 2005;35(4):214–219

Nakamoto Y, Tatsumi M, Hammoud D, Cohade C, Osman MM, Wahl RL. Normal FDG distribution patterns in the head and neck: PET/CT evaluation. Radiology 2005;234(3):879–885

Vermeersch H, Loose D, Ham H, Otte A, Van de Wiele C. Nuclear medicine imaging for the assessment of primary and recurrent head and neck carcinoma using routinely available tracers. Eur J Nucl Med Mol Imaging 2003;30(12):1689–1700

CASE 83

Clinical Presentation

A 63-year-old woman has been shown to have an unknown primary malignancy on the basis of tiny lung metastases seen on a CT scan. PET is requested to search for the primary malignancy.

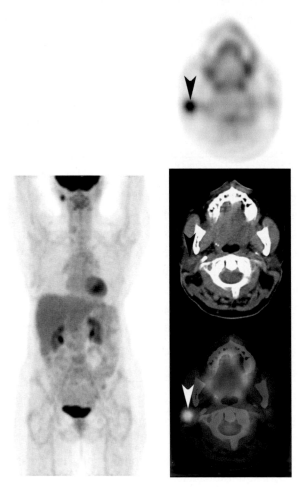

Fig. 83.1   **Fig. 83.2**

Technique

- The patient is instructed to avoid vigorous exercise for 24 hours prior to the scan, fast for at least 4 hours before the study, drink water during the fasting and uptake periods, and void prior to the scan
- A venous serum glucose sample is obtained prior to the injection of ^{18}F-FDG (reference range is < 120 mg/dl for non-diabetic patients and < 200 mg/dl for diabetic patients), and the patient's height and weight are recorded
- A 10–20 mCi dose of ^{18}F-FDG is injected intravenously (in a dimly lit quiet room for brain PET scans), and the patient is asked to rest comfortably in a room that is kept warm

- Most PET scans are now acquired on a hybrid PET/CT scanner, and a low dose spiral CT is acquired for attenuation correction of the PET images and for anatomic localization. Some centers may choose to perform oral and/or intravenous contrast-enhanced diagnostic CT as part of the PET/CT examination
- Sixty minutes following the ^{18}F-FDG injection, the spiral CT is performed using a weight-based algorithm from the skull base to the upper thighs (for most oncologic indications), or from the vertex to the feet, or centered over the brain depending on the tumor being evaluated
- A 2D or 3D PET acquisition (depending on the manufacturer) is then performed over the same region(s), and all PET images are corrected for attenuation, detector efficiency, scatter, decay, and random coincidences
- Consistency in ^{18}F-FDG injected dose, scan acquisition time relative to the injection time, and acquisition and reconstruction protocols is important when performing serial scanning on the same patient

Image Interpretation

An anterior maximum-intensity projection (MIP) image (**Fig. 83.1**) identifies a solitary focus of uptake in the neck on the right. The tiny lung metastases are not identified because they are below the resolution of the PET scan. Axial images (**Fig. 83.2**) reveal the uptake (*arrowheads*) to be within a nodule in the right parotid gland.

Differential Diagnosis

- Sialadenitis
- Primary salivary gland tumor

Diagnosis and Clinical Follow-Up

Primary salivary gland tumor. Diagnosis final, no clinical follow-up.

Discussion

Although there generally is not a role for PET in the initial diagnosis of head and neck cancers, an exception is in the setting of a cervical metastasis of an unknown primary. Here, PET can be helpful in identifying the site of the primary malignancy when an otherwise complete workup, including physical examination, endoscopy, and anatomic imaging (CT/MRI), fails to identify the primary. Failure to identify the primary may result from its small size, submucosal location, or location inaccessible to endoscopy or difficult to evaluate with cross-sectional imaging. Presumptive radiation therapy is often undertaken if the primary tumor cannot be identified, with extensive radiation fields involving the entire pharyngeal mucosa, larynx, and both sides of the neck . However, if the primary can be identified, surgery or directed radiation therapy may be used, resulting in reduced morbidity.

PET would appear to be an ideal imaging modality in this setting, given the high ^{18}F-FDG avidity of many tumors and the ability to image the entire body. One-third of cervical metastases are found to originate below the clavicles, with approximately half of these originating in the lungs.

Rusthoven et al. (2004) reviewed 16 studies involving 302 patients undergoing PET evaluation for cervical lymph node metastases after conventional workup failed to identify the primary malignancy. PET identified the primary lesion in 24.5% of patients, and 24% of the primary tumors were located below the clavicle. Among head and neck primaries, tumors of the tonsils and base of tongue were the most prevalent. The highest accuracy was in tumors of the hypopharynx and larynx. The most common site of false-negative results was the base of tongue, attributed to the high baseline ^{18}F-FDG uptake as a result of speech and swallowing. The tonsils were the most common site of false-positive findings, which the authors attributed to the influence of inflammation. This review also found that PET discovered unsuspected regional or distant metastases in 27% of patients. Such information can lead to a change in patient management, from intent to cure to palliation. Overall, PET led to changes in treatment in 24.7% of patients in the six studies that reported this end point.

PEARLS AND PITFALLS

- In the setting of a cervical metastasis of an unknown primary, PET identifies the primary in approximately one-fourth of cases following a failed traditional workup.
- Advantages of PET include the high ^{18}F-FDG avidity of most tumors that metastasize to the cervical region and the nearly whole-body field of view of PET; approximately one-third of primaries will be located below the clavicles.
- Identification of the primary leads to more directed therapy, resulting in reduced morbidity.
- In this setting, the most common site of a false-negative PET result is the tongue base, and the most common site of a false-positive result is the tonsils.

Suggested Reading

Rohren EM, Turkington TG, Coleman RE. Clinical applications of PET in oncology. Radiology 2004;231(2):305–332

Rusthoven KE, Koshy M, Paulino AC. The role of fluorodeoxyglucose positron emission tomography in cervical lymph node metastases from an unknown primary tumor. Cancer 2004;101(11):2641–2649

CASE 84

Clinical Presentation

A 53-year-old man has a diagnosis of squamous cell carcinoma of the base of tongue with neck nodal metastases. PET is requested for the purpose of planning radiation therapy.

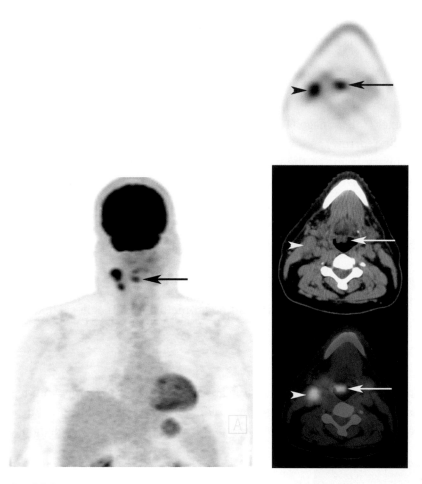

Fig. 84.1   **Fig. 84.2**

Technique

- The patient is instructed to avoid vigorous exercise for 24 hours prior to the scan, fast for at least 4 hours before the study, drink water during the fasting and uptake periods, and void prior to the scan
- A venous serum glucose sample is obtained prior to the injection of ^{18}F-FDG (reference range is < 120 mg/dl for non-diabetic patients and < 200 mg/dl for diabetic patients), and the patient's height and weight are recorded
- A 10–20 mCi dose of ^{18}F-FDG is injected intravenously (in a dimly lit quiet room for brain PET scans), and the patient is asked to rest comfortably in a room that is kept warm

- Most PET scans are now acquired on a hybrid PET/CT scanner, and a low dose spiral CT is acquired for attenuation correction of the PET images and for anatomic localization. Some centers may choose to perform oral and/or intravenous contrast-enhanced diagnostic CT as part of the PET/CT examination
- Sixty minutes following the ^{18}F-FDG injection, the spiral CT is performed using a weight-based algorithm from the skull base to the upper thighs (for most oncologic indications), or from the vertex to the feet, or centered over the brain depending on the tumor being evaluated
- A 2D or 3D PET acquisition (depending on the manufacturer) is then performed over the same region(s), and all PET images are corrected for attenuation, detector efficiency, scatter, decay, and random coincidences
- Consistency in ^{18}F-FDG injected dose, scan acquisition time relative to the injection time, and acquisition and reconstruction protocols is important when performing serial scanning on the same patient

Image Interpretation

An anterior maximum-intensity pixel (MIP) image (**Fig. 84.1**) demonstrates uptake within the primary tumor just to the right of midline (*arrow*) and within two right-sided lymph nodes. Axial images (**Fig. 84.2**) reveal uptake in the primary lesion at the base of the tongue (*arrows*) and in one of the lymph nodes (*arrowheads*). The other involved node is at a different axial level.

Differential Diagnosis

Squamous cell carcinoma of the base of tongue with ipsilateral nodal metastases

Diagnosis and Clinical Follow-Up

Squamous cell carcinoma of the base of tongue with ipsilateral nodal metastases. Diagnosis final, no clinical follow-up.

Discussion

The process of radiotherapy planning begins with careful identification of the cancerous target volumes as well as avoidance of structures that are sensitive to high-dose radiation. The selection and delineation of target volumes take into account the natural history and patterns of spread of the malignancy

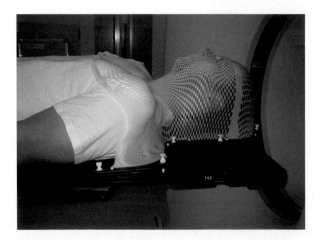

Fig. 84.3

specific to the site, subsite, stage, and histology. For each individual patient and tumor configuration, the target volumes are outlined in detail with anatomic imaging (CT and MRI) and more recently with complementary functional imaging information from ^{18}F-FDG-PET. Head and neck malignancies are treated with highly accurate, conformal radiotherapy techniques like intensity-modulated radiotherapy (IMRT), which require the patient to be placed in a plastic custom-fitted immobilization shell (**Fig. 84.3**). This allows the precise localization required for carefully aimed radiotherapy beams and for exact reproducibility during multiple fractions of radiation given daily over several weeks. The determination of which neck lymph node regions should receive high-dose radiation (areas of known gross disease) versus low-dose radiation (areas at risk for occult microscopic disease) is based on clinical and imaging information. In this regard, the more sensitive and specific functional information derived from PET can aid in determining the nature of an otherwise equivocal lymph node by CT or MRI criteria. In the current case, PET guided radiotherapy planning by confidently including the two ^{18}F-FDG–positive lymph nodes along with the primary right tongue base tumor in the high-dose radiation target volume, and placing the left neck lymph nodes in the lower-dose radiation target volume.

In a review, Menda and Graham (2005) identified five articles that reported gross tumor volume (GTV) changes as a result of incorporating PET data in the planning regimen. The use of PET data resulted in an increase in GTV in 18% and a decrease in GTV in 49% of patients, for an overall change in target volume in 67% of patients. Although less commonly available, other PET radiopharmaceuticals may be used to further refine radiation therapy planning. ^{18}F-FDG-MISO is an example of an agent that images tumor hypoxia. ^{18}F-MISO diffuses into cells and is retained intracellularly when the oxygen tension is low. Hypoxic tumor cells are more resistant to radiotherapy. Knowledge of the presence and location of areas of hypoxia allows radiation therapy planners to selectively increase the dose delivered to the hypoxic areas.

^{18}F-FDG-PET is also effective in evaluating the post-therapy neck for residual disease. Evaluation of the post-therapy neck with both clinical and anatomic imaging (CT, MRI) is limited by edema, inflammation, and tissue distortion. PET has generally been shown to be more sensitive and specific in this setting, with a very high negative predictive value that generally obviates the need for a repeated biopsy. However, increased benign ^{18}F-FDG uptake early in the post-radiation period due to inflammation can lead to false-positive studies. Most authors advocate waiting 2 to 3 months after therapy to perform follow-up PET.

PEARLS AND PITFALLS

- Molecular imaging data obtained with PET complement anatomic information from CT and MRI in radiation therapy planning. This is particularly important in the setting of new radiation therapy techniques such as IMRT, which allow the anatomically precise delivery of radiation.
- PET frequently establishes that otherwise equivocal lymph nodes are not involved, allowing the selection of smaller radiation target volumes with resultant lower morbidity rates. Less often, the converse occurs, and PET identifies areas of tumor involvement not otherwise appreciated, resulting in increased target volumes and appropriate treatment of all tumor.
- New PET tracers, such as the hypoxia-imaging agent ^{18}F-MISO, have the potential to further refine radiation planning by identifying tumor areas that will be more resistant to radiotherapy, allowing higher radiation doses to be directed to these areas.
- Following radiation therapy planning, PET is accurate in assessing for residual or recurrent disease, although if undertaken within 2 to 3 months after therapy, false-positive results may occur.

Suggested Reading

Greven KM, Williams DW III, McGuirt WF Sr, Harkness BA, D'Agostino RB Jr, Watson NE Jr. Serial positron emission tomography scans following radiation therapy of patients with head and neck cancer. Head Neck 2001;23(11):942–946

Menda Y, Graham MM. Update on ^{18}F-fluorodeoxyglucose/positron emission tomography and positron emission tomography/computed tomography imaging of squamous head and neck cancers. Semin Nucl Med 2005;35(4):214–219

Padhani AR, Krohn KA, Lewis JS, Alber M. Imaging oxygenation of human tumours. Eur Radiol 2007;17(4):861–872

Terhaard CH, Bongers V, van Rijk PP, Hordijk GJ. ^{18}F-fluoro-deoxy-glucose positron-emission tomography scanning in detection of local recurrence after radiotherapy for laryngeal/pharyngeal cancer. Head Neck 2001;23(11):933–941

Zimmer LA, Branstetter BF, Nayak JV, Johnson JT. Current use of ^{18}F-fluorodeoxyglucose positron emission tomography and combined positron emission tomography and computed tomography in squamous cell carcinoma of the head and neck. Laryngoscope 2005;115(11):2029–2034

CASE 85

Clinical Presentation

A 55-year-old woman undergoes resection of a glioblastoma multiforme from her right frontal lobe, followed by radiation therapy. Monitoring for tumor recurrence is performed with MRI and PET shortly (**Fig. 85.1**) and five months (**Fig. 85.2**) after treatment.

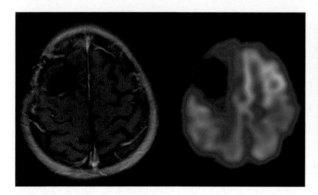

Fig. 85.1

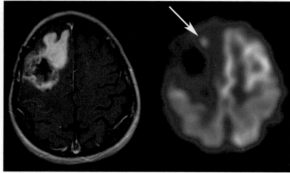

Fig. 85.2

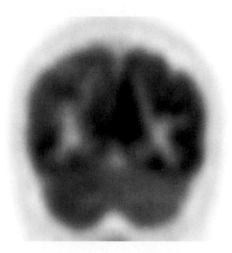

Fig. 85.3

Technique

- The patient is instructed to avoid vigorous exercise for 24 hours prior to the scan, fast for at least 4 hours before the study, drink water during the fasting and uptake periods, and void prior to the scan
- A venous serum glucose sample is obtained prior to the injection of ^{18}F-FDG (reference range is < 120 mg/dl for non-diabetic patients and < 200 mg/dl for diabetic patients), and the patient's height and weight are recorded

- A 10–20 mCi dose of ^{18}F-FDG is injected intravenously (in a dimly lit quiet room for brain PET scans), and the patient is asked to rest comfortably in a room that is kept warm
- Most PET scans are now acquired on a hybrid PET/CT scanner, and a low dose spiral CT is acquired for attenuation correction of the PET images and for anatomic localization. Some centers may choose to perform oral and/or intravenous contrast-enhanced diagnostic CT as part of the PET/CT examination
- Sixty minutes following the ^{18}F-FDG injection, the spiral CT is performed using a weight-based algorithm from the skull base to the upper thighs (for most oncologic indications), or from the vertex to the feet, or centered over the brain depending on the tumor being evaluated
- A 2D or 3D PET acquisition (depending on the manufacturer) is then performed over the same region(s), and all PET images are corrected for attenuation, detector efficiency, scatter, decay, and random coincidences
- Consistency in ^{18}F-FDG injected dose, scan acquisition time relative to the injection time, and acquisition and reconstruction protocols is important when performing serial scanning on the same patient
- Gadolinium-enhanced MRI is also performed. T1-weighted post-contrast images are coregistered and fused with the PET data set.

Image Interpretation

Axial MRI and corresponding PET image shortly after surgery and radiation therapy (**Fig. 85.1**) demonstrate absent ^{18}F-FDG uptake in the site of surgical resection and decreased uptake in adjacent brain parenchyma secondary to radiation and edema. On follow-up MRI 5 months later (**Fig. 85.2**), there is marked contrast enhancement around the resection site, which is a typical and nonspecific finding. However, on the corresponding PET scan, there is a new focus of increased ^{18}F-FDG uptake (*arrow*) anterior to the resection site.

An interesting finding is revealed on a coronal PET slice (**Fig. 85.3**). There is decreased ^{18}F-FDG uptake throughout a portion of the right cerebral hemisphere as a result of the therapy. However, there is also decreased uptake within the contralateral cerebellar hemisphere.

Differential Diagnosis

- Recurrent tumor
- Seizure
- Infection

Diagnosis and Clinical Follow-Up

Recurrent tumor. Diagnosis final, no clinical follow-up.

Discussion

The brain normally demonstrates high physiologic uptake of ^{18}F-FDG, much greater in gray matter than in white matter. Nonetheless, ^{18}F-FDG-PET has proved effective in assessing brain tumors in several scenarios.

In general, PET is not indicated in the initial diagnosis of a brain tumor because the physiologic uptake within brain and the limited spatial resolution result in a lower sensitivity for detection in comparison with CT or MRI. However, once a brain lesion is discovered, there are some niche applications for PET in the initial evaluation. First, a PET scan may be requested to aid in determining the grade of a tumor discovered in an area difficult to biopsy, as the degree of uptake of ^{18}F-FDG has been shown to correlate well with tumor grade. Second, PET may be used to help guide biopsy by demonstrating which parts of a tumor have the highest metabolic rate. These typically represent the most aggressive areas and are the areas that should be biopsied to best direct patient management. Finally, PET may be used in the setting of discovery of an enhancing brain lesion in a patient infected with human immunodeficiency virus (HIV). The main differential in this scenario is between primary central nervous system lymphoma and infection, typically toxoplasmosis. ^{18}F-FDG-PET has proved effective in distinguishing between the two entities; lymphoma demonstrates increased uptake, which is not the case with toxoplasmosis.

The main application of PET in brain tumors is in the assessment of residual or recurrent malignancy following therapy. Therapy typically consists of surgical removal of the tumor, often followed by radiation therapy. These interventions result in decreased ^{18}F-FDG uptake in the brain in the region of the previous tumor and thus a high sensitivity of 80 to 90% for the detection of recurrent disease. MRI and CT are of limited value in this scenario because there is inevitably contrast enhancement throughout the area, as in the current case, which may be due to benign radiation damage and reactive gliosis, or potentially to recurrent tumor. These benign post-therapy changes do not routinely elicit increased ^{18}F-FDG uptake, although rarely there may be false-positive results following intense focal radiation therapy, such as with gamma-knife therapy. Conversely, tumor recurrence demonstrates increased uptake, typically equal to or greater than that in gray matter. Because the degree of ^{18}F-FDG uptake correlates with tumor grade, false-negative studies may occur in the setting of low-grade tumors.

Given the high physiologic ^{18}F-FDG uptake in the brain, other PET agents have been applied to the assessment of brain tumors. An amino acid labeled with ^{11}C, ^{11}C-MET, has been the most commonly used. Most brain tumors, including low-grade tumors, overexpress L-amino acid transporters, resulting in increased ^{11}C-MET uptake. Also, there is better tumor delineation than with ^{18}F-FDG because of the significantly lower background brain activity. However, it appears that ^{11}C-MET is less reliable than ^{18}F-FDG in predicting tumor grade. The proliferation agent ^{18}F-tyrosine, although less widely studied at this point, is also showing promising results. Clearly, both agents are less widely available than ^{18}F-FDG.

The decreased uptake in the contralateral cerebellar hemisphere in this case is known as crossed cerebellar diaschisis. It is due to decreased function of the neurons in the opposite cerebral hemisphere. It is not specific to tumor therapy and may result as well from conditions such as stroke or injury. It is also seen in brain imaging with SPECT.

PEARLS AND PITFALLS

- PET is not indicated for the routine detection of brain tumors because the high physiologic uptake of ^{18}F-FDG in the brain and the lower resolution render it less sensitive than anatomic imaging with CT or MRI. Furthermore, most institutions will not include the brain on PET scans obtained for the assessment of extracranial malignancies; if brain metastases are suspected, imaging of the brain should be performed with CT or MRI.
- When a brain tumor is discovered, ^{18}F-FDG-PET is occasionally indicated to help establish the grade of the tumor when biopsy is deemed difficult. As the degree of ^{18}F-FDG uptake is related to grade, ^{18}F-FDG-PET may also be used to follow a low-grade tumor for degeneration to a higher grade.
- ^{18}F-FDG-PET may also be used at the time of diagnosis to direct biopsy to the most aggressive portion of the tumor.
- The major application of PET in brain tumors is in the evaluation of recurrent malignancy. In this scenario, PET is sensitive and specific, whereas assessment by MRI is limited by nonspecific enhancement arising from post-therapy inflammation.

- Potential causes of false-positive studies include abscess, seizure, and recent intensive focal radiation therapy (gamma knife). The ideal time to wait following radiation therapy has not been firmly established, but it appears that a minimum of 3 to 4 months will limit false-positive results.
- False-negative studies can occur because of low-grade tumors and small tumor size.

Suggested Reading

Hustinx R, Pourdehnad M, Kaschten B, Alavi A. PET imaging for differentiating recurrent brain tumor from radiation necrosis. Radiol Clin North Am 2005;43(1):35–47

Langleben DD, Segall GM. PET in differentiation of recurrent brain tumor from radiation injury. J Nucl Med 2000;41(11):1861–1867

Minn H. PET and SPECT in low-grade glioma. Eur J Radiol 2005;56(2):171–178

Schaller BJ, Modo M, Buchfelder M. Molecular imaging of brain tumors: a bridge between clinical and molecular medicine? Mol Imaging Biol 2007;9(2):60–71

CASE 86

Clinical Presentation

A 49-year-old woman develops post-transplant lymphoproliferative disease following a liver transplant for Wilson disease. PET is requested for further evaluation.

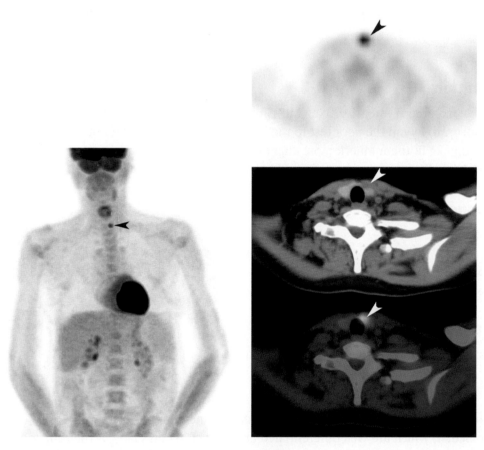

Fig. 86.1   Fig. 86.2

Technique

- The patient is instructed to avoid vigorous exercise for 24 hours prior to the scan, fast for at least 4 hours before the study, drink water during the fasting and uptake periods, and void prior to the scan
- A venous serum glucose sample is obtained prior to the injection of ¹⁸F-FDG (reference range is < 120 mg/dl for non-diabetic patients and < 200 mg/dl for diabetic patients), and the patient's height and weight are recorded
- A 10–20 mCi dose of ¹⁸F-FDG is injected intravenously (in a dimly lit quiet room for brain PET scans), and the patient is asked to rest comfortably in a room that is kept warm
- Most PET scans are now acquired on a hybrid PET/CT scanner, and a low dose spiral CT is acquired for attenuation correction of the PET images and for anatomic localization. Some centers may

269

choose to perform oral and/or intravenous contrast-enhanced diagnostic CT as part of the PET/CT examination

- Sixty minutes following the ^{18}F-FDG injection, the spiral CT is performed using a weight-based algorithm from the skull base to the upper thighs (for most oncologic indications), or from the vertex to the feet, or centered over the brain depending on the tumor being evaluated

- A 2D or 3D PET acquisition (depending on the manufacturer) is then performed over the same region(s), and all PET images are corrected for attenuation, detector efficiency, scatter, decay, and random coincidences

- Consistency in ^{18}F-FDG injected dose, scan acquisition time relative to the injection time, and acquisition and reconstruction protocols is important when performing serial scanning on the same patient

Image Interpretation

The three-dimensional maximum-intensity pixel (MIP) image (**Fig. 86.1**) demonstrates a small focus of ^{18}F-FDG uptake (*arrowhead*) low in the neck just to the left of midline. There are no other abnormalities; a larger area of uptake in the midneck more superiorly is physiologic uptake within the larynx. Axial images (**Fig. 86.2**) confirm that the uptake is within a thyroid nodule (*arrowheads*).

Differential Diagnosis

- Thyroid adenoma
- Thyroid cancer
- Thyroid lymphoma
- Focal thyroiditis

Diagnosis and Clinical Follow-Up

Papillary thyroid cancer. Diagnosis final, no clinical follow-up.

Discussion

Primary thyroid cancers include papillary, follicular, medullary, and anaplastic forms. The majority are papillary and follicular, which are well differentiated and as such retain many of the functions of normal thyroid tissue, including the ability to concentrate iodine via the sodium iodide symporter. Furthermore, well-differentiated thyroid cancers demonstrate low rates of glycolysis and thus usually do not show increased uptake of ^{18}F-FDG. For this reason, the majority of thyroid cancers are better assessed with the traditional ^{131}I or ^{123}I scan. However, less well differentiated thyroid cancers behave less like native thyroid tissue and lose the ability to concentrate iodine. Conversely, they tend to be more aggressive and have higher glycolytic rates, so they tend to take up ^{18}F-FDG. Thus, thyroid cancers usually will take up either radioiodine or ^{18}F-FDG but not the other, the so-called flip-flop phenomenon. Thyroid cancers may be less well differentiated at diagnosis or become so following radioiodine therapy.

The main use of PET in thyroid cancer is to assess for disease recurrence when the radioiodine scan is negative and recurrence is suspected, typically because of a rising serum level of thyroglobulin. The sensitivity of ^{18}F-FDG-PET is as high as 85% in the setting of a negative radioiodine scan. The avidity of a thyroid cancer for ^{18}F-FDG is predictive of resistance to radioiodine therapy, and an inverse correlation has been shown between the burden of ^{18}F-FDG–avid disease and survival.

Focal uptake in the thyroid may be an incidental finding in patients undergoing ^{18}F-FDG-PET for an unrelated indication, as in the index case. It is important to note that ^{18}F-FDG uptake in a thyroid nodule is not necessarily indicative of malignancy, as adenomas and focal thyroiditis may also demonstrate increased uptake. However, malignancy must be excluded, and further workup is indicated.

Because the majority of thyroid cancers are iodine-avid, it is of interest to note that PET can be performed with [124]I, a positron-emitting isotope of iodine. However, this isotope is not widely available, and it decays primarily by gamma emission (only 24% of its emitted particles are positrons), which degrades the images. It has been used primarily in selected centers to perform dosimetry calculations.

PEARLS AND PITFALLS_____

- The majority of thyroid cancers are well differentiated and should be imaged with radioiodine rather than PET.
- Less well differentiated thyroid cancers are less likely to concentrate iodine and more likely to concentrate ^{18}F-FDG.
- When thyroid cancer recurrence is suspected (eg, in the setting of a rising serum thyroglobulin level) and radioiodine imaging is negative, ^{18}F-FDG-PET should be considered to assess for recurrent disease.
- Preparation for ^{18}F-FDG-PET in a patient being followed for thyroid cancer does not necessarily require elevating the patient's thyroid-stimulating hormone (TSH) level, as is done before radioiodine imaging. However, evidence suggests that there is benefit in doing so, particularly through the use of recombinant TSH rather than thyroid hormone withdrawal.
- Focal uptake in the thyroid may be an incidental finding in patients undergoing PET for an unrelated indication. This does not necessarily represent malignancy, as benign thyroid nodules may demonstrate increased ^{18}F-FDG uptake, but further evaluation is certainly required to exclude malignancy.

Suggested Reading

Cohen MS, Arslan N, Dehdashti F, Doherty GM, Lairmore TC, Brunt LM, Moley JF. Risk of malignancy in thyroid incidentalomas identified by fluorodeoxyglucose-positron emission tomography. Surgery 2001;130(6):941–946

Feine U, Lietzenmayer R, Hanke JP, Held J, Wöhrle H, Müller-Schauenburg W. ^{18}F-FDG and ^{131}I-iodide uptake in thyroid cancer. J Nucl Med 1996;37(9):1468–1472

Kolbert KS, Pentlow KS, Pearson JR, Sheikh A, Finn RD, Humm JL, Larson SM. Prediction of absorbed dose to normal organs in thyroid cancer patients treated with 131I by use of 124I PET and 3-dimensional internal dosimetry software. J Nucl Med 2007;48(1):143–149

Schöder H, Yeung HWD. Positron emission imaging of head and neck cancer, including thyroid carcinoma. Semin Nucl Med 2004;34(3):180–197

Wang W, Larson SM, Fazzari M, Tickoo SK, Kolbert K, Sgouros G, Yeung H, Macapiniac H, Rosai J, Robbins RJ. Prognostic value of [^{18}F]fluorodeoxyglucose positron emission tomographic scanning in patients with thyroid cancer. J Clin Endocrinol Metab 2000;85(3):1107–1113

Zhuang H, Kumar R, Mandel S, Alavi A. Investigation of thyroid, head, and neck cancers with PET. Radiol Clin North Am 2004;42(6):1101–1111, viii

CASE 87

Clinical Presentation

A 34-year-old man who had a malignant melanoma excised from the left forearm has clinically bulky left axillary lymphadenopathy. A staging PET examination is performed.

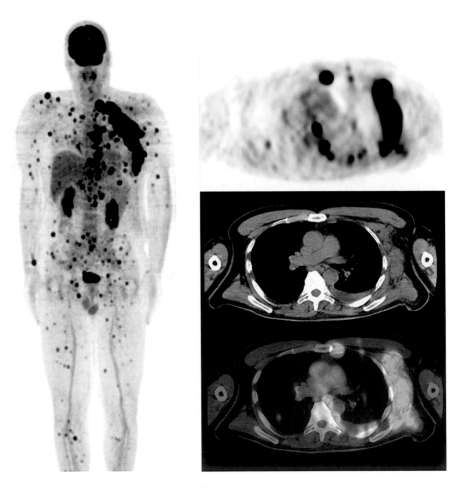

Fig. 87.1   **Fig. 87.2**

Technique

- The patient is instructed to avoid vigorous exercise for 24 hours prior to the scan, fast for at least 4 hours before the study, drink water during the fasting and uptake periods, and void prior to the scan
- A venous serum glucose sample is obtained prior to the injection of ^{18}F-FDG (reference range is < 120 mg/dl for non-diabetic patients and < 200 mg/dl for diabetic patients), and the patient's height and weight are recorded
- A 10-20 mCi dose of ^{18}F-FDG is injected intravenously (in a dimly lit quiet room for brain PET scans), and the patient is asked to rest comfortably in a room that is kept warm

- Most PET scans are now acquired on a hybrid PET/CT scanner, and a low dose spiral CT is acquired for attenuation correction of the PET images and for anatomic localization. Some centers may choose to perform oral and/or intravenous contrast-enhanced diagnostic CT as part of the PET/CT examination
- Sixty minutes following the ^{18}F-FDG injection, the spiral CT is performed using a weight-based algorithm from the skull base to the upper thighs (for most oncologic indications), or from the vertex to the feet, or centered over the brain depending on the tumor being evaluated
- A 2D or 3D PET acquisition (depending on the manufacturer) is then performed over the same region(s), and all PET images are corrected for attenuation, detector efficiency, scatter, decay, and random coincidences
- Consistency in ^{18}F-FDG injected dose, scan acquisition time relative to the injection time, and acquisition and reconstruction protocols is important when performing serial scanning on the same patient

Image Interpretation

Anterior maximum-intensity pixel (MIP) image (**Fig. 87.1**) and axial images (**Fig. 87.2**) at the level of the upper thorax show extensive, disseminated ^{18}F-FDG–avid disease, particularly in the left axilla, where there is intensely ^{18}F-FDG–avid bulky lymphadenopathy. There are numerous pulmonary, pleural, nodal, cutaneous, and muscular metastases, in addition to ^{18}F-FDG–avid hepatic and splenic metastases.

Differential Diagnosis

Metastatic malignant melanoma

Diagnosis and Clinical Follow-Up

This patient had disseminated malignant melanoma. Consequently, regional lymph node dissection was canceled, and the patient was enrolled in a regimen involving systemic chemotherapy.

Discussion

Melanoma is one of the most metabolically active tumors. Although melanoma is curable when diagnosed early, disseminated melanoma is generally poorly responsive to treatment. However, up to 20% of patients with isolated nodal metastases may respond to surgical resection and lymph node dissection. Therefore, it is important to differentiate patients with only local metastases from those with multiple distal metastases.

PET has limited sensitivity for the detection of regional lymph node metastases in clinically normal lymph nodes and cannot replace sentinel lymph node imaging and biopsy. However, if there are clinically enlarged lymph nodes, PET may be used to assess disease activity and extent with much greater sensitivity.

The sensitivity of PET for metastatic disease is greater than 80%. However, lesions smaller than 1 cm may be missed. Because of the possibility of disseminated skin metastases, PET/CT scans in patients with melanoma normally evaluate the entire body, whereas a more limited field of view from the skull base to the upper thighs is obtained in most other oncology PET/CT scans.

PEARLS AND PITFALLS

- In melanoma, ^{18}F-FDG-PET imaging should include the whole body.
- In patients with bulky regional lymphadenopathy, ^{18}F-FDG-PET may have a role to assess for metastatic involvement instead of sentinel node imaging and biopsy.
- In melanoma, ^{18}F-FDG-PET imaging may also be used before the surgical resection of an apparently isolated metastasis to exclude additional subclinical metastatic disease.

Suggested Reading

Acland KM, Healy C, Calonje E, O'Doherty M, Nunan T, Page C, Higgins E, Russell-Jones R. Comparison of positron emission tomography scanning and sentinel node biopsy in the detection of micrometastases of primary cutaneous malignant melanoma. J Clin Oncol 2001;19(10):2674–2678

Prichard RS, Hill AD, Skehan SJ, O'Higgins NJ. Positron emission tomography for staging and management of malignant melanoma. Br J Surg 2002;89(4):389–396

Swetter SM, Carroll LA, Johnson DL, Segall GM. Positron emission tomography is superior to computed tomography for metastatic detection in melanoma patients. Ann Surg Oncol 2002;9(7):646–653

CASE 88

Clinical Presentation

A 56-year-old woman has a prior history of ovarian cancer. She has been asymptomatic, but levels of the tumor marker cancer antigen (CA)-125 are rising. PET is requested to assess for tumor recurrence.

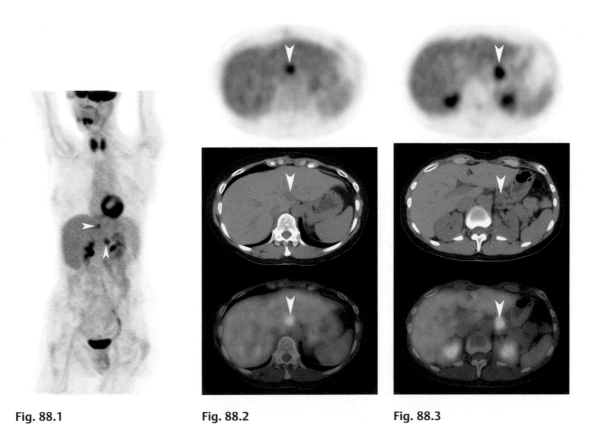

Fig. 88.1   Fig. 88.2   Fig. 88.3

Technique

- The patient is instructed to avoid vigorous exercise for 24 hours prior to the scan, fast for at least 4 hours before the study, drink water during the fasting and uptake periods, and void prior to the scan
- A venous serum glucose sample is obtained prior to the injection of ^{18}F-FDG (reference range is < 120 mg/dl for non-diabetic patients and < 200 mg/dl for diabetic patients), and the patient's height and weight are recorded
- A 10–20 mCi dose of ^{18}F-FDG is injected intravenously (in a dimly lit quiet room for brain PET scans), and the patient is asked to rest comfortably in a room that is kept warm
- Most PET scans are now acquired on a hybrid PET/CT scanner, and a low dose spiral CT is acquired for attenuation correction of the PET images and for anatomic localization. Some centers may

275

choose to perform oral and/or intravenous contrast-enhanced diagnostic CT as part of the PET/CT examination

- Sixty minutes following the ^{18}F-FDG injection, the spiral CT is performed using a weight-based algorithm from the skull base to the upper thighs (for most oncologic indications), or from the vertex to the feet, or centered over the brain depending on the tumor being evaluated
- A 2D or 3D PET acquisition (depending on the manufacturer) is then performed over the same region(s), and all PET images are corrected for attenuation, detector efficiency, scatter, decay, and random coincidences
- Consistency in ^{18}F-FDG injected dose, scan acquisition time relative to the injection time, and acquisition and reconstruction protocols is important when performing serial scanning on the same patient

Image Interpretation

A left anterior oblique view from the maximum-intensity pixel (MIP) data set (**Fig. 88.1**) reveals two foci of abnormal uptake (*arrowheads*) in the upper abdomen. Axial images demonstrate one to be in the liver (**Fig. 88.2**, *arrowheads*) and the other in the gastrohepatic ligament (**Fig. 88.3**, *arrowheads*). There is also intense uptake throughout the thyroid.

Differential Diagnosis

- Thyroid cancer with metastases
- Recurrence of ovarian cancer
- Hepatocellular carcinoma with metastasis

Diagnosis and Clinical Follow-Up

Recurrence of ovarian cancer in the liver and the gastrohepatic ligament. The cause of the thyroid uptake was not determined in this patient. Most commonly, such diffuse uptake would be on the basis of Graves disease or thyroiditis. Diagnosis final, no clinical follow-up.

Discussion

Ovarian cancer has the highest mortality rate of the gynecologic malignancies. Symptoms are rare early in the course of the disease and there is no effective screening test, so most patients present with stage III or IV disease. Metastasis is often through direct spread within the peritoneal cavity, with tumor cells traveling up the paracolic gutters and depositing on the surfaces of organs, including the peritoneal surface, right hemidiaphragm, liver, bowel, and omentum. Initial therapy consists of surgery to remove the bulk of the tumor (cytoreductive surgery), followed by chemotherapy and possibly external beam radiotherapy.

As with most malignancies, PET is not routinely indicated in the initial diagnosis of ovarian cancer. It is not sufficiently sensitive (small tumors and low-grade malignancies may be negative on PET) or sufficiently specific (several benign lesions may be positive on PET). However, increased uptake may be discovered in the ovary as an incidental finding in patients undergoing PET for another indication. Although this is not necessarily indicative of malignancy, further workup is indicated, especially for postmenopausal women, in whom increased uptake in an ovary is very likely to represent malignancy.

PET may be effective in the staging of ovarian cancer. Staging is conventionally based on laparotomy and CT. In a comparison of PET plus CT with CT alone, the scheme using PET correlated with postoperative staging 87% of the time, versus 53% for CT alone. The main effects of PET were to detect disease outside the pelvis and to clarify the status of patients with stage III or IV disease by distinguishing

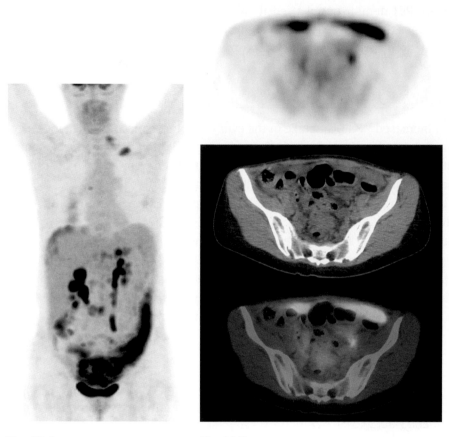

Fig. 88.4   **Fig. 88.5**

whether metastases were within liver parenchyma or implants on the surface and by demonstrating that subcentimeter lymph nodes were positive in some cases. **Figures 88.4** and **88.5** are from a different patient undergoing staging for ovarian cancer. The MIP image (**Fig. 88.4**) reveals widespread metastases, including extensive peritoneal implantation, best appreciated in the left lower quadrant and over the dome of the liver. There has also been metastatic spread to a left supraclavicular node (Virchow node), a left subpectoral node, and the right side of the thorax. Axial images through the pelvis (**Fig. 88.5**) confirm uptake in the thickened peritoneum, consistent with peritoneal carcinomatosis.

Following initial therapy, patients typically undergo a second-look laparotomy to assess for residual disease, which may mandate further therapy. Conventional imaging with CT has been shown to be insufficiently sensitive to obviate surgery in this scenario. However, initial studies with PET have shown it to be similar to second-look laparotomy in detecting residual disease, so it may be possible to replace second-look laparotomy with this less invasive technique, although this needs to be confirmed with larger studies.

The main application of PET in ovarian cancer has been in detecting recurrent disease. Ovarian cancer has a propensity to recur; up to 75% of patients will present with recurrent disease, so that close follow-up is indicated. The tumor marker CA-125 is monitored to assess for recurrence. It is, of course, unable to determine the location of recurrence, and a rise in CA-125 above nadir level leads to a search for the site of recurrence, which will govern further therapy. PET has consistently outperformed CT and MRI, the conventional imaging modalities, in detecting recurrence. Pooled data have shown sensitivities and specificities of 90% and 86%, respectively, for PET versus 68% and 58%, respectively, for conventional imaging. In a study of patients with rising carcinoembryonic antigen but negative or equivocal CT scans, PET demonstrated a sensitivity of 83% and a positive predictive value of 94% for recurrent disease larger than 1 cm. In another study, PET led to an intermodality change in therapy in 44% of patients compared with conventional workup.

PEARLS AND PITFALLS _____

- The incidental finding of increased ^{18}F-FDG uptake in the ovary is not specific for malignancy; several benign entities may demonstrate increased uptake, including inflammatory processes, benign tumors, and corpus luteal cysts. However, further workup is warranted, especially in postmenopausal women, in whom ovarian uptake on PET is strongly associated with malignancy.
- PET is more accurate than CT in staging ovarian cancer. In particular, PET finds significantly more disease outside the pelvis.
- Although studies are limited, PET may be able to replace the second-look laparotomy as a means of assessing residual malignancy following initial therapy.
- The best-established application of PET in ovarian cancer is in the assessment of recurrent disease, particularly in the setting of a rising CA-125 tumor marker. PET has consistently outperformed anatomic imaging and has led to changes in therapy in a significant number of patients.

Suggested Reading

Bristow RE, del Carmen MG, Pannu HK, Cohade C, Zahurak ML, Fishman EK, Wahl RL, Montz FJ. Clinically occult recurrent ovarian cancer: patient selection for secondary cytoreductive surgery using combined PET/CT. Gynecol Oncol 2003;90(3):519–528

Chung HH, Kang WJ, Kim JW, Park NH, Song YS, Chung JK, Kang SB, Lee HP. Role of [^{18}F]FDG PET/CT in the assessment of suspected recurrent ovarian cancer: correlation with clinical or histological findings. Eur J Nucl Med Mol Imaging 2007;34(4):480–486

Fenchel S, Grab D, Nuessle K, Kotzerke J, Rieber A, Kreienberg R, Brambs HJ, Reske SM. Asymptomatic adnexal masses: correlation of FDG PET and histopathologic findings. Radiology 2002;223(3):780–788

Havrilesky LJ, Kulasingam SL, Matchar DB, Myers ER. FDG-PET for management of cervical and ovarian cancer. Gynecol Oncol 2005;97(1):183–191

Kim S, Chung JK, Kang SB, Kim MH, Jeong JM, Lee DS, Lee MC. [^{18}F]FDG PET as a substitute for second-look laparotomy in patients with advanced ovarian carcinoma. Eur J Nucl Med Mol Imaging 2004;31(2):196–201

Mangili G, Picchio M, Sironi S, Viganò R, Rabaiotti E, Bornaghi D, Bettinardi V, Crivellaro C, Messa C, Fazio F. Integrated PET/CT as a first-line re-staging modality in patients with suspected recurrence of ovarian cancer. Eur J Nucl Med Mol Imaging 2007;34(5):658–666

Yoshida Y, Kurokawa T, Kawahara K, Tsuchida T, Okazawa H, Fujibayashi Y, Yonekura Y, Kotsuji F. Incremental benefits of FDG positron emission tomography over CT alone for the preoperative staging of ovarian cancer. AJR Am J Roentgenol 2004;182(1):227–233

CASE 89

Clinical Presentation

A female patient with a Ewing sarcoma of the right ulna received standard multiple-agent chemo-therapy and local radiotherapy at age 11. As a young adult, she underwent amputation and chemo-therapy (**Fig. 89.1**) for a secondary cancer of the arm. Seven years later, she undergoes ¹⁸F-FDG-PET (**Fig. 89.2**) imaging following a routine bone scan to assess for recurrence.

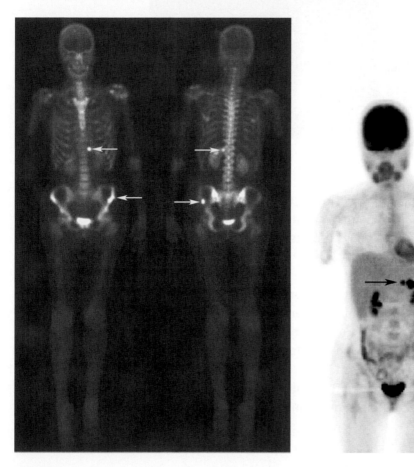

Fig. 89.1   Fig. 89.2

Technique

* The patient is instructed to avoid vigorous exercise for 24 hours prior to the scan, fast for at least 4 hours before the study, drink water during the fasting and uptake periods, and void prior to the scan
* A venous serum glucose sample is obtained prior to the injection of ¹⁸F-FDG (reference range is < 120 mg/dl for non-diabetic patients and < 200 mg/dl for diabetic patients), and the patient's height and weight are recorded
* A 10–20 mCi dose of ¹⁸F-FDG is injected intravenously (in a dimly lit quiet room for brain PET scans), and the patient is asked to rest comfortably in a room that is kept warm

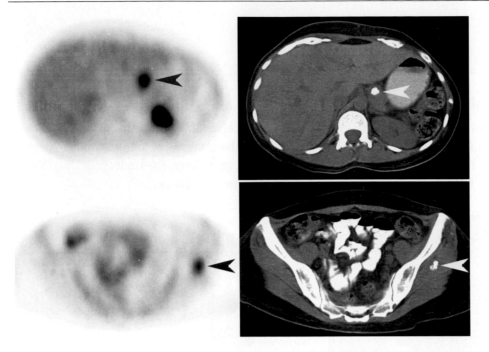

Fig. 89.3

- Most PET scans are now acquired on a hybrid PET/CT scanner, and a low dose spiral CT is acquired for attenuation correction of the PET images and for anatomic localization. Some centers may choose to perform oral and/or intravenous contrast-enhanced diagnostic CT as part of the PET/CT examination
- Sixty minutes following the ^{18}F-FDG injection, the spiral CT is performed using a weight-based algorithm from the skull base to the upper thighs (for most oncologic indications), or from the vertex to the feet, or centered over the brain depending on the tumor being evaluated
- A 2D or 3D PET acquisition (depending on the manufacturer) is then performed over the same region(s), and all PET images are corrected for attenuation, detector efficiency, scatter, decay, and random coincidences
- Consistency in ^{18}F-FDG injected dose, scan acquisition time relative to the injection time, and acquisition and reconstruction protocols is important when performing serial scanning on the same patient

Image Interpretation

The ^{99m}Tc-MDP bone scan (**Fig. 89.1**) reveals two foci of soft tissue uptake (*arrows*), one just to the left of the lower thoracic spine and one in the left buttock. There are no osseous metastases. An anterior maximum-intensity pixel (MIP) image from the ^{18}F-FDG-PET scan (**Fig. 89.2**) demonstrates focal uptake in the same two spots (*arrows*), with no additional sites of abnormal uptake. Axial slices from the PET scan and corresponding CT slices at two levels (**Fig. 89.3**) reveal the abnormal uptake to be within calcified lesions in the pancreas and left buttock muscles (*arrowheads*).

Differential Diagnosis

- Metastases from osteosarcoma
- Metastases from Ewing sarcoma
- Inflammatory lesions

Diagnosis and Clinical Follow-Up

Metastases from osteosarcoma. Diagnosis final, no clinical follow-up.

Discussion

Sarcomas make up a heterogeneous group of tumors arising from mesenchymal tissue. They represent approximately 1% of all malignant tumors. Metastatic spread is usually hematogenous, mainly to lung but also to bone. Definitive therapy is tumor- and stage-dependent. It typically involves timed surgical resection and systemic chemotherapy with or without local radiotherapy. Sarcomas may arise from bone or soft tissue. Osteosarcomas may be primary or secondary to a variety of processes, including radiation therapy (as in this case), Paget disease, and certain benign tumors. Osteosarcoma soft tissue metastases typically show uptake on bone scans. PET has shown significant early promise in the management of patients with sarcoma in several settings.

In a meta-analysis of 1,163 patients, ^{18}F-FDG-PET was found to have a sensitivity of 91% and specificity of 85% in the detection of sarcomas. The mean ^{18}F-FDG uptake, as reflected in the standardized uptake value (SUV), was statistically higher in the sarcomas than in benign tumors. However, there is some overlap, as low-grade tumors may exhibit low levels of ^{18}F-FDG uptake, and it is not recommended that PET replace biopsy. Still, there may be a role for PET at the time of diagnosis; many sarcomas are heterogeneous, and ^{18}F-FDG can be used to help direct the biopsy. For example, ^{18}F-FDG uptake is often greatest at the periphery, corresponding to areas with the most aggressive histology, and it is these areas that should be sampled to ensure the most clinically valid tumor assessment.

The staging workup of sarcomas typically includes a radiograph and MRI of the primary site to evaluate local tumor extent, CT of the chest to assess for pulmonary metastases, and a bone scan to evaluate for osseous metastases. ^{18}F-FDG-PET has not been shown to be superior to the conventional workup, so there is no present indication for its routine use in sarcoma staging. It may be indicated in selected cases—for example, to assess equivocal lung lesions, provided they are of the order of 1 cm or greater.

The response of sarcomas to neoadjuvant chemotherapy is an important prognostic indicator. A means of assessing response in vivo may help direct management—for example, by minimizing ineffective chemotherapy and its associated morbidity or by switching to other, active agents. It is believed that biochemical changes may occur earlier than morphologic changes. ^{18}F-FDG-PET has been shown to be a good means of assessing response; changes in ^{18}F-FDG uptake have correlated with histologic response, probability of disease recurrence, and outcomes. The optimal timing for PET in this scenario has not been established.

PET has also proved efficacious in monitoring for disease recurrence. Patients with sarcomas may be at high risk for recurrence, both locally at the primary site and distally. PET has been shown to be better at detecting distal sites of disease than conventional imaging is, in part because of the larger field of view used in PET. An exception is in the lungs, where CT is more sensitive in detecting small lesions. Both MRI and PET are effective in assessing the primary site for recurrence, although MRI assessment may be hindered by hardware-induced artifact, and PET may be better in this setting. A suggested monitoring algorithm includes CT of the chest, MRI of the primary site, and whole-body ^{18}F-FDG-PET.

PEARLS AND PITFALLS_____

- ^{18}F-FDG-PET can be useful in guiding the biopsy of a suspected sarcoma to ensure that the area of greatest metabolic activity is sampled.

- ^{18}F-FDG-PET is helpful in assessing the response to neoadjuvant chemotherapy.
- ^{18}F-FDG-PET is useful in distinguishing postoperative change from residual tumor at the primary site.
- ^{18}F-FDG-PET is complementary to CT and MRI in monitoring for recurrent disease.

Suggested Reading

Bastiaannet E, Groen H, Jager PL, Cobben DC, van der Graaf WT, Vaalburg W, Hoekstra HJ. The value of FDG-PET in the detection, grading and response to therapy of soft tissue and bone sarcomas; a systematic review and meta-analysis. Cancer Treat Rev 2004;30(1):83–101

Brenner W, Bohuslavizki KH, Eary JF. PET imaging of osteosarcoma. J Nucl Med 2003;44(6):930–942

Johnson GR, Zhuang H, Khan J, Chiang SB, Alavi A. Roles of positron emission tomography with ^{18}F-deoxyglucose in the detection of local recurrent and distant metastatic sarcoma. Clin Nucl Med 2003;28(10):815–820

Schuetze SM. Utility of positron emission tomography in sarcomas. Curr Opin Oncol 2006;18(4):369–373

CASE 90

Clinical Presentation

A 49-year-old man in whom a malignancy has recently been diagnosed undergoes PET requested for purposes of staging.

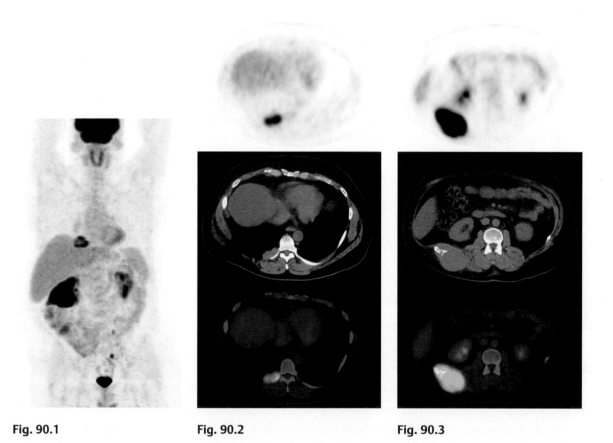

Fig. 90.1   Fig. 90.2   Fig. 90.3

Technique

- The patient is instructed to avoid vigorous exercise for 24 hours prior to the scan, fast for at least 4 hours before the study, drink water during the fasting and uptake periods, and void prior to the scan
- A venous serum glucose sample is obtained prior to the injection of ^{18}F-FDG (reference range is < 120 mg/dl for non-diabetic patients and < 200 mg/dl for diabetic patients), and the patient's height and weight are recorded
- A 10-20 mCi dose of ^{18}F-FDG is injected intravenously (in a dimly lit quiet room for brain PET scans), and the patient is asked to rest comfortably in a room that is kept warm

- Most PET scans are now acquired on a hybrid PET/CT scanner, and a low dose spiral CT is acquired for attenuation correction of the PET images and for anatomic localization. Some centers may choose to perform oral and/or intravenous contrast-enhanced diagnostic CT as part of the PET/CT examination
- Sixty minutes following the ^{18}F-FDG injection, the spiral CT is performed using a weight-based algorithm from the skull base to the upper thighs (for most oncologic indications), or from the vertex to the feet, or centered over the brain depending on the tumor being evaluated
- A 2D or 3D PET acquisition (depending on the manufacturer) is then performed over the same region(s), and all PET images are corrected for attenuation, detector efficiency, scatter, decay, and random coincidences
- Consistency in ^{18}F-FDG injected dose, scan acquisition time relative to the injection time, and acquisition and reconstruction protocols is important when performing serial scanning on the same patient

Image Interpretation

An anterior maximum-intensity pixel (MIP) view (**Fig. 90.1**) demonstrates a large area of intensely increased ^{18}F-FDG uptake to the right of midline in the upper abdomen and a smaller focus more superiorly on the right. Axial images at the level of the smaller focus (**Fig. 90.2**) demonstrate the uptake to be within the seventh rib and an associated soft tissue mass, and axial images at the level of the larger focus (**Fig. 90.3**) reveal that activity to be within the twelfth rib and a large soft tissue mass.

Differential Diagnosis

- Osseous metastases
- Multiple myeloma
- Multifocal osteosarcoma

Diagnosis and Clinical Follow-Up

Multiple myeloma. Diagnosis final, no clinical follow-up.

Discussion

Multiple myeloma is a B-cell hematologic malignancy, characterized by the proliferation and accumulation of plasma cells in bone marrow and the overproduction of monoclonal immunoglobulins. The peak incidence is in the seventh decade. The diagnosis is based on the identification of plasma cell infiltration in the bone marrow, monoclonal paraproteins, and osteolytic bone lesions. The extent of the bone lesions influences management and prognosis. With new therapies, correct determination of the extent of disease and monitoring of the response to therapy is increasingly important.

The diagnostic imaging assessment of multiple myeloma has been suboptimal. The nuclear medicine bone scan, so useful in evaluating the entire skeleton for metastases in most other cancers, is insensitive in the setting of multiple myeloma. The radiographic skeletal survey has been the traditional modality but has been shown to be of limited sensitivity in evaluating early disease and has been replaced by MRI in many institutions. However, MRI also suffers from some limitations, including a limited field of view, the inability to scan some patients because of claustrophobia or implants, and the inability to reliably distinguish active from adequately treated lesions. Although the literature on the use of PET in multiple myeloma is limited, it would appear to offer several advantages. Studies to date have indicated high sensitivities and specificities, better than those of the radiographic skeletal survey and generally on a par with, or better than, those of MRI. PET has been shown to change patient management in some cases. One particular advantage has been the ability to document active disease, which has been reliably accomplished in the setting of focal disease. However, when there is diffuse myelomatous infiltration of the spine, PET has been less successful. Investigators have recently reported on the use of ^{11}C-choline PET in multiple myeloma. Compared with ^{18}F-FDG-PET, ^{11}C-choline-PET identified more lesions, and the lesions had higher standardized uptake values (SUVs).

PEARLS AND PITFALLS_____

- PET offers advantages over MRI in the assessment of multiple myeloma, including a larger field of view and a better ability to distinguish active from fibrotic disease.
- Both MRI and PET may be indicated for optimal evaluation of the diffusely infiltrated spine.

Suggested Reading

Bredella MA, Steinbach L, Caputo G, Segall G, Hawkins R. Value of FDG PET in the assessment of patients with multiple myeloma. AJR Am J Roentgenol 2005;184(4):1199–1204

Nanni C, Zamagni E, Farsad M, Castellucci P, Tosi P, Cangini D, Salizzoni E, Lanini R, Cavo M, Fanti S. Role of ^{18}F-FDG PET/CT in the assessment of bone involvement in newly diagnosed multiple myeloma: preliminary results. Eur J Nucl Med Mol Imaging 2006;33(5):525–531

Nanni C, Zamagni E, Cavo M, Rubello D, Tacchetti P, Pettinato C, Farsad M, Castellucci P, Ambrosini V, Montini GC, Al-Nahhas A, Franchi R, Fanti S. 11C-choline vs. ^{18}F-FDG PET/CT in assessing bone involvement in patients with multiple myeloma. World J Surg Oncol 2007;5:68

Schirrmeister H, Bommer M, Buck AK, et al. Initial results in the assessment of multiple myeloma using ^{18}F-FDG PET. Eur J Nucl Med Mol Imaging 2002;29(3):361–366

Part B Neuroendocrine Imaging

Steven C. Burrell

CASE 91

Clinical Presentation

A 61-year-old woman presents with cramping and watery diarrhea that began 2 years earlier. More recently, she has experienced marked shortness of breath on exertion. CT of the chest, done for recurrent infections, reveals a large liver mass, biopsy of which leads to the investigations outlined below. She also undergoes echocardiography, which demonstrates marked thickening of the leaflets

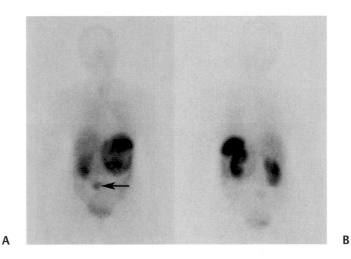

Fig. 91.1

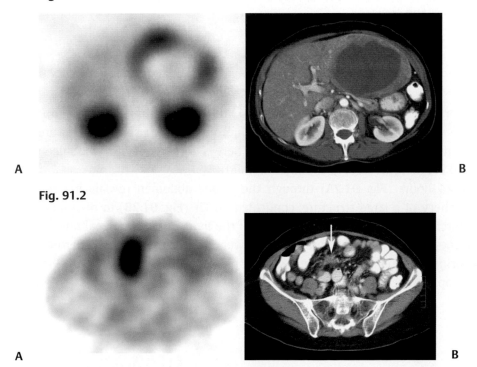

Fig. 91.2

Fig. 91.3

of the tricuspid and pulmonary valves with associated regurgitation, in addition to a dilated right ventricle with poor systolic function.

Technique

- ^{111}In-pentetreotide

- If possible, withhold nonradiolabeled octreotide before the scan: withhold 24 hours for short-acting octreotide and 3 to 4 weeks for long-acting formulations.

- The patient should be well hydrated to enhance renal clearance.

- If the patient has an insulinoma, a glucose infusion should be available to treat paradoxical hypo-glycemia.

- 6 mCi (222 MBq)

- Slow intravenous injection over 1 minute

- Medium-energy collimator

- 172- and 247-keV photopeaks, 20% window

- Planar: anterior and posterior views from head to pelvis at 4 and 24 hours

- SPECT: abdomen and pelvis at 4 hours

- SPECT: chest, abdomen, and pelvis at 24 hours

- Additional images can be obtained at 48 hours if there is uncertainty whether abdominal activity represents pathologic or physiologic uptake.

Image Interpretation

Anterior (**Fig. 91.1A**) and posterior (**Fig. 91.1B**) planar images at 24 hours demonstrate abnormal up-take in a large structure in the upper abdomen to the left of midline, and within a smaller structure lower in the abdomen (arrow) immediately to the right of midline. There is normal uptake in the spleen and kidneys (intense), liver and bladder (moderate), and thyroid (mild).

An axial SPECT image at 24 hours (**Fig. 91.2A**) through the upper abdomen reveals marked pathologic uptake in the periphery of a large structure, confirmed on CT (**Fig. 91.2B**) to be a large metastasis with a necrotic center replacing most of the left lobe of the liver. There is normal intense physiologic activity in the kidneys. A SPECT image through the lower abdomen (**Fig. 91.3A**) demon-strates intense uptake in the primary tumor. This correlates with a spiculated mass (arrow) on CT (**Fig. 91.3B**) and an associated desmoplastic reaction in the mesentery.

Differential Diagnosis

- Neuroendocrine tumor with a liver metastasis

- Other malignancies expressing somatostatin receptors (eg, melanoma or breast carcinomas)

- Inflammatory conditions expressing somatostatin receptors (eg, granulomatous diseases)

Diagnosis and Clinical Follow-Up

- Midgut carcinoid tumor with a solitary metastasis to the liver

Discussion

Neuroendocrine tumors, including carcinoids, are a diverse group of tumors arising from neuroendocrine cells. They may arise either from neural crest cells that migrate during embryologic development into different tissues or from pluripotent stem cells within the source organ. Characteristically, tumors in this family take up amine precursors, and synthesize and store bioactive compounds in vesicles or neurosecretory granules. The release of these metabolically active compounds, which may be monitored in the blood or urine, results in most of the symptomatology. Neuroendocrine tumors can be classified based on their cell of origin, including gut and lung neuroendocrine cells (carcinoid, small-cell lung cancer), islet cells (insulinoma, gastrinoma, glucagonoma, and others), sympatho-adrenal stem cells (pheochromocytoma, paraganglioma, neuroblastoma), the C cells of the thyroid (medullary thyroid carcinoma), and Merkel cells of the skin (Merkel cell tumors).

Carcinoids are carcinoma-like neoplasms arising from neuroendocrine cells, predominantly of the gastrointestinal tract. Sixty to eighty percent of carcinoids arise in the midgut, most commonly the appendix or terminal ileum. All carcinoids are potentially malignant, with the likelihood varying according to location; ileal, gastric, and colonic carcinoids are frequently malignant, and a large proportion of these have already metastasized when they are detected. Like many other neuroendocrine tumors, carcinoids are capable of producing a variety of syndromes as a result of the overproduction and release of peptide hormones. Serotonin is the dominant secretory product of carcinoids and is responsible for the *carcinoid syndrome*: intestinal hypermotility (diarrhea, cramping, nausea, and vomiting); vasomotor instability (flushing, cyanosis, dermatitis); bronchoconstriction (wheezing, dyspnea); and right-sided heart problems. The latter occur in 50% of patients with carcinoid syndrome and typically consist of tricuspid regurgitation, pulmonic stenosis, and endocardial fibrosis, resulting from a desmoplastic reaction to serotonin. Serotonin is metabolized in the liver and lungs into 5-hydroxyindoleacetic acid (5-HIAA), which is excreted in the urine. Thus, for a gastrointestinal carcinoid to produce the carcinoid syndrome, there must be liver metastases that produce serotonin and release it directly into the systemic circulation. Hepatic metastases frequently attain sizes much greater than that of the primary. A CT hallmark of the primary carcinoid tumor is the presence of a desmoplastic reaction in the mesentery.

Several radiopharmaceuticals are available for imaging neuroendocrine tumors, based mainly on the uptake characteristics of the tumors (eg, ^{123}I-MIBG or ^{131}I-MIBG) or the cell receptors of these tumors (eg, ^{111}In-pentetreotide). ^{111}In-Pentetreotide is a conjugate of octreotide, an analog of somatostatin. Somatatostatin is a small (14 amino acids) regulatory neuropeptide present in neurons and endocrine cells. The half-life of somatostatin is only 1 to 3 minutes, so the analog octreotide (eight amino acids) was developed; with its 90- to 120-minute half-life, it is more appropriate for imaging and therapeutic use. In ^{111}In-pentetreotide, octreotide is bound to ^{111}In via a DTPA (diethylene-triamine-penta-aceti acid) bridge. Tumors derived from neuroendocrine tissue tend to have high concentrations of somatostatin receptors, making ^{111}In-pentetreotide an effective imaging agent. ^{111}In-pentetreotide binds mainly to somatostatin receptor subtypes 2 and 5.

Imaging with ^{111}In-pentetreotide has a high sensitivity for most neuroendocrine tumors, including 86–95% in carcinoids. In addition to neuroendocrine tumors, ^{111}In-pentetreotide may be taken up in other tumors expressing high levels of somatostatin receptors (eg, lymphoma, melanoma, and breast cancer) as well as in some inflammatory conditions (eg, granulomatous and autoimmune diseases). Applications of ^{111}In-pentetreotide imaging in neuroendocrine tumors include localizing the primary lesion when other modalities are unable to do so, staging, assessing response to therapy, assessing for recurrence, aiding intraoperative tumor localization with a gamma probe, and establishing somatostatin receptor status in vivo for potential therapy with somatostatin analogs.

PEARLS AND PITFALLS

- Many neuroendocrine tumors express somatostatin receptors in high numbers and are thus amenable to imaging with the somatostatin analog ^{111}In-pentetreotide.
- Although ^{111}In-pentetreotide is the preferred radiopharmaceutical for imaging most neuroendocrine tumors, MIBG tagged with radioactive iodine is preferred for pheochromcytomas and neuroblastomas. Furthermore, there may be a complementary role for these two tracers in any given patient because some tumors may be positive with one tracer but not the other.
- If possible, octreotide should be withheld from patients being treated with this agent before they undergo ^{111}In-pentetreotide imaging: for at least 1 day with short-acting formulations and for 3 to 4 weeks with long-acting formulations.
- Normal sites of uptake include the spleen, kidneys, liver, bladder, thyroid, gastrointestinal tract (although rarely on the early 4-hour images), and occasionally the pituitary, breasts, and gallbladder.
- Bowel excretion is seen mainly at 24 hours. Therefore, SPECT of the abdomen is recommended at 4 and 24 hours, especially when abdominal tumors are being evaluated. It can always be repeated at 48 hours if necessary. SPECT of the chest should be performed at 24 hours, when the blood pool activity has cleared.
- Because the main route of excretion is renal, impaired renal function can cause an increase in background activity.
- False-positive activity can be seen in the nasal region and pulmonary hila as a result of respiratory infections, throughout the lungs following bleomycin or radiation therapy, and at sites of recent surgery. Occasional physiologic activity in the gallbladder may be mistaken for disease; delayed images may demonstrate migration into the small bowel.

Suggested Reading

Balon HR, Goldsmith SJ, Siegel PA, et al. Society of Nuclear Medicine Procedure Guideline for Somatostatin Receptor Scintigraphy with In-11 Pentetreotide version 1.0, approved February 21, 2001. http://interactive.snm.org/docs/pg_ch27_0403.pdf. Accessed April 17, 2010

Cotran RS, Kumar V, Robbins SL. Robbins Pathologic Basis of Disease. Philadelphia, PA: WB Saunders; 1989:872–875

Hoefnagel CA. Metaiodobenzylguanidine and somatostatin in oncology: role in the management of neural crest tumours. Eur J Nucl Med 1994;21(6):561–581

Kaltsas GA, Mukherjee JJ, Grossman AB. The value of radiolabelled MIBG and octreotide in the diagnosis and management of neuroendocrine tumours. Ann Oncol 2001;12(Suppl 2):S47–S50

Kwekkeboom D, Krenning EP, de Jong M. Peptide receptor imaging and therapy. J Nucl Med 2000;41(10):1704–1713

Seregni E, Chiti A, Bombardieri E. Radionuclide imaging of neuroendocrine tumours: biological basis and diagnostic results. Eur J Nucl Med 1998;25(6):639–658

CASE 92

Clinical Presentation

A 41-year-old woman presents with palpitations associated with nausea and severe headaches. At the time of assessment, her blood pressure is normal at 126/78 mm Hg, and her heart rate is normal at 84 beats/min. Laboratory workup demonstrates significantly elevated levels of urinary vanillyl-mandelic acid, epinephrine, and norepinephrine.

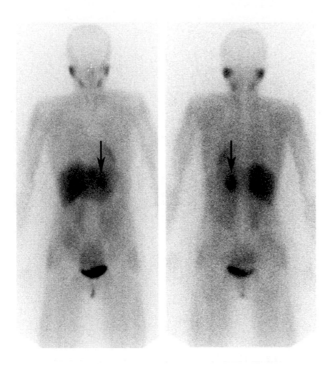

A   B

Fig. 92.1

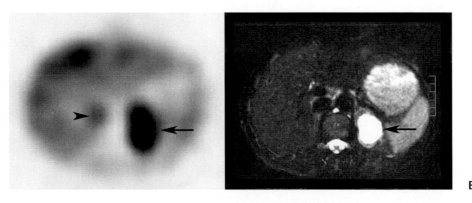

A   B

Fig. 92.2

Technique

- ¹²³I-MIBG
- The patient should be well hydrated.
- Drugs known or expected to interfere with MIBG uptake should be withheld. These include some β-blockers (in particular, labetalol), catecholamine agonists including oral decongestants, antipsychotics, tricyclic antidepressants, some calcium channel blockers, and cocaine. A more detailed list, along with the recommended withholding period, is provided in Bombardieri et al. (2003).
- Thyroid blockade should be performed with saturated potassium iodide three times daily, three drops each time, beginning on the day before the injection and continuing for a total of 3 days (¹²³I-MIBG) or 5 days (¹³¹I-MIBG).
- 5 mCi
- Slow intravenous injection over 5 minutes
- Low-energy, high-resolution collimator
- 159-keV photopeak, 20% window
- Planar: anterior and posterior views from head to pelvis at 4 and 24 hours
- SPECT: abdomen and pelvis at 4 hours
- SPECT: chest, abdomen, and pelvis at 24 hours

Image Interpretation

Anterior (**Fig. 92.1A**) and posterior (**Fig. 92.1B**) planar images from a ¹²³I-MIBG scan demonstrate markedly increased uptake in a structure (arrow) in the left upper abdomen posteriorly. There are no other abnormalities. There is normal physiologic uptake within the liver, heart, salivary glands, and bladder. An axial slice from the ¹²³I-MIBG SPECT acquisition (**Fig. 92.2A**) confirms intense uptake in a structure (arrow) in the left retroperitoneum. There is very mild uptake in the right retroperitoneum associated with the adrenal gland (arrow-head). The corresponding MRI (**Fig. 92.2B**) demonstrates intense signal on T2 sequence in the structure in the left retroperitoneum. There is no MRI abnormality in the vicinity of the right adrenal gland.

Differential Diagnosis

- Pheochromocytoma
- Ganglioneuroma
- Carcinoid

Diagnosis and Clinical Follow-Up

Left adrenal pheochromocytoma. Normal mild uptake in right adrenal gland.

The patient underwent left adrenalectomy, including removal of a 3.7-cm pheochromocytoma. She has remained asymptomatic since, and urinary catecholamine levels have repeatedly been normal.

Discussion

Pheochromocytomas are neuroendocrine tumors arising from chromaffin cells. Strictly speaking, only those originating within the adrenal medulla (70–90%) are referred to as *pheochromocytomas*, whereas those arising elsewhere are known as *paragangliomas*. Eighty to ninety percent occur spontaneously; the remainder are associated with familial syndromes, including familial predisposition to pheochromocytomas, multiple endocrine neoplasia (MEN 2a and 2b), tuberous sclerosis, neurofibromatosis, and von Hippel-Lindau disease. About 5 to 10% of pheochromocytomas are malignant, which is reliably established only by the presence of metastases. Most pheochromocytomas secrete norepinephrine and epinephrine, leading most notably to hypertension, which may be accentuated by paroxysmal attacks. Sudden catecholamine release may also result in headache, anxiety, perspiration, tremor, fatigue, nausea and vomiting, abdominal pain, and visual disturbances.

MIBG is a combination of the benzyl group of bretylium and the guanidine group of guanethidine. MIBG is similar in structure and function to norepinephrine, and consequently MIBG is taken up in cells of neural crest origin. Uptake is predominantly via an active uptake-1 mechanism, and once inside the cytoplasm, MIBG is stored in vesicles, from which it may be released and become available for reuptake by the same mechanism. When radiolabeled with ^{123}I or ^{131}I, MIBG is an effective imaging agent for tumors derived from neural crest cells, including pheochromocytomas, ganglioneuromas, and neuroblastomas. Other neuroendocrine tumors, including paragangliomas, medullary thyroid carcinomas, and carcinoid tumors, may also be positive on MIBG scans, although less frequently.

The shorter half-life of ^{123}I (13.0 hours vs. 8.1 days) allows a much larger activity of ^{123}I-MIBG to be given compared with ^{131}I-MIBG for the same radiation dose. This, along with the favorable detector parameters of the 159-keV photons of ^{123}I, yields considerably higher-quality images with ^{123}I-MIBG than with ^{131}I-MIBG. It also allows SPECT imaging to be performed with ^{123}I-MIBG. ^{123}I-MIBG detects more sites of disease than ^{131}I-MIBG but is not as widely available. **Figure 92.3** contrasts an anterior ^{123}I-MIBG scan (**Fig. 92.3A**) and a ^{131}I-MIBG scan (**Fig. 92.3B**) obtained 1 year apart in a 49-year-old man.

MIBG imaging accurately detects pheochromocytomas, with a sensitivity of 88% and specificity of 99% in the appropriate clinical setting. In comparison with CT and MRI, MIBG imaging is more specific and allows imaging of the entire body for metastases. An interesting finding on MIBG scans in the setting of a pheochromocytoma is that cardiac uptake may be reduced, roughly in proportion to the level of circulating catecholamines. In fact, another application of MIBG imaging is the assessment of cardiac sympathetic innervation; this has been undertaken in the setting of heart failure, certain arrhythmic conditions, and denervation secondary to diabetes and cardiac transplant.

^{131}I-MIBG may be used in high doses as therapy for metastatic pheochromocytoma. ^{131}I-MIBG has been shown to induce objective remissions, assessed by reductions in tumor volumes or in catecholamine secretions, in 25 to 50% of treated patients. Side effects have been minimal.

PET with ^{18}F-FDG has undergone exponential growth for tumor imaging in recent years. However, MIBG imaging has generally proved better for depicting pheochromocytomas. Consequently ^{18}F-FDG-PET would generally be reserved for patients whose pheochromocytomas are not MIBG-avid. Initial studies with less common PET radiopharmaceuticals, including ^{18}F-DOPA and ^{11}C-hydroxyephedrine, have proved quite accurate in the assessment of pheochromocytomas, but their clinical role has yet to be established.

PEARLS AND PITFALLS _____

• MIBG is a norepinephrine analog effective in imaging tumors derived from neural crest cells, including pheochromocytomas, neuroblastomas, and ganglioneuromas. Other neuroendocrine tumors may also be imaged with MIBG, although ^{111}In pentetreotide is generally a better imaging agent for those tumors. However, there may be a complementary role for these two tracers in any given patient, as some neuroendocrine tumors may be positive with one tracer but not the other.

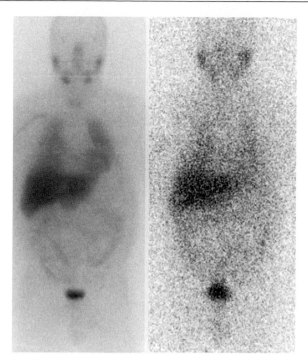

A   B

Fig. 92.3

- MIBG is labeled with either ^{123}I or [131]I. Higher-quality images are obtained with ^{123}I-MIBG, although it is not as widely available as ^{131}I-MIBG.
- Normal uptake on MIBG scans is seen in the salivary glands, nasopharynx, myocardium, liver, and bladder. Fainter or more variable uptake may be seen in the gut, blocked thyroid gland, normal adrenal glands, spleen, uterus, and lung bases. Mild uptake is frequently seen in the low neck in children.
- Normal adrenal gland uptake must not be mistaken for pathology. Normal adrenal uptake is seen more commonly with ^{123}I-MIBG than with ^{131}I-MIBG.
- Proper patient preparation includes administering saturated potassium iodide to protect the thyroid from free radioiodine, and withholding medications known or expected to interfere with MIBG uptake.
- ^{131}I-MIBG may be used in high doses as therapy for metastatic pheochromocytomas and other MIBG-avid neuro-endocrine tumors.
- PET with ^{18}F-FDG is less sensitive overall than MIBG imaging for pheochromocytomas, but it may be helpful in selected patients with MIBG-negative pheochromocytomas.

Suggested Reading

Bombardieri E, Aktolun C, Baum RP, et al. [131]I/^{123}I-metaiodobenzylguanidine (MIBG) scintigraphy: procedure guidelines for tumour imaging. Eur J Nucl Med Mol Imaging 2003;30(12):BP132–BP139

Cotran RS, Kumar V, Robbins SL. Robbins Pathologic Basis of Disease. Philadelphia, PA: WB Saunders; 1989:1263–1265

Hoefnagel CA. Metaiodobenzylguanidine and somatostatin in oncology: role in the management of neural crest tumours. Eur J Nucl Med 1994;21(6):561–581

Shulkin BL, Thompson NW, Shapiro B, Francis IR, Sisson JC. Pheochromocytomas: imaging with 2-[^{18}F]fluoro-2-deoxy-D-glucose PET. Radiology 1999;212(1):35–41

Wiseman GA, Kvols LK. Therapy of neuroendocrine tumors with radiolabeled MIBG and somatostatin analogues. Semin Nucl Med 1995;25(3):272–278

CASE 93

Clinical Presentation

A 61-year-old man presents with recurrent duodenal ulcers and duodenitis.

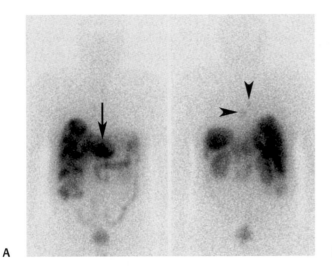

A   B

Fig. 93.1

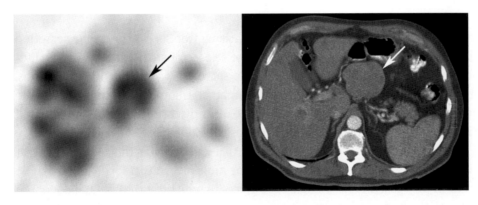

A   B

Fig. 93.2

Technique

- ^{111}In-pentetreotide
- If possible, withhold nonradiolabeled octreotide before the scan: withhold 24 hours for short-acting octreotide and 3 to 4 weeks for long-acting formulations.
- The patient should be well hydrated to enhance renal clearance.
- If the patient has an insulinoma, a glucose infusion should be available to treat paradoxical hypoglycemia.
- 6 mCi (222 MBq)
- Slow intravenous injection over 1 minute

299

- Medium-energy collimator
- 172- and 247-keV photopeaks, 20% window
- Planar: anterior and posterior views from head to pelvis at 4 and 24 hours
- SPECT: abdomen and pelvis at 4 hours
- SPECT: chest, abdomen, and pelvis at 24 hours
- Additional images can be obtained at 48 hours if there is uncertainty whether abdominal activity represents pathologic or physiologic uptake.

Image Interpretation

Anterior (**Fig. 93.1A**) and posterior (**Fig. 93.1B**) planar images at 24 hours demonstrate a large focus of intense uptake in the central abdomen, numerous foci of uptake throughout the liver, and foci of faint uptake in the thorax. A SPECT image (**Fig. 93.2A**) and corresponding CT slice (**Fig. 93.2B**) confirm uptake in a large mass arising from the head of the pancreas and within several liver lesions.

Differential Diagnosis

- Gastrinoma with metastases
- Other enteropancreatic tumor with metastases
- Other malignancies expressing somatostatin receptors (eg, melanoma or breast carcinoma)

Diagnosis and Clinical Follow-Up

Pancreatic gastrinoma with metastases to the liver, thoracic lymph nodes, and retroperitoneal lymph nodes. Diagnosis final, no clinical follow-up.

Discussion

Neuroendocrine tumors of the pancreas often cause symptoms arising from excess hormone secretion rather than invasion. Although the tumors are slow-growing, the release of such products can be life-threatening. These tumors are named according to the peptide secreted: gastrinomas, insulinomas, VIPomas (vasoactive intestinal peptide), glucagonomas, and somatostatinomas. Gastrinomas are the most common, and patients typically present with severe peptic ulcer disease resulting from elevated gastric acid production in response to the high gastrin secretion. The Zollinger-Ellison syndrome may result and is diagnosed when a patient has a fasting serum gastrin level greater than 1000 pg/mL or a positive secretin test. Gastrinomas are often extrapancreatic or multiple, so that localization can be difficult. The majority occur in the "gastrinoma triangle," the apices of which are the confluences of the cystic and common bile ducts, the body and tail of the pancreas, and the second and third portions of the duodenum.

In the setting of a pancreatic islet cell tumor, ^{111}In-pentetreotide imaging can be useful in locating the primary tumor, staging, assessing response to therapy, assessing for recurrence, and aiding intraoperative tumor localization with a gamma probe.

Imaging with ^{111}In-pentetreotide can also be used to establish somatostatin receptor status in vivo for potential therapy with somatostatin analogs. Nonradiolabeled octreotide can control symptoms from islet cell tumors by inhibiting peptide release. In some centers, radioisotope therapy is performed with radiolabeled octreotide. High doses of ^{111}In-pentetreotide have been used, with tumor cell damage achieved via the release of auger electrons. More recently, the β⁻ emitter ^{90}Y has been used, coupled to octreotide via DOTA (1,4,7,10-tetraazacyclododecane-1,4,7,10-tetra-acetic acid). The longer path length of the β^- electron compared with that of the auger electron allows better tumor penetration.

PEARLS AND PITFALLS

- Gastrinomas are the most common enteropancreatic islet cell tumors.
- The majority of gastrinomas are actually located adjacent to the pancreas.
- Imaging of neuroendocrine tumors with ^{111}In-pentetreotide can be used to establish somatostatin receptor (subtypes 2 and 5) avidity in vivo, which is useful when therapy with somatostatin analogs is being considered. Therapy may consist of unlabeled octreotide or radiolabeled octreotide with high doses of ^{111}In-pentetreotide or ^{90}Y-DOTA-octreotide.

Suggested Reading

Balon HR, Goldsmith SJ, Siegel PA, et al. Society of Nuclear Medicine Procedure Guideline for Somatostatin Receptor Scintigraphy with In-11 Pentetreotide version 1.0, approved February 21, 2001. http://interactive.snm.org/docs/pg_ch27_0403.pdf. Accessed April 17, 2010

Buetow PC, Miller DL, Parrino TV, Buck JL. Islet cell tumors of the pancreas: clinical, radiologic, and pathologic correlation in diagnosis and localization. Radiographics 1997;17(2):453–472, quiz 472A–472B

Hoefnagel CA. Metaiodobenzylguanidine and somatostatin in oncology: role in the management of neural crest tumours. Eur J Nucl Med 1994;21(6):561–581

Kaltsas GA, Mukherjee JJ, Grossman AB. The value of radiolabelled MIBG and octreotide in the diagnosis and management of neuroendocrine tumours. Ann Oncol 2001;12(Suppl 2):S47–S50

Kaplan LM. Endocrine tumors of the gastrointestinal tract and pancreas. In: Isselbacher KJ, Braunwald E, Martin JB, Fauci AS, Wilson JD, Kasper DL, eds. Harrison's Principles of Internal Medicine. 13th ed. New York, NY: McGraw-Hill; 1994:1535–1542

Kwekkeboom D, Krenning EP, de Jong M. Peptide receptor imaging and therapy. J Nucl Med 2000;41(10):1704–1713

CASE 94

Clinical Presentation

A 15-month-old girl has symptoms of an upper respiratory infection. A chest radiograph demonstrates a posterior mediastinal mass. She is referred for further evaluation of the mass.

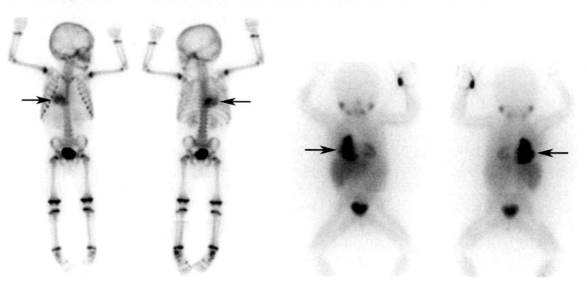

Fig. 94.1   Fig. 94.2

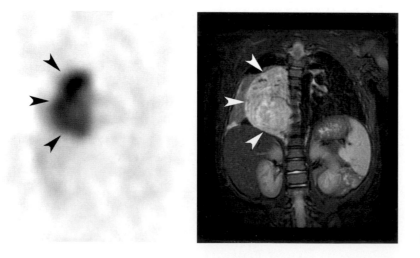

A   B

Fig. 94.3

Technique

Bone Scan (also see below for ^{123}I-MIBG Scan)

- ^{99m}Tc-HDP
- No specific preparation

- 6 mCi

- Intravenous injection

- Low-energy, high-resolution collimator

- 140-keV photopeak, 20% window

- Flow and pool images of chest, abdomen, and pelvis

- Static images at 2 hours of entire skeleton

Technique

^{123}I-MIBG

- The patient should be well hydrated.

- Drugs known or expected to interfere with MIBG uptake should be withheld. These include some β-blockers (in particular, labetalol), catecholamine agonists including oral decongestants, antipsychotics, tricyclic antidepressants, some calcium channel blockers, and cocaine. A more detailed list, along with the recommended withholding period, is provided in Bombardieri et al. (2003).

- Thyroid blockade should be performed with the administration of a saturated potassium iodide tablet, 65 mg once per day (pediatric dose), beginning on the day before the injection and continuing for a total of 3 days.

- 1 mCi

- Slow intravenous injection over 5 minutes

- Low-energy, high-resolution collimator

- 159-keV photopeak, 20% window

- Static images at 18 hours of entire body

- SPECT images of thorax and abdomen

Image Interpretation

Anterior (**Fig. 94.1A**) and posterior (**Fig. 94.1B**) planar images from the bone scan demonstrate markedly increased uptake in the right mediastinal soft tissue mass, but no osseous abnormalities.

Anterior (**Fig. 94.2A**) and posterior (**Fig. 94.2B**) planar images from the ^{123}I-MIBG scan (**Fig. 94.2**) demonstrate intense accumulation of ^{123}I-MIBG in the mass, with no other areas of abnormal uptake. (Activity in the left wrist is at the injection site.) A coronal image from the SPECT acquisition (**Fig. 94.3A**) correlates with an 8-cm paraspinal mass on MRI (**Fig. 94.3B**).

Differential Diagnosis

- Neuroblastoma
- Ganglioneuroma
- Pheochromocytoma

Diagnosis and Clinical Follow-Up

Neuroblastoma, stage IIB (in addition to the mass, a positive 7-mm intercostal lymph node was resected at surgery). Diagnosis final, no clinical follow-up.

Discussion

Neuroblastoma is the third most common malignancy in childhood, after brain tumors and leukemia. Neuroblastomas arise from neural crest cells, with 50 to 80% occurring in the adrenal medulla or adjacent retroperitoneum. Eighty percent present in children younger than 5 years. Neuroblastomas may be associated with the rare opsoclonus-myoclonus syndrome. Approximately 85% are associated with urinary excretion of catecholamines or catecholamine metabolites. There is actually a spectrum of disease, in which neuroblastomas, the most common, are the most immature and malignant, ganglioneuromas the most mature and benign, and ganglioneuroblastomas intermediate in aggressiveness. Metastases occur in the majority of cases of neuroblastoma. The prognosis depends on various factors, most notably age and stage of disease.

MIBG scans are positive in most children with neuroblastoma, with sensitivities of 90% or higher in most studies. MIBG accurately depicts the primary tumor, as well as local and distant metastases. In the appropriate clinical setting the specificity is very high, typically above 95%. The pediatric tumors that might otherwise be confused with neuroblastoma, Wilms tumors and sarcomas, do not demonstrate significant MIBG uptake. Pheochromocytomas, although MIBG-avid, are rare in the pediatric population and are readily distinguished from neuroblastomas on clinical grounds. The high specificity renders MIBG imaging effective in establishing a diagnosis, which may be useful preoperatively. Greater utility lies in staging the disease; in many patients, MIBG detects more sites of tumor involvement than do all other imaging modalities combined. Further clinical benefit is seen in the post-therapy setting, with MIBG a sensitive and specific indicator of residual or recurrent disease.

Because of the tendency of neuroblastoma to metastasize to bone marrow, patients have traditionally undergone bone scanning for staging purposes. Many primary neuroblastomas take up bone scanning agents such as ^{99m}Tc-MDP, and in fact neuroblastoma is a common cause of nonosseous uptake on bone scans. The sensitivity of bone scans for osseous metastases may be reduced because of their propensity to metastasize to the bone marrow (and so not elicit cortical osteoneogenesis detectable on bone scan) and to the metaphyses of the long bones (where activity may be obscured by intense physiologic uptake in the adjacent physes). MIBG imaging frequently detects more osseous metastases than does the bone scan, although occasionally the bone scan will detect lesions not seen on the MIBG scan. In the post-therapy setting, MIBG is typically more specific, as increased activity may be seen on the bone scan arising from the osseous reparative process, even if the tumor has been eradicated.

Radioisotope therapy of neuroblastoma with high doses of ^{131}I-MIBG has been performed in several centers, with cell damage occurring through the emission of β^- by the ^{131}I isotope. Favorable dosimetry is afforded by the high uptake of MIBG in tumors and the prolonged half-life in tumors relative to that in background tissue. ^{131}I-MIBG therapy of neuroblastomas has been undertaken predominantly in patients who have been extensively treated with, and failed, other therapies. In this population, many patients have had partial remission, although often short-lived. There have been a relatively small number of complete remissions. More recently, there has been a move toward using ^{131}I-MIBG earlier in the therapy regimen. The most common significant complication has been myelosuppression.

PET with ^{18}F-FDG has undergone exponential growth in tumor imaging in recent years. However, MIBG imaging has generally proved better for depicting the primary tumor and metastases, both before and after therapy, in patients with neuroblastoma. Consequently ^{18}F-FDG-PET would generally be reserved for the rare patient whose neuroblastoma is not MIBG-avid.

PEARLS AND PITFALLS_____

- Normal uptake on MIBG scans is seen in the salivary glands, nasopharynx, myocardium, liver, and bladder. Fainter or more variable uptake may be seen in the gut, blocked thyroid gland, normal adrenal glands, spleen, uterus, and lung bases. Mild uptake is frequently seen in the low neck in children.

- Proper patient preparation includes administering saturated potassium iodine to protect the thyroid from free radioiodine, and withholding medications known or expected to interfere with MIBG uptake.

- MIBG imaging is sensitive and specific in the setting of a known neuroblastoma. Sources of false-positive findings have included physiologic gastrointestinal and genitourinary uptake, and uptake in tumors that have matured to ganglioneuromas.

- Nonosseous neuroblastomas frequently demonstrate uptake on bone scans. MIBG imaging may detect more osseous metastases than do bone scans, but occasionally the bone scan detects lesions not seen on MIBG imaging.

- High doses of ^{131}I-MIBG may be used for neuroblastoma therapy. All known lesions should be demonstrated to be MIBG-avid before radioisotope therapy with MIBG is undertaken. Post-therapy scans with the large therapy dose may demonstrate more sites of disease than were seen on the pre-therapy scans.

Suggested Reading

Bombardieri E, Aktolun C, Baum RP, et al. [131]I/^{123}I-metaiodobenzylguanidine (MIBG) scintigraphy: procedure guidelines for tumour imaging. Eur J Nucl Med Mol Imaging 2003;30(12):BP132–BP139

Cotran RS, Kumar V, Robbins SL. Robbins Pathologic Basis of Disease. Philadelphia, PA: WB Saunders; 1989:1265–1267

Gelfand MJ. Meta-iodobenzylguanidine in children. Semin Nucl Med 1993;23(3):231–242

Shulkin BL, Shapiro B. Current concepts on the diagnostic use of MIBG in children. J Nucl Med 1998;39(4):679–688

CASE 95

Clinical Presentation

A 64-year-old man presents with weight loss, night sweats, and episodic dizziness. Routine blood work reveals a critically low glucose level of 1.0 mmol/L (18 mg/dL). Fasting blood work is subsequently ordered, yielding a glucose level of 1.2 mmol/L (21 mg/dL) coincident with a serum insulin level of 267 pmol/L (normal, 14–145 pmol/L). While fasting, the patient becomes clammy, sweaty, and generally unwell. He is instructed to consume frequent meals as well as orange juice mixed with sugar. These measures result in a significant reduction in his symptoms.

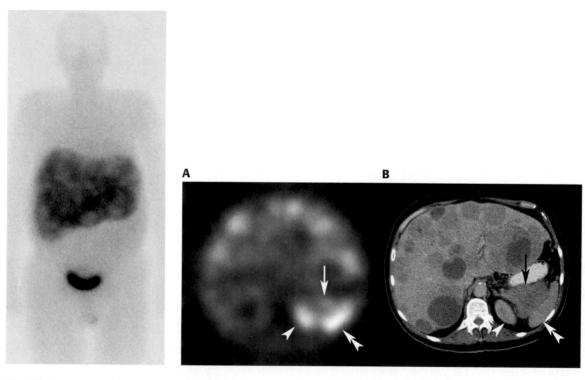

Fig. 95.1   Fig. 95.2

Technique

- ^{111}In-pentetreotide
- If possible, withhold nonradiolabeled octreotide before the scan: withhold 24 hours for short-acting octreotide and 3 to 4 weeks for long-acting formulations.
- The patient should be well hydrated to enhance renal clearance.
- If the patient has an insulinoma, a glucose infusion should be available to treat paradoxical hypoglycemia.
- 6 mCi (222 MBq)
- Slow intravenous injection over 1 minute
- Medium-energy collimator
- 172- and 247-keV photopeaks, 20% window

- Planar: anterior and posterior views from head to pelvis at 4 and 24 hours
- SPECT: abdomen and pelvis at 4 hours
- SPECT: chest, abdomen, and pelvis at 24 hours
- Additional images can be obtained at 48 hours if there is uncertainty whether abdominal activity represents pathologic or physiologic uptake.

Image Interpretation

Planar image at 24 hours (**Fig. 95.1**) demonstrates markedly abnormal heterogeneous uptake throughout the enlarged liver. An axial SPECT image at 24 hours (**Fig. 95.2A**) and CT scan (**Fig. 95.2B**) demonstrate multiple ^{111}In-pentetreotide–avid lesions within the liver. Several lesions, particularly posteriorly, demonstrate reduced ^{111}In-pentetreotide uptake, consistent with necrosis. There is a separate mass arising from the tail of the pancreas. On the CT scan, it is seen in the region of the splenic hilum. It demonstrates moderately increased uptake on the ^{111}In-pentetreotide scan, adjacent to the intense physiologic uptake in the spleen and left kidney.

Differential Diagnosis

- Neuroendocrine tumor with liver metastases
- Other malignancies expressing somatostatin receptors (eg, melanoma, breast carcinoma)

Diagnosis and Clinical Follow-Up

Insulinoma arising from the tail of the pancreas with multiple metastases to the liver. Diagnosis final.

After the octreotide avidity of the tumor was demonstrated through in vivo imaging, the patient was treated with nonradiolabeled octreotide. This resulted in good glycemic control and significant relief of symptoms and improvement in quality of life.

Discussion

Insulinomas, which arise from the pancreatic β- cells, are the second most common islet cell tumors. Hypersecretion of insulin results in the classic clinical presentation known as the Whipple triad, which consists of fasting hypoglycemia, hypoglycemic symptoms, and immediate relief of symptoms following intravenous administration of glucose. Only about 10% of insulinomas are malignant, whereas the majority of other islet cell tumors are malignant. However, the sensitivity of ^{111}In-pentetreotide imaging is lower for insulinomas (50–60%) than for other islet cell tumors (75–100%), likely a reflection of the fact that insulinomas express low levels of somatostatin receptor subtypes 2 and 5. Because most insulinomas are small, only about half are detected by CT. Thus ^{111}In-pentetreotide imaging can be useful in locating the primary tumor. As with other islet cell tumors, it can also be useful in staging, assessing response to therapy, assessing for recurrence, and aiding intraoperative tumor localization with a gamma probe.

In patients with an insulinoma, the injection of octreotide, whether radiolabeled or unlabeled, can result in severe hypoglycemia, likely due to the inhibition of glucagon secretion. Thus, it is necessary to have an intravenous infusion of glucose available.

PEARLS AND PITFALLS_____

- Insulinomas are the second most common pancreatic islet cell tumor.
- Whereas most islet cell tumors are malignant, 90% of insulinomas are benign.

- The sensitivity of ^{111}In-pentetreotide imaging is lower for insulinomas (50–60%) than for other islet cell tumors (75–100%).
- When a patient is suspected of having an insulinoma, an intravenous infusion of glucose should be available before ^{111}In-pentetreotide is injected because of the potential for inducing severe paradoxical hypoglycemia.
- Imaging of neuroendocrine tumors with ^{111}In-pentetreotide can be used to establish somatostatin receptor (subtypes 2 and 5) avidity in vivo, which is useful when therapy with somatostatin analogs is being considered.

Suggested Reading

Balon HR, Goldsmith SJ, Siegel PA, et al. Society of Nuclear Medicine Procedure Guideline for Somatostatin Receptor Scintigraphy with In-11 Pentetreotide version 1.0, approved February 21, 2001. http://interactive.snm.org/docs/pg_ch27_0403.pdf. Accessed April 17, 2010

Hoefnagel CA. Metaiodobenzylguanidine and somatostatin in oncology: role in the management of neural crest tumours. Eur J Nucl Med 1994;21(6):561–581

Kaltsas GA, Mukherjee JJ, Grossman AB. The value of radiolabelled MIBG and octreotide in the diagnosis and management of neuroendocrine tumours. Ann Oncol 2001;12(Suppl 2):S47–S50

Kaplan LM. Endocrine tumors of the gastrointestinal tract and pancreas. In: Isselbacher KJ, Braunwald E, Martin JB, Fauci AS, Wilson JD, Kasper DL, eds. Harrison's Principles of Internal Medicine. 13th ed. New York, NY: McGraw-Hill; 1994:1535–1542

Kwekkeboom D, Krenning EP, de Jong M. Peptide receptor imaging and therapy. J Nucl Med 2000;41(10):1704–1713

CASE 96

Clinical Presentation

Two years ago, a 30-year-old gravida 1, para 0 woman presented with severely labile hypertension during pregnancy, which continued into the postpartum period. Now she presents with elevated calcium, parathyroid hormone, and calcitonin.

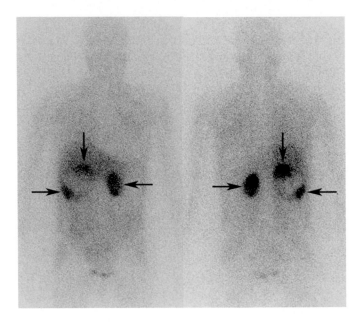

Fig. 96.1

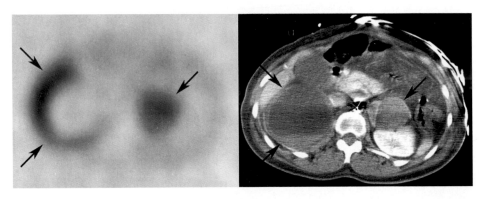

A   **B**

Fig. 96.2

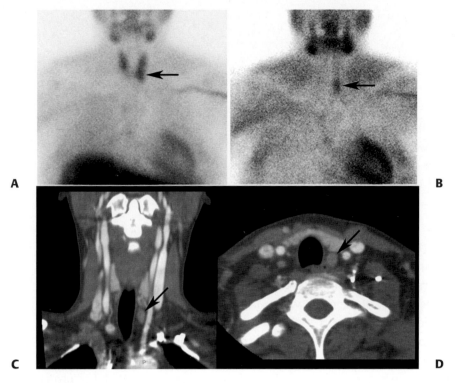

Fig. 96.3

Technique

^{111}In-Pentetreotide Scan (also see ^{99m}Tc-Sestamibi Scan)

- If possible, withhold nonradiolabeled octreotide before the scan; withhold 24 hours for short-acting octreotide and 3 to 4 weeks for long-acting formulations.
- The patient should be well hydrated to enhance renal clearance.
- If the patient has an insulinoma, a glucose infusion should be available to treat paradoxical hypoglycemia.
- 6 mCi (222 MBq)
- Slow intravenous injection over 1 minute
- Medium-energy collimator
- 172- and 247-keV photopeaks, 20% window
- Planar: anterior and posterior views from head to pelvis at 4 and 24 hours
- SPECT: abdomen and pelvis at 4 hours
- SPECT: chest, abdomen, and pelvis at 24 hours
- Additional images can be obtained at 48 hours if there is uncertainty whether abdominal activity represents pathologic or physiologic uptake.

Technique

⁹⁹ᵐTc-Sestamibi Scan

- None
- 30 mCi (1110 MBq)
- Intravenous injection
- Low-energy, high-resolution collimator
- 140-keV photopeak, 20% window
- Planar: anterior neck and upper chest at 10 to 15 minutes and again at 3 to 4 hours (**Fig. 96.3A**)
- SPECT: neck and upper chest at 10 to 15 minutes and again at 3 to 4 hours (**Fig. 96.3B**)

Image Interpretation

Anterior (**Fig. 96.1A**) and posterior (**Fig. 96.1B**) planar ¹¹¹In-pentetreotide images demonstrate large areas of abnormal uptake in the upper abdomen bilaterally. An axial SPECT image (**Fig. 96.2A**) and corresponding CT scan (**Fig. 96.2B**) confirm intense uptake in large retroperitoneal structures bilaterally. The activity on the right is within the periphery of the mass, with a large amount of necrosis centrally.

Following the second presentation 2 years later, a ⁹⁹ᵐTc-sestamibi scan was obtained, with planar images at 15 minutes (**Fig. 96.3A**) and 3 hours (**Fig. 96.3B**). On the early images, there is normal uptake throughout the thyroid gland, with more focal uptake in the vicinity of the left lower lobe. Following clearance from the thyroid, the delayed images confirm a solitary focus of uptake on the left. Coronal (**Fig. 96.3C**) and axial (**Fig. 96.3D**) slices from a CT scan reveal a small nodule posterior and inferior to the thyroid gland, correlating with the focus of ⁹⁹ᵐTc-sestamibi uptake.

Differential Diagnosis

- Bilateral pheochromocytomas
- Bilateral pheochromocytomas plus parathyroid adenoma
- Bilateral pheochromocytomas plus parathyroid adenoma plus medullary thyroid cancer (MTC)

Diagnosis and Clinical Follow-Up

Bilateral pheochromocytomas plus parathyroid adenoma plus MTC: multiple endocrine neoplasia (MEN) 2a. Diagnosis final. (Although it was not evident on imaging, the presence of MTC was known from the elevated serum calcitonin and confirmed pathologically following thyroidectomy.)

Discussion

MEN syndromes are hereditary cancer syndromes characterized by the occurrence of two or more endocrine tumors. There are two categories, MEN 1 and MEN 2.

MEN 1 is associated with more than 20 possible endocrine and non-endocrine tumors. A practical definition is a case with two of the three main tumors: parathyroid adenoma, enteropancreatic endocrine tumor, and pituitary tumor. Parathyroid adenomas are the most common, present in 90% of cases, and the resultant hyperparathyroidism is the most frequent and usually the earliest manifestation. Gastrinomas (40% of MEN 1 cases) are the most common enteropancreatic tumor, and prolactinomas (20% of MEN 1 cases) are the most common pituitary tumor.

MEN 2 comprises a variety of syndromes, all with a high penetrance of MTC. There are several subtypes, including MEN 2a (MTC, 90%; pheochromocytoma, 50%; parathyroid tumors, 20–30%) and MEN 2b (MTC, pheochromocytoma, marfanoid habitus, mucosal and intestinal ganglioneuromatosis). The main cause of death in patients with MEN 2 is MTC.

PEARLS AND PITFALLS

- Although MEN 1 syndromes are most commonly associated with tumors arising from the "three *P's*" (parathyroid, enteropancreatic, and pituitary), there are actually associations with more than 20 possible different endocrine and non-endocrine tumors.
- All variants of MEN 2 are associated with a high incidence of MTC.
- The evaluation of patients with a known or suspected MEN syndrome requires a multidisciplinary approach involving endocrinologists, surgeons, oncologists, radiologists, nuclear medicine physicians, and pathologists.
- The large range of tumor types and organs requires the radiologist and nuclear medicine physician to be familiar with the role of various imaging modalities in the assessment of patients with MEN.

Suggested Reading

Brandi ML, Gagel RF, Angeli A, et al. Guidelines for diagnosis and therapy of MEN type 1 and type 2. J Clin Endocrinol Metab 2001;86(12):5658–5671

Scarsbrook AF, Thakker RV, Wass JA, Gleeson FV, Phillips RR. Multiple endocrine neoplasia: spectrum of radiologic appearances and discussion of a multitechnique imaging approach. Radiographics 2006;26(2):433–451

CASE 97

Clinical Presentation

A 70-year-old woman presents with mild diplopia and a lateral gaze. Twenty-eight years previously, she underwent resection of an olfactory esthesioneuroblastoma; two recurrences were also resected.

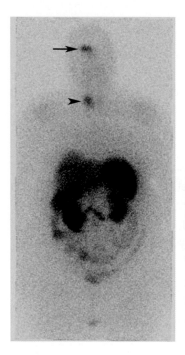

Fig. 97.1

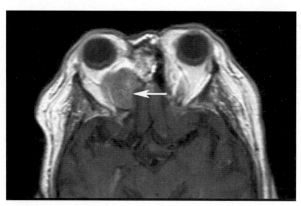

Fig. 97.2

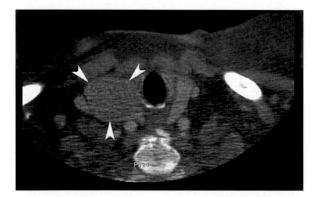

Fig. 97.3

Technique

- ^{111}In-pentetreotide
- If possible, withhold nonradiolabeled octreotide before the scan: withhold 24 hours for short-acting octreotide and 3 to 4 weeks for long-acting formulations.
- The patient should be well hydrated to enhance renal clearance.
- If the patient has an insulinoma, a glucose infusion should be available to treat paradoxical hypoglycemia.
- 6 mCi (222 MBq)
- Slow intravenous injection over 1 minute
- Medium-energy collimator
- 172- and 247-keV photopeaks, 20% window
- Planar: anterior and posterior views from head to pelvis at 4 and 24 hours
- SPECT: abdomen and pelvis at 4 hours
- SPECT: chest, abdomen, and pelvis at 24 hours
- Additional images can be obtained at 48 hours if there is uncertainty whether abdominal activity represents pathologic or physiologic uptake.

Image Interpretation

Anterior planar image at 24 hours (**Fig. 97.1**) demonstrates a focus of intense uptake corresponding to the right orbital mass demonstrated on MRI (**Fig. 97.2**). The ^{111}In-pentetreotide scan also demonstrates a focus of uptake in the thyroid. Review of a recent CT scan (**Fig. 97.3**) reveals a 3-cm mass in the right lobe of the thyroid.

Because this is the 24-hour image, there is extensive physiologic uptake of ^{111}In-pentetreotide uptake within the bowel, as well as within the spleen, kidneys, bladder, and liver.

Differential Diagnosis

- Recurrent esthesioneuroblastoma with a thyroid metastasis
- Recurrent esthesioneuroblastoma with medullary thyroid carcinoma
- Recurrent esthesioneuroblastoma with some other thyroid cancer

Diagnosis and Clinical Follow-Up

Recurrent esthesioneuroblastoma with a Hürthle cell thyroid neoplasm. Diagnosis final, no clinical follow-up.

Discussion

Esthesioneuroblastoma is a rare tumor of the nasal vault, believed to arise from olfactory epithelium. These tumors show varying biological activity, from indolent growth with long-term survival, as in this case, to highly aggressive neoplasms with survival limited to a few months. Although the literature is limited because of the rarity of this tumor, there are reports of ^{111}In-pentetreotide uptake in primary tumors and metastases, suggesting that this modality may play a valuable role in the management of patients with esthesioneuroblastoma.

Hürthle cell carcinomas comprise approximately 3% of all thyroid malignancies. They are composed largely of oncocytic follicular cells. Among the thyroid neoplasms, somatostatin receptor expression has been most highly associated with medullary thyroid cancer, a neuroendocrine tumor. However, it has been shown that a variety of thyroid neoplasms, including Hürthle cell, papillary, and follicular tumors, can demonstrate prominent ^{111}In-pentetreotide uptake. Thus, ^{111}In-pentetreotide imaging may be useful in the evaluation of patients with thyroid tumors of varying cell lines that are not radioiodine-avid.

PEARLS AND PITFALLS_____

- Esthesioneuroblastomas are rare tumors arising from the nasal vault. They can express somatostatin receptors, so that ^{111}In-pentetreotide imaging can be useful in their management. Potential roles may include staging, assessing for residual tumor following therapy, and assessing for recurrence.
- A variety of thyroid neoplasms other than medullary thyroid cancer may express somatostatin receptors and be visualized on ^{111}In-pentetreotide imaging. Therefore, ^{111}In-pentetreotide scanning may be helpful in patients with thyroid tumors that are not radioiodine-avid, particularly if ^{18}F-FDG-PET is not available.

Suggested Reading

Bustillo A, Telischi F, Weed D, et al. Octreotide scintigraphy in the head and neck. Laryngoscope 2004;114(3):434–440

Dulguerov P, Allal AS, Calcaterra TC. Esthesioneuroblastoma: a meta-analysis and review. Lancet Oncol 2001;2(11):683–690

Görges R, Kahaly G, Müller-Brand J, Mäcke H, Roser HW, Bockisch A. Radionuclide-labeled somatostatin analogues for diagnostic and therapeutic purposes in nonmedullary thyroid cancer. Thyroid 2001;11(7):647–659

Ramsay HA, Kairemo KJA, Jekunen AP. Somatostatin receptor imaging of olfactory neuroblastoma. J Laryngol Otol 1996;110(12):1161–1163

Rostomily RC, Elias M, Deng M, et al. Clinical utility of somatostatin receptor scintigraphic imaging (octreoscan) in esthesioneuroblastoma: a case study and survey of somatostatin receptor subtype expression. Head Neck 2006;28(4):305–312

Section VI

Radioisotope Therapy

Steven C. Burrell and Annick D. Van den Abbeele

CASE 98

Clinical Presentation

A 34-year-old woman presents with a lump in her neck (**Figs. 98.1**).

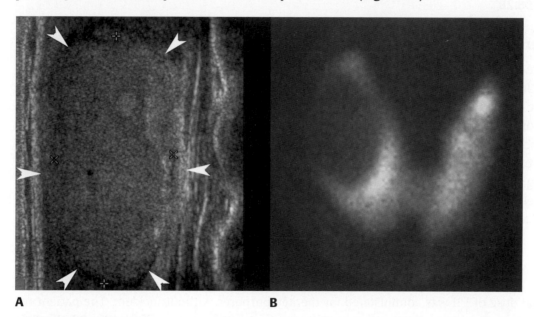

Fig. 98.1

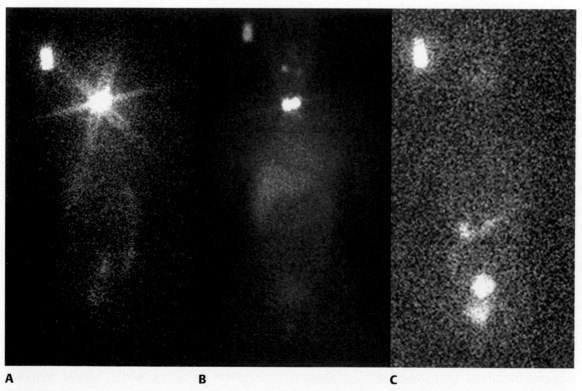

Fig. 98.2

319

Technique

- ⁹⁹ᵐTc-pertechnetate, 10 mCi (370 MBq) intravenously. Planar imaging of the neck with a pinhole collimator 20 minutes later (**Fig. 98.1B**).
- ¹³¹I, 2 mCi (74 MBq) orally. Planar imaging with a high-energy collimator 2 days later (**Fig. 98.2A, C**).
- ¹³¹I, 100 mCi (3700 MBq) orally (therapy dose). Planar imaging with a high-energy collimator 7 days later (**Fig. 98.2B**).

Image Interpretation

Coronal image from thyroid ultrasound (**Fig. 98.1A**) reveals a 3.5-cm mildly heterogeneous nodule (*arrowheads*) in the right lobe. ⁹⁹ᵐTC scan (**Fig. 98.1B**) demonstrates very little uptake in the nodule ("cold" nodule). The incidence of malignancy in cold nodules is 15 to 20%, so a fine-needle aspiration biopsy is performed, diagnosing papillary thyroid cancer. The patient undergoes thyroidectomy and is referred to nuclear medicine for therapy with ¹³¹I. A pre-therapy scan is performed (**Fig. 98.2A**) 2 days following the oral administration of ¹³¹I, 2 mCi. As expected, there is intense uptake in the thyroid remnant, resulting in some star artifact as a result of collimator penetration. There is physiologic uptake in the liver, bowel, and bladder, with no evidence of iodine-avid metastases. A rectangular area of activity to the right of the head is within a standard of known activity placed next to the patient for calculation purposes.

Therapy

A 100 mCi oral dose of ¹³¹I was administered for therapy purposes without incident. The patient returned 1 week later for a post-therapy scan with the on-board therapy dose of ¹³¹I (**Fig. 98.2B**). This confirmed the absence of metastases. A follow-up diagnostic scan (2 mCi) 6 months later (**Fig. 98.2C**) demonstrates successful ablation of the thyroid remnants and no metastases; there is physiologic uptake in the colon, bladder, and (mild uptake) in salivary glands.

Discussion

Most thyroid cancers are papillary and follicular cancers. The vast majority of these are well differentiated and as such retain many of the properties of native thyroid tissue, including the ability to concentrate iodine. This makes thyroid cancer amenable to both imaging and therapy with radioactive iodine. Imaging may be performed with either ¹²³I, which emits a 159-keV photon, or ¹³¹I, which emits a 364-keV photon. Therapy is performed with ¹³¹I via its β⁻ particle, with a maximum energy of 0.61 MeV and a half-life of 8.06 days. The evaluation of the thyroid with radioiodine was actually the first clinical application of nuclear medicine; thyroid uptake of radioiodine was measured in animals with ¹²⁸I in 1928, thyroid cancer metastases were assessed with ¹³⁰I in 1931, and the first radioisotope therapy was performed with ¹³⁰I in 1942.

The standard therapy for well-differentiated thyroid cancers is near-total or total thyroidectomy; this is followed by therapy with oral ¹³¹I because recurrence rates are higher in patients treated with surgery alone. The radioiodine therapy is administered (1) to ablate the normal thyroid gland remnants that inevitably remain following thyroidectomy and limit the sensitivity of subsequent monitoring with radioiodine imaging and the serum tumor marker thyroglobulin and (2) as adjuvant therapy for any metastases that may be present. Although no randomized, controlled studies have compared the different treatment approaches, large, retrospective, long-term follow-up studies have shown that ¹³¹I therapy results in lower recurrence rates and improved survival. An exception is in the very low-risk patient (young person with a tumor < 1.5 cm confined to the thyroid gland), in whom ^{131}I therapy has not been shown to confer a clear advantage.

The uptake of ^{131}I within thyroid cancer metastases depends on the following:

- Size of metastatic lesion
- Iodine avidity of metastasis
- Iodine turnover rate in metastasis
- Level of circulating thyroid-stimulating hormone (TSH; a higher TSH level results in greater radioiodine uptake in tumor)
- Endogenous pool of inorganic iodine (higher levels of stable iodine result in less radioiodine uptake in tumor).

Of these, the last two are modifiable, and their optimization is an essential aspect of preparation for radioiodine scanning and radioiodine therapy for thyroid cancer. Conventionally, the TSH level is maximized by inducing a hypothyroid state, which results in elevation of the endogenous TSH level through negative feedback. A hypothyroid state is achieved by withholding thyroid replacement hormone in these patients, whose thyroid glands have been removed. Replacement thyroxine (T_4) is withheld for at least 4 weeks, and replacement triiodothyronine (T_3) for at least 2 weeks. More recently, recombinant TSH has been introduced as a means of elevating circulating TSH levels without inducing a hypothyroid state, which is advantageous in certain patients—those in whom hypothyroidism is not well tolerated or is frankly dangerous because of comorbidities, and those whose TSH levels do not rise adequately in response to induced hypothyroidism. Recombinant TSH is generally approved for use in preparation for radioiodine scanning and in some guidelines for thyroid remnant ablation, but its use in preparation for the therapy of metastases is still under review. The minimization of circulating levels of stable iodine is achieved by avoiding any large iodine loads, such as radiographic contrast, for a period of about 6 weeks, and by introducing a low-iodine diet for 2 weeks before therapy; it has been shown that a low-iodine diet can double the dose of ^{131}I delivered to the thyroid gland.

PEARLS AND PITFALLS _____

- Well-differentiated thyroid cancers generally retain the ability to concentrate iodine, facilitating both imaging and therapy with radioactive iodine.
- Following surgical thyroidectomy, radioactive iodine therapy is generally indicated to ablate residual thyroid tissue and destroy any metastases, although this treatment may not be indicated in very low risk patients.
- Preparation for radioiodine scanning or therapy includes maximization of the TSH level, traditionally through the inducement of a hypothyroid state and more recently through the administration of recombinant TSH.
- Preparation also includes minimization of the endogenous iodine pool through a low-iodine diet and the avoidance of large iodine loads, such as radiographic contrast.

Suggested Reading

Cooper DS, Doherty GM, Haugen BR, et al. American Thyroid Association management guidelines for patients with thyroid nodules and differentiated thyroid cancer. Thyroid 2009;19(11):1167–1214

Dietlein M, Moka D, Schicha H. Radioiodine therapy for thyroid cancer. In: Biersack H-J, Grunwald F, eds. Thyroid Cancer. Berlin, Germany: Springer Verlag; 2005:95–126

Mazzafari EL, Kloos RT. Carcinoma of follicular epithelium: radioiodine and other treatments and outcomes. In: Braverman LE, Utiger RD, eds. The Thyroid. Philadelphia, PA: Lippincott Williams & Wilkins; 2005:934–966

Mazzaferri EL, Jhiang SM. Long-term impact of initial surgical and medical therapy on papillary and follicular thyroid cancer. Am J Med 1994;97(5):418–428

CASE 99

Clinical Presentation

A 24-year-old woman presents with palpable right-sided neck nodes. A CT scan is requested for further assessment.

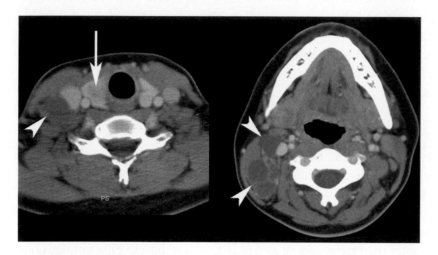

Fig. 99.1

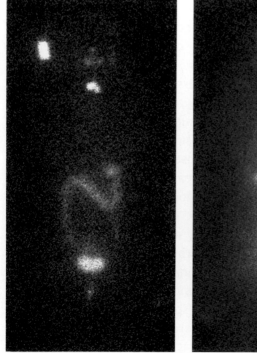

Fig. 99.2 Initial whole body scan.

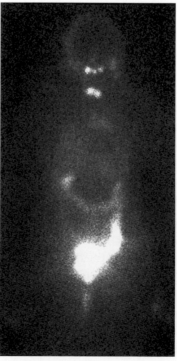

Fig. 99.3 Post-therapy scan.

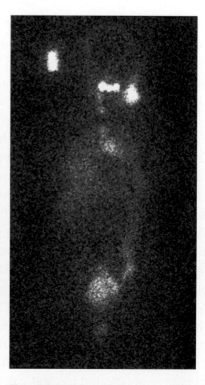

Fig. 99.4 Three years later: whole body scan.

323

Technique

- ^{131}I, 2 mCi (74 MBq) orally. Planar imaging with a high-energy collimator 2 days later (**Figs. 99.2** and **99.4**).
- ^{131}I, 150 mCi (5550 MBq) orally (therapy dose). Planar imaging with a high-energy collimator 7 days later (**Fig. 99.3**).

Image Interpretation

CT images at two levels through the neck (**Fig. 99.1**) demonstrate multiple rim-enhancing enlarged lymph nodes (*arrowheads*), many with cystic centers. A low-density lesion is also seen in the right lobe of the thyroid (*arrow*). This is biopsied and shown to be papillary thyroid cancer. Following thyroidectomy, a ^{131}I scan is performed (**Fig. 99.2**) in preparation for radioiodine therapy. This demonstrates uptake in the thyroid remnants, with no metastases identified. A rectangular area of activity to the right of the head (**Figs. 99.2** and **99.4**) is within a standard of known activity placed next to the patient for uptake calcification purposes.

Therapy

The patient was administered an oral dose of 150 mCi of ^{131}I for thyroid ablation and adjuvant therapy. A post-therapy scan 1 week later (**Fig. 99.3**) revealed diffuse uptake in the lungs and focal uptake in the mediastinum, consistent with metastases. A follow-up study 6 months later (not shown) demonstrated ongoing lung uptake, and she was re-treated with 200 mCi of ^{131}I. Subsequent scans initially showed resolution of the lung uptake. However, a follow-up scan 3 years later (**Fig. 99.4**) showed recurrence, with bilateral neck uptake, left greater than right, as well as mediastinal and diffuse lung uptake. Consequently, she was re-treated with 150 mCi of ^{131}I.

Discussion

An interesting observation in the scintigraphic imaging of thyroid cancer is that well-differentiated thyroid cancers appear as photopenic ("cold") nodules on thyroid gland scans with ^{123}I or ^{99m}Tc-pertechnetate, as in Case 98, yet appear as areas of increased uptake ("hot spots") on ^{123}I or ^{131}I scans for thyroid metastases (**Figs. 99.3** and **99.4**). This apparent paradox is readily understood by recognizing that thyroid cancer has some iodine uptake, although less than that of native thyroid tissue. As a result, thyroid cancer appears decreased against the background of native thyroid tissue on a thyroid gland scan, but increased relative to most tissues on a whole-body scan following TSH stimulation.

The ^{131}I whole body radioiodine scan is typically performed with a dose of 2 mCi. Larger doses (5–10 mCi) have been shown to cause "thyroid stunning," resulting in decreased uptake in metastases on subsequent radioiodine therapy. In addition to the pre-therapy low-dose diagnostic scan, scans are also obtained following therapy by using the large therapy dose of ^{131}I. As a result of the larger dose, the post-therapy scan may identify metastases not seen on the pre-therapy scan, as in the index case.

Several approaches have been used to determine the dose of ^{131}I for therapy. A frequently used protocol prescribes fixed empiric doses, such as 100 mCi for disease confined to the thyroid, 150 mCi in the setting of local nodal spread, and 200 mCi when there are distal metastases. More sophisticated methods include calculation of the administered activity to deliver a specified radiation dose to the mestastases, which requires an assessment of the rate of iodine turnover by the metastases and therefore serial imaging on several days following the administration of a tracer dose of radioiodine. In another more sophisticated method, calculation of the maximum tolerable dose is based on the radiation dose delivered to the bone marrow (200-rad limit), lungs (< 3 GBq when there is diffuse pulmonary uptake), or whole body (< 4.5 GBq retained at 48 hours). However, there is no convincing evidence that outcome improves in the routine scenario with the use of these analytic approaches.

In the longer term after therapy, the radioiodine scan is used to monitor the disease status. Protocols vary, but the first follow-up scan is often obtained 6 months following therapy. This scan should demonstrate successful ablation of the thyroid remnants, as in the index case. Failure to achieve ablation, often defined as more than 1% of the administered dose localizing to the thyroid bed, should lead to repeated radioiodine therapy because of the potential for residual normal thyroid tissue to limit the sensitivity of monitoring with radioiodine scans and serum thyroglobulin. Observance of metastases on radioiodine scans is also an indication for re-treatment.

PEARLS AND PITFALLS

- Radioiodine therapy for thyroid cancer was traditionally performed on an in-patient basis to limit exposure to family members and the general public. Recently, many jurisdictions have allowed therapy on an outpatient basis when it can be demonstrated that the exposure to others is minimal.
- The most common side effects of the therapy include nausea, radiation-induced inflammation, and sialadenitis.
- In patients with lung metastases, the prognosis is best when the metastases are seen only on ^{131}I images and not on radiographs or CT scans, implying very small metastases.
- The follow-up of patients with thyroid cancer includes whole-body ^{131}I scanning to assess for residual or recurrent disease, and monitoring of the serum tumor marker thyroglobulin.

Suggested Reading

Comtois R, Thériault C, Del Vecchio P. Assessment of the efficacy of iodine-131 for thyroid ablation. J Nucl Med 1993;34(11):1927–1930

Cooper DS, Doherty GM, Haugen BR, et al. American Thyroid Association management guidelines for patients with thyroid nodules and differentiated thyroid cancer. Thyroid 2009;19(11):1167–1214

Dietlein M, Moka D, Schicha H. Radioiodine therapy for thyroid cancer. In: Biersack H-J, Grunwald F, eds. Thyroid Cancer. Berlin, Germany: Springer Verlag; 2005:95–126

Mazzaferri EL, Jhiang SM. Long-term impact of initial surgical and medical therapy on papillary and follicular thyroid cancer. Am J Med 1994;97(5):418–428

Mazzafari EL, Kloos RT. Carcinoma of follicular epithelium: radioiodine and other treatments and outcomes. In: Braverman LE, Utiger RD, eds. The Thyroid. Philadelphia, PA: Lippincott Williams & Wilkins; 2005:934–966

CASE 100

Clinical Presentation

A 26-year-old woman presents with clinical and biochemical evidence of hyperthyroidism.

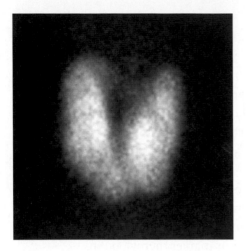

Fig. 100.1

Technique

- 99mTc-pertechnetate, 10 mCi (370 MBq) intravenously.
- Planar imaging of the neck with a pinhole collimator 20 minutes later (**Figs. 100.1** and **100.2**).

Image Interpretation

Anterior view from the 99mTc-pertechnetate scan, with pinhole collimator 4 cm from the neck (**Fig. 100.1**), demonstrates intense, increased uptake throughout the substantially enlarged thyroid. The intense uptake in the thyroid results in little visualization of the background tissues. A pyramidal lobe is appreciated extending superiorly from the upper aspect of the left lobe. A 6-hour radioiodine uptake assessment earlier the same day revealed a markedly elevated uptake of 80% (normal, 5–20%). The uptake and scan findings are consistent with Graves disease.

Therapy

An oral dose of 13 mCi of 131I was administered. The patient was still hyperthyroid 10 months later and was referred back to nuclear medicine. The repeated scan (**Fig. 100.2**) again demonstrated intense uptake throughout an enlarged thyroid, although it was smaller than on the initial study. There was again visualization of a pyramidal lobe and little visualization of the background tissues. Repeated 6-hour radioiodine uptake was 47%, significantly less than on the original study, but still elevated. She was retreated with 9 mCi of 131I, and her hyperthyroidism has not recurred.

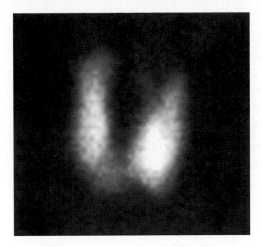

Fig. 100.2

Discussion

The treatment of hyperthyroidism with ^{131}I is the most commonly performed therapy in nuclear medicine. It has been successfully used for this purpose for more than 60 years and is the most widely used treatment modality for the definitive therapy of hyperthyroidism. It is effective, safe, and relatively inexpensive. In the majority of patients with Graves disease, a single treatment with ^{131}I is successful in eliminating thyrotoxicosis. Although many patients may become euthyroid in the short term, ultimately most proceed to hypothyroidism. If hyperthyroidism persists, the treatment can be repeated as needed. Many clinicians will initially treat Graves disease with antithyroid medications in the hope of a spontaneous remission, but ultimately most patients proceed to definitive therapy with [131]I. Radioiodine therapy is also the primary treatment of choice in toxic nodular goiter. An exception is in patients who have a large multinodular goiter with tracheal compression, in whom surgical resection is indicated.

To maximize the efficacy of ^{131}I therapy, antithyroid medications must be withheld for 4 days (this may vary somewhat with local practice) before treatment and for several days afterward. Many patients are on β-blocker therapy to mitigate the effects of hyperthyroidism, and these drugs need not be withheld. Large amounts of iodine should be avoided before therapy; most notably, iodinated radiographic contrast should not be administered within 6 weeks before therapy.

Orally administered radioiodine is incorporated into the thyroid gland and deposited at the cell–colloid interface, where the emission of β⁻ particles inhibits follicular cell function and damages reproduction mechanisms. The radiation dose delivered to the thyroid gland depends largely on the orally administered activity of ^{131}I, the subsequent uptake within the gland, the size of the gland, and the residence time in the gland. Several approaches have been used to determine the activity administered for radioiodine therapy. They can be grouped into three general categories, listed in increasing level of complexity:

1. A fixed dose is given to all patients.
2. The size of the gland and the radioiodine uptake are incorporated into the plan. The larger the gland, the greater the amount of activity required to deliver the same dose on a volumetric basis,

and the greater the percentage of uptake, the smaller the administered activity required to deliver the same scheme uses the following formula or a similar variant:

A. Administered Activity (mCi) = $\dfrac{0.1 \text{ mCi/g} \times \text{Size of Thyroid Gland (g)} \times 100\%}{\text{Radioiodine Uptake (\%)}}$

B. The size of the thyroid gland is typically estimated through palpation, and the gland size is expressed as a multiple of normal, with a normal size of the gland taken to be 20 g.

3. The residence time in the gland can be incorporated into the analysis by administering a tracer dose of ^{131}I and performing scans on several subsequent days with measurement of the rate of clearance from the gland. This level of complexity is not generally warranted.

PEARLS AND PITFALLS

- Antithyroid medications should be withheld for at least 4 days before therapy.
- Pregnancy and breast-feeding are contraindications to the administration of [131]I.
- Primary side effects include the induction of hypothyroidism, radiation-induced sore throat, and a transient increase in hyperthyroidism secondary to the release of preformed thyroid hormone. In the extreme case, this can result in thyroid storm, which is extremely rare. Patients should be alerted to watch for increasing symptoms and to seek medical attention if symptoms increase significantly.
- The induction of hypothyroidism is a frequent consequence of radioiodine therapy, and patients must be advised of the potential need for lifelong replacement thyroid hormone and medical follow-up.
- Therapy for hyperthyroidism is typically performed on an outpatient basis. Patient education is required to ensure minimization of radiation exposure to family members and the general public in accordance with local practice.
- The majority of patients will be rendered euthyroid or hypothyroid with a single dose of [131]I. Because of the delayed effects of the therapy, a period of at least 3 months should be allowed before repeated treatment for persistent hyperthyroidism is undertaken.

Suggested Reading

Cooper DS. Treatment of thyrotoxicosis. In: Braverman LE, Utiger RD, eds. The Thyroid. Philadelphia, PA: Lippincott Williams & Wilkins; 2005:665–694

Maurer AH, Charkes ND. Radioiodine treatment for nontoxic multinodular goiter. J Nucl Med 1999;40(8):1313–1316

Tuttle RM, Becker DV, Hurley JR. Radioiodine treatment of thyroid disease. In: Sandler MP, Coleman RE, Patton JA, Wackers FJTh, Gottschalk A, eds. Diagnostic Nuclear Medicine. Philadelphia, PA: Lippincott Williams & Wilkins; 2003:653–670

CASE 101

Clinical Presentation

A 30-year-old man with refractory low-grade non-Hodgkin lymphoma is referred to nuclear medicine for radioimmunotherapy.

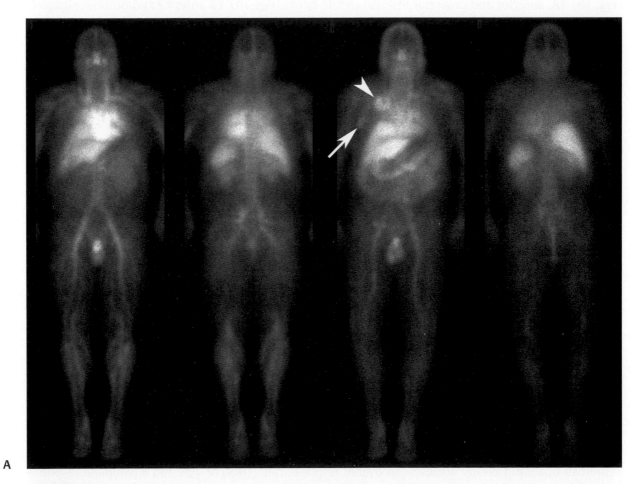

Fig. 101.1

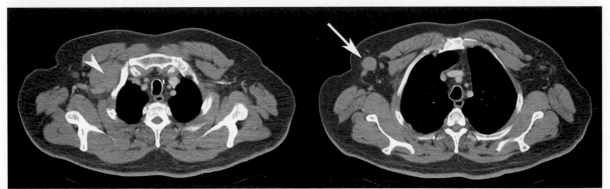

Fig. 101.2

Technique

- ^{111}In-ibritumomab tiuxetan 5 mCi intravenously. Planar imaging with a medium-energy collimator at 2 hours (**Fig. 101.1A**) and 48 hours (**Fig. 101.1B**).

Image Interpretation

The patient was administered unlabeled rituximab, 250 mg/m^2, to bind peripheral binding sites. He was then administered ^{111}In-ibritumomab tiuxetan, 5 mCi, and imaging was performed at 2 hours (**Fig. 101.1A,** anterior and posterior images) and 48 hours (**Fig. 101.1B** anterior and posterior images) to confirm appropriate biodistribution. This was indeed demonstrated, with uptake predominantly in the blood pool, liver, and spleen on the early images, and less blood pool activity (e.g., see the heart) and persistent liver and spleen uptake on the delayed images. In addition, the delayed images reveal uptake in two sites of disease, (**A**) a right supraclavicular lymph node (*arrowhead*) and (**B**) a right axillary lymph node (*arrow*), also shown on the CT scan (**Fig. 101.2**).

Therapy

Seven days following the administration of the ^{111}In-ibritumomab tiuxetan, the patient was again administered unlabeled rituximab, 250 mg/m^2, to bind peripheral binding sites. This was followed by the administration of a therapy dose of ibritumomab tiuxetan labeled with the β$^-$ emitter ^{90}Y-ibritumomab, 0.4 mCi/kg, by slow intravenous injection over 10 minutes.

Discussion

In the past few years, therapies have been developed that use monoclonal antibodies as vehicles to deliver radioisotopes to surface receptors on tumor cells, a process known as radioimmumotherapy. The premise is that radioactivity can be targeted to disseminated tumor sites while radiation to nontarget organs is minimized. Numerous radiolabeled antibodies have been developed for both hematologic and solid tumors. The most successful have been two agents directed at the CD20 antigen of B-cell lymphomas, ^{90}Y-ibritumomab tiuxetan (Zevalin, Spectrum Pharmaceuticals) and ^{131}I-tositumomab (Bexxar, GlaxoSmithKline). Both are registered for the treatment of relapsed or refractory low-grade, follicular, or transformed non-Hodgkin lymphoma, including rituximab-refractory disease.

The nonradiolabeled anti-CD20 monoclonal antibody rituximab has become a widely used therapy for patients with non-Hodgkin lymphoma. In patients with disease refractory to rituximab, ^{90}Y-ibritumomab tiuxetan therapy achieved an overall response rate (ORR) of 74% and a complete response rate (CRR) of 15% (Witzig, Flinn, et al., 2002). Similar results have been found with ^{131}I-tositumomab (Horning et al., 2005). In a phase III randomized, controlled trial of rituximab versus ^{90}Y-ibritumomab tiuxetan, the radiolabeled monoclonal antibody achieved a significantly higher ORR (80% vs 56%) and CRR (30% vs 16%) than did the unlabeled version, confirming the additional benefit derived from the local delivery of radiotherapy beyond that provided by the monoclonal antibody alone (Witzig, Gordon, et al., 2002).

Practically speaking, there are several similarities and several differences between the two agents. Both ibritumomab and tositumomab are murine antibodies. Both are used in a regimen in which the patient first receives nonradiolabeled ("cold") anti-CD20 to occupy CD20 receptors on circulating B cells and in the spleen, thus enhancing delivery of the radiolabeled monoclonal antibody to tumor cells. For ^{131}I-tositumomab, the cold anti-CD20 is also tositumomab (murine), whereas for ^{90}Y-ibritumomab, the cold anti-CD20 is rituximab, a chimeric antibody. Patients being treated with ^{131}I-tositumomab require thyroid blockade with Lugol solution or the equivalent to avoid thyroid damage from free ^{131}I. As ^{131}I is both a β- and a gamma emitter, additional radiation safety precautions are required following therapy with ^{131}I-tositumomab.

For ^{131}I-tositumomab, patient-specific dosimetry calculations are done the week before the planned therapy by administering a low dose of ^{131}I-tositumomab and performing whole-body scans at three time points over the ensuing days to calculate the rate of clearance. For ^{90}Y-ibritumomab tiuxetan, the dose is based on the patient's weight, without assessment of individual clearance. The dose is reduced for both agents if the platelet counts are low. Some jurisdictions, including the United States, require pre-therapy scans to be obtained when ^{90}Y-ibritumomab tiuxetan is used; these assess for altered biodistribution, which is a contraindication to therapy. As ^{90}Y does not emit gamma photons for imaging, the pre-therapy scan is performed with ^{111}In-ibritumomab tiuxetan. Imaging is performed at 2 to 24 hours and at 48 to 72 hours following administration, with an optional third scan at 90 to 120 hours. Examples of altered biodistribution include accelerated clearance from the blood pool with poor visualization of the blood pool on the 2- to 24-hour scan, and uptake in kidneys, lungs, or bowel greater than liver uptake on the later images. As in the index case, uptake in tumor sites is frequently seen on the delayed images, although this is not a prerequisite for therapy.

As with many forms of radioisotope therapy, marrow suppression and resultant decreases in platelets and white blood cells are common side effects, and nadirs are reached at about 4 to 6 weeks. Therefore, close hematologic follow-up is necessary. Common side effects include fever, chills, and asthenia. These can often be mitigated by slowing the rate of infusion. Severe hypersensitivity reactions are uncommon but must be anticipated, and the therapy should be administered only in a setting where management of such a response is possible. Side effects can be reduced by first treating with diphenhydramine and acetaminophen. HAMA (human anti-mouse antibody) and HACA (human anti-chimeric antibody) responses can occur and may interfere with or preclude subsequent diagnostic or therapeutic studies with monoclonal antibodies.

PEARLS AND PITFALLS

- Radioimmunotherapy involves the delivery of systemic radiotherapy to disseminated tumor sites via the administration of a therapeutic radioisotope attached to a monoclonal antibody directed at a surface antigen on tumor cells.
- The most successful agents to date, ^{90}Y-ibritumomab tiuxetan and ^{131}I-tositumomab, use antibodies directed at CD20 antigens, which occur on normal B cells and more than 90% of lymphomas derived from B cells.
- Both agents have demonstrated significant efficacy in the setting of relapsed or refractory low-grade lymphoma. The role of these agents earlier in the course of the disease is still being developed, with encouraging initial results.
- Contraindications include myelosuppression (platelet count < 100,000/mm^3) or expectation of myelosuppression (> 25% marrow involvement), known type 1 hypersensitivity or anaphylactic reaction to murine proteins or to any component of the therapeutic regimen, and pregnancy.
- Additional radiolabeled monoclonal antibodies directed at hematologic malignancies and solid tumors are under investigation.

Suggested Reading

Horning SJ, Younes A, Jain V, et al. Efficacy and safety of tositumomab and iodine-131 tositumomab (Bexxar) in B-cell lymphoma, progressive after rituximab. J Clin Oncol 2005;23(4):712–719

Kaminski MS, Zelenetz AD, Press OW, et al. Pivotal study of iodine I 131 tositumomab for chemotherapy-refractory low-grade or transformed low-grade B-cell non-Hodgkin's lymphomas. J Clin Oncol 2001;19(19):3918–3928

Wahl RL. Tositumomab and (131)I therapy in non-Hodgkin's lymphoma. J Nucl Med 2005;46(Suppl 1):128S–140S

Witzig TE, Flinn IW, Gordon LI, et al. Treatment with ibritumomab tiuxetan radioimmunotherapy in patients with rituximab-refractory follicular non-Hodgkin's lymphoma. J Clin Oncol 2002;20(15): 3262–3269

Witzig TE, Gordon LI, Cabanillas F, et al. Randomized controlled trial of yttrium-90-labeled ibritumomab tiuxetan radioimmunotherapy versus rituximab immunotherapy for patients with relapsed or refractory low-grade, follicular, or transformed B-cell non-Hodgkin's lymphoma. J Clin Oncol 2002;20(10):2453–2463

CASE 102

Clinical Presentation

A 76-year-old man with prostate cancer and pain from bone metastases undergoes palliative external beam radiotherapy to his left hip with symptomatic relief. However, the symptoms recur and involve multiple sites despite optimal medical treatment. He is deemed not to be a candidate for further external beam radiotherapy because of the multifocal nature of his symptoms, and he is referred to nuclear medicine for systemic radioisotope therapy.

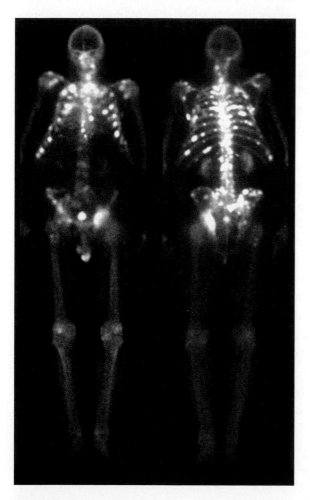

Fig. 102.1

Technique

- ^{99m}Tc-MDP, 25 mCi (925 MBq) intravenously. Planar imaging with a low-energy, high-resolution collimator 3 hours later (**Figs. 102.1** and **102.2A**).
- ^{89}Sr (148 MBq) intravenously (therapy dose).

Image Interpretation

The ^{99m}Tc-MDP bone scan (**Fig. 102.1**) reveals numerous sites of metastatic disease, predominantly within the axial skeleton.

Therapy

The patient was administered ^{89}Sr, 4 mCi, by slow intravenous injection over 2 minutes. Following therapy, he became pain free for a period of about 8 months. His pain subsequently recurred. Given the favorable response to the initial ^{89}Sr therapy, this treatment was repeated.

Discussion

In the later stages of malignancy, pain from bone metastases is a common symptom and often adversely affects the quality of life. When disseminated metastases result in multiple sites of bone pain, external beam radiotherapy is no longer practical. In this setting, radiotherapy with systemically administered radiopharmaceuticals has proved successful in alleviating bone pain. Originally performed with sodium phosphate ^{32}P, the most commonly used agents today are: ^{89}Sr, administered as strontium chloride ^{89}Sr; ^{153}Sm, administered as ^{153}Sm-EDTMP (ethylene diamine tetramethylene phosphonate); and less commonly, ^{186}Re, administered as ^{186}Re-etidronate (^{186}Re-HEDP [hydroxyethylene diphosphonate]). All are incorporated into bone similarly to bone-scanning agents and so are preferentially concentrated at areas of increased bone turnover, such as sites of metastatic disease. These agents are β$^-$ emitters and as such deliver local β$^-$ radiation at sites of osseous metastatic disease throughout the body. Recently, α particle emitters such as ^{223}Ra have been investigated. Compared with therapy with β$^-$ emitters, therapy with α emitters is expected to have the advantages of greater tumor damage, due to higher linear energy transfer (LET), and less bone marrow suppression, as the very short particle range leads to less cross fire into bone marrow from the sites of radiopharmaceutical deposition in cortical bone. The key physical parameters of these radioisotopes are listed in **Table 102.1**.

In addition to being a β$^-$ emitter, ^{153}Sm is also a gamma emitter, which allows imaging with a standard gamma camera. Because of similarities in mechanism of uptake, the image generated will generally mirror the bone scan obtained with a ^{99m}Tc-labeled diphosphonate, such as ^{99m}Tc-MDP. **Figure 102.2** demonstrates this in a different patient (**Fig. 102.2A**, ^{99m}Tc-MDP bone scan; **Fig. 102.2B**, scan with therapy dose of ^{153}Sm). However, the gamma emission does lead to additional radiation protection issues with respect to persons exposed to the patient.

The therapy is intended as a palliative treatment of the bone pain and has not been shown to increase survival. Therapy should be undertaken in the setting of a multidisciplinary and multimodality approach to pain management. Response rates range from 60 to 84%, and the mean duration of response typically ranges from 2 to 5 months. The onset of pain relief is 7 to 14 days, so this therapy is not indicated for acute pain relief. Patients should have a life expectancy of at least 2 months. Patients whose symptoms are relieved and subsequently recur may be re-treated, as in the index case. The most common side effect is bone marrow suppression. Platelet levels and white blood cell counts should be checked before therapy and monitored every 2 weeks for 8 weeks following therapy, as the nadir typically occurs about 6 weeks following treatment. Some patients may experience a temporary increase in pain within the first few days following therapy. This flare response is usually mild and can be managed with an increase in analgesics. A standard dose of 4 mCi is usually administered for ^{89}Sr, and 1 mCi/kg for ^{153}Sm.

Table 102.1 Physical Properties of Key Radioisotopes Used in Metastatic Bone Pain Therapy

Radioisotope	Half-Life	Maximum Energy, MeV	Maximum Range
Phosphorus 32	14.3 d	1.71 (β^-)	8.5 mm
Strontium 89	50.5 d	1.46 (β^-)	7 mm
Samarium 153	46.3 h	0.81 (β^-)	4 mm
Rhenium 186	16.9 h	1.07 (β^-)	10 mm
Radium 223	11.4 d	5.78 (α, average)	< 10 μm

PEARLS AND PITFALLS

- Radioisotope therapy of bone metastases provides some reduction in pain in approximately 75% of patients.
- Patients should have bony pain at multiple sites, corresponding with uptake on a recent bone scan, to be considered for treatment.
- The most common side effect is marrow suppression. Patients should have adequate platelet and white blood cell levels in blood obtained no more than 7 days before therapy.
- Radioisotope therapy is not indicated for the treatment of pain arising from spinal cord compression or pathologic fracture. When these processes are present or felt to be impending, radioisotope therapy for other sites of pain should be undertaken only in conjunction with management directed at these processes and only after acute issues have been dealt with.

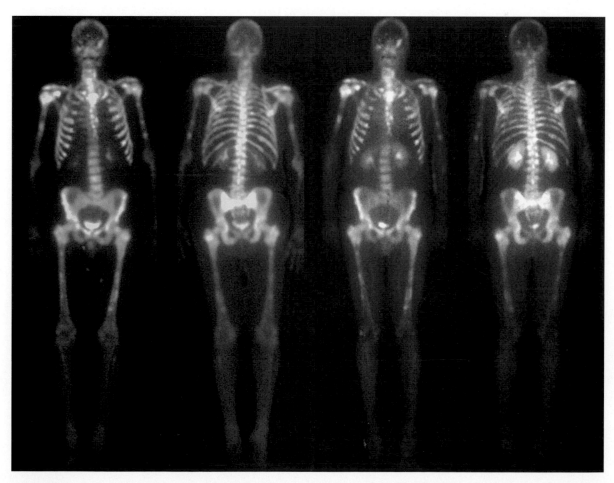

A   B

Fig. 102.2

Suggested Reading

Bodei L, Lam M, Chiesa C, et al. European Association of Nuclear Medicine (EANM). EANM procedure guideline for treatment of refractory metastatic bone pain. Eur J Nucl Med Mol Imaging 2008;35(10):1934–1940

Lewington VJ. Bone-seeking radionuclides for therapy. J Nucl Med 2005;46(1, Suppl 1):38S–47S

McEwan AJB. Unsealed source therapy of painful bone metastases: an update. Semin Nucl Med 1997;27(2):165–182

Nilsson S, Franzén L, Parker C, et al. Bone-targeted radium-223 in symptomatic, hormone-refractory prostate cancer: a randomised, multicentre, placebo-controlled phase II study. Lancet Oncol 2007;8(7):587–594

Pandit-Taskar N, Batraki M, Divgi CR. Radiopharmaceutical therapy for palliation of bone pain from osseous metastases. J Nucl Med 2004;45(8):1358–1365

Society of Nuclear Medicine Procedure Guideline for Palliative Treatment of Painful Bone Metastases version 3.0, approved January 25, 2003. http://interactive.snm.org/docs/pg_ch25_0403.pdf. Accessed April 21, 2010

CASE 103

Clinical Presentation

A 56-year-old man with rheumatoid arthritis presents with right knee pain refractory to conventional therapy.

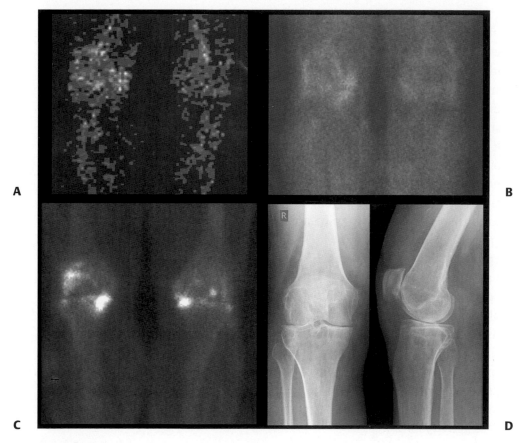

Fig. 103.1

Technique

- ^{99m}Tc-MDP, 25 mCi (925 MBq) intravenously, followed by 60-second dynamic flow (**Fig. 103.1A**), 60-second pool (**Fig. 103.1B**), and bone phase imaging 3 hours later (**Fig. 103.1C**).

Image Interpretation

Flow (**Fig. 103.1A**) and pool (**Fig. 103.1B**) images from a ^{99m}Tc-MDP bone scan demonstrate significantly increased blood flow to the right knee due to inflammation. The delayed bone phase image from the bone scan (**Fig. 103.1C**) demonstrates increased uptake, particularly in the medial compartment and the patellofemoral joint. There is increased uptake to a lesser extent in the left knee. Anterior and lateral radiographs (**Fig. 103.1D**) reveal marked joint space narrowing with minimal osseous proliferation as well as a joint effusion, consistent with the rheumatoid arthritis.

337

Therapy

Following local anesthesia and sterile preparation, a 22-gauge needle was used to enter the knee compartment from a patellofemoral approach. Straw-colored fluid was aspirated. One milliliter of radiographic contrast was injected, and fluoroscopy was performed to confirm the intra-articular position. ^{90}Y, 5 mCi, was then injected into the joint, along with 1 mL of 0.5% bupivacaine and 80 mg of depomethylprednisolone.

Discussion

Radiosynovectomy, first performed in 1952, is an effective therapy for pain, swelling, and stiffness due to arthritis associated with synovial hypertrophy. The technique has most commonly been used in the knees, but it has also been used in many other joints, including the hips, shoulders, elbows, and small joints of the fingers. Radiosynovectomy may be considered when patients fail to respond to systemic therapies and local (intra-articular) corticosteroid therapy. In this setting, surgical synovectomy has traditionally been performed, but radiosynovectomy is an equally effective option with a lower cost, less invasiveness, and shorter rehabilitation time. Radiosynovectomy has most commonly been performed in patients with rheumatoid arthritis, but it is also effective in patients with seronegative and crystalline arthritides, pigmented villonodular synovitis, or hemarthrosis and synovitis associated with hemophilia. Although not indicated routinely in osteoarthritis, radiosynovectomy is also effective in this entity when it is significantly associated with synovial inflammation. Radiosynovectomy should be undertaken within a multidisciplinary approach to pain management that includes rheumatology or orthopedics along with nuclear medicine.

Following sterile preparation and local anesthesia, the joint is entered with standard aspiration/injection techniques; typically, a 22-gauge needle is used. Most physicians will use fluoroscopy and the injection of radiographic contrast to confirm that the joint has been entered, as it is important not to inject the radiopharmaceutical into surrounding tissues. The intra-articular position can also be confirmed through aspiration of joint fluid or by injection of ^{99m}Tc sulfur colloid with imaging in the nuclear medicine suite. Following injection of the therapy radiopharmaceutical, a steroid such as depo-methylprednisolone is typically injected to help prevent radiation-induced synovitis and to relieve pain. Pain is also relieved by the intra-articular injection of a local anesthetic such as bupivacaine. After therapy, the patient is placed on bed rest for 2 days to immobilize the joint and limit lymphatic uptake, followed by limited activity for 2 weeks.

The injected radiopharmaceutical rapidly undergoes phagocytosis by synoviocytes lining the surface of the synovium. ^{90}Y has generally replaced chromic phosphate ^{32}P as the agent of choice. In some jurisdictions, additional agents, such as ^{186}Re and ^{169}Er are available. The use of different radiopharmaceuticals with different energies and path lengths makes it possible to tailor the agent to the size of the joint, with ^{90}Y-colloid used for the knee joint, ^{186}Re for medium-size joints, and ^{169}Er for small joints, such as those of the hand. The intent in this regimen is to match the radiation path length to the thickness of the synovium, to maximize synovial exposure while limiting damage to the underlying cartilage.

Radiosynovectomy has proved to be an effective therapy. In a review of 53 studies in patients with rheumatoid arthritis, 1-year follow-up revealed good or excellent results in 60 to 80% of patients. Similar result rates have been seen in other diseases. Many patients will experience rapid pain relief, likely a consequence of the injected steroids and local anesthetic. Conversely, there may be a short-term increase in pain as a result of radiation-induced synovitis. Symptomatic improvement attributable to the radiopharmaceutical may be delayed up to 1 month, with further decreases in symptoms out to

6 months. If the therapy is successful but symptoms recur, the treatment can be repeated, with at least 6 months allowed between therapies.

PEARLS AND PITFALLS _____

- Radiosynovectomy is an effective therapy for patients with pain associated with synovial inflammation in rheumatoid and other forms of arthritis.
- The procedure is indicated in patients whose pain is refractory to conventional systemic therapies and intra-articular steroid injections.
- Contraindications include pregnancy or breast-feeding; infection of the joint, periarticular tissues, or overlying skin; a ruptured Baker cyst; massive hemarthrosis; and intra-articular fracture.
- Potential side effects include those associated with joint aspiration (infection, bleeding), deep venous thrombosis resulting from bed rest, and rarely radiation necrosis.
- If symptoms recur, the treatment can be repeated 6 months or more following initial therapy.

Suggested Reading

Clunie G, Fischer M; EANM. EANM procedure guidelines for radiosynovectomy. Eur J Nucl Med Mol Imaging 2003;30(3):BP12–BP16

Deutsch E, Brodack JW, Deutsch KF. Radiation synovectomy revisited. Eur J Nucl Med 1993;20(11): 1113–1127

Schneider P, Farahati J, Reiners C. Radiosynovectomy in rheumatology, orthopedics, and hemophilia. J Nucl Med 2005;46(1, Suppl 1):48S–54S

CASE 104

Clinical Presentation

A 45-year-old woman presents with a carcinoid tumor and multiple liver metastases. Because of the multifocal nature of her disease and subacutely progressive symptoms despite optimal chemotherapy, she is referred to Nuclear Medicine for consideration of systemic radioisotope therapy.

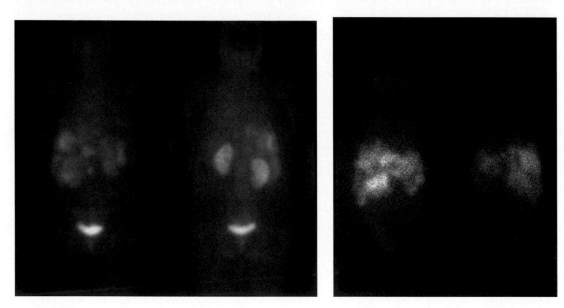

Fig. 104.1   Fig. 104.2

Technique

- ^{111}In-pentetreotide, 3 mCi (111 MBq) intravenously. Planar imaging with a medium-energy collimator 48 hours after injection (**Fig. 104.1**).
- ^{131}I-MIBG, 0.5 mCi (18 MBq) intravenously. Planar imaging with a high-energy collimator 48 hours after injection (**Fig. 104.2**).
- ^{123}I-MIBG, 6 mCi (222 MBq) intravenously. Planar imaging with a low-energy, high-resolution collimator 24 hours after injection (**Fig. 104.3**).

Image Interpretation

The original ^{111}In-pentetreotide scan (**Fig. 104.1**) reveals numerous areas of increased and decreased uptake throughout the liver, in keeping with active and necrotic carcinoid metastases, respectively. Because therapy with ^{131}I-MIBG is being considered, it is necessary to demonstrate that all active tumor sites are MIBG-avid, and consequently a ^{131}I-MIBG scan is performed (**Fig. 104.2**), confirming that this is the case.

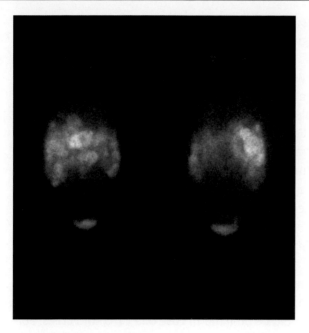

Fig. 104.3

Therapy

The patient was administered a slow intravenous infusion of 150 mCi of ^{131}I-MIBG without any immediate side effects. Her platelet count decreased from 215,000/mm³ before therapy to a nadir of 94,000/mm³ 8 weeks later, then rebounded to 351,000/mm³ another 8 weeks later. She subsequently reported mild relief of her symptoms. A follow-up MIBG scan 3 months after therapy, this time labeled with ^{123}I rather than [131]I (because of a change in institutional procedure) demonstrated stability of her disease (**Fig. 104.3**). There was no significant change in size of the metastases on CT. She was then re-treated with ^{131}I-MIBG as the next step in a multiple-dose regimen.

Discussion

Tumors arising from the neuroendocrine system are often treated surgically. However, when there is disseminated disease, treatment options include chemotherapy and octreotide therapy. Carcinoid tumors in particular often present with extensive metastatic disease. When conventional therapies are no longer effective, treatment with high doses of ^{131}I-MIBG may offer beneficial palliative effects. MIBG is a combination of the benzyl group of bretylium and the guanidine group of guanethidine. It is similar in structure and function to norepinephrine, and consequently MIBG is taken up in cells of neural crest origin, including pheochromocytomas, paragangliomas, and neuroblastomas. Uptake may also be seen in other neuroendocrine tumors, such as carcinoid tumors and medullary thyroid cancer. MIBG can be labeled with either ^{131}I or ^{123}I, allowing gamma imaging of neuroendocrine tumors. However, ^{131}I is also a β⁻ emitter (half-life of 8.04 days, maximum energy of 0.61 MeV, and mean particle range of 0.45 mm), and the administration of large doses of ^{131}I-MIBG allows radioisotope therapy of disseminated metastases.

Not all of the above tumors will necessarily concentrate MIBG in any given patient, and consequently it is necessary to obtain a ^{123}I-MIBG or ^{131}I-MIBG scan before therapy to ascertain that all known sites of disease are MIBG-avid. The primary aims of the therapy are palliative. In a review of 98 patients who underwent ^{131}I-MIBG for progressive metastatic carcinoid tumor, Safford et al. (1988) reported a decrease in symptoms (flushing, diarrhea) in 49%. A survival increase was reported in those who had a decrease in symptoms. It is uncommon to elicit a significant reduction in tumor size; CT has shown a reduction in only 10 to 15% of patients.

Several different protocols have been used. Most use an initial dose of 100 to 300 mCi of ^{131}I-MIBG, with subsequent treatments at 3- to 6-month intervals as long as there are beneficial results and marrow suppression and other side effects are acceptable. A maximum cumulative dose of 1.0 to 1.2 Ci is recommended to avoid permanent marrow toxicity. Patient preparation includes stopping medications that can interfere with MIBG uptake. The list of such medications is extensive (Giammarile et al., 2008). Because of the potential for permanent thyroid damage from free ^{131}I, thyroid blockade procedures must be instituted, typically with potassium iodide capsules or Lugol solution, beginning 24 to 48 hours before therapy and continuing for 10 to 15 days after treatment. The most common short-term side effects are nausea and emesis, and prophylactic antiemetics are advised. Therapy should be performed by physicians, technicians, nurses, and radiation safety personnel familiar with the procedure and potential side-effects. The radiopharmaceutical is infused slowly over 45 minutes to 4 hours. Vital signs must be monitored throughout. MIBG-induced hypertension can often be managed by simply stopping the infusion. However, α- or β-blockers may be required and should be on hand before therapy is started. When carcinoids are treated, octreotide should be on hand in case of a carcinoid crisis. Following therapy, a whole-body scan may be obtained with the on-board therapy dose of ^{131}I-MIBG a few days later. Weekly blood work should be followed for 8 weeks to monitor for suppression of platelets and white blood cells. Radiation safety precautions must be observed by caregivers and family members in the first few days following therapy in accordance with local guidelines.

Many neuroendocrine tumors will concentrate the somatostatin analog ^{111}In-pentetreotide but not ^{131}I-MIBG, so there is interest in performing radioisotope therapy with radiolabeled somatostatin agents. Unlike ^{131}I, ^{111}In is not a β- emitter. Therapy with ^{111}In-pentetreotide relies on radiation from auger and conversion electrons, which have a much shorter particle range and hence lower tissue penetration. More recently, somatostatin analogs labeled with β- emitters have been developed, including ^{90}Y-DOTA-Tyr[3]-octreotide, ^{90}Y-DOTA-lanreotide, and ^{177}Lu-DOTA-Tyr[3]-octreotate.

PEARLS AND PITFALLS

- The administration of ^{131}I-MIBG to patients with neuroendocrine tumors is intended as a symptomatic treatment for those whose known neuroendocrine tumors sites have all been shown to accumulate ^{131}I-MIBG on a pre-therapy scan.
- Numerous medications may interfere with the uptake of ^{131}I-MIBG and must be stopped before therapy. Thyroid blockade is also necessary before treatment.
- Vital signs must be carefully monitored as MIBG administration can result in unstable blood pressure. Short-acting α- or β-blockers should be on hand when catecholamine-secreting tumors are treated, and (nonradiolabeled) octreotide should be available when carcinoid tumors are treated.
- Common side effects are nausea and vomiting as well as bone marrow suppression. Marrow suppression typically reaches a nadir about 6 weeks after therapy. Marrow suppression is particularly prevalent when bone marrow is involved by tumor.
- Therapy with ^{131}I-MIBG is usually undertaken in a regimen of repeated doses, with a few months between doses to allow bone marrow recovery.

Suggested Reading

Giammarile F, Chiti A, Lassmann M, Brans B, Flux G; EANM. EANM procedure guidelines for 131I-meta-iodobenzylguanidine (131I-mIBG) therapy. Eur J Nucl Med Mol Imaging 2008;35(5):1039–1047

Kaltsas G, Rockall A, Papadogias D, Reznek R, Grossman AB. Recent advances in radiological and radio-nuclide imaging and therapy of neuroendocrine tumours. Eur J Endocrinol 2004;151(1):15–27

Pashankar FD, O'Dorisio MS, Menda Y. MIBG and somatostatin receptor analogs in children: current concepts on diagnostic and therapeutic use. J Nucl Med 2005;46(Suppl 1):55S–61S

Safford SD, Coleman RE, Gockerman JP, et al. Iodine-131 metaiodobenzylguanidine treatment for meta-static carcinoid: results in 98 patients. Cancer 2004;101(9):1987–1993

Section VII

Inflammation/Infection Imaging

M. Elizabeth Oates

CASE 105

Clinical Presentation

A 68-year-old woman presents with fever of unknown origin. Because of limited venous access, ^{67}Ga is selected as the radiopharmaceutical of choice for evaluation.

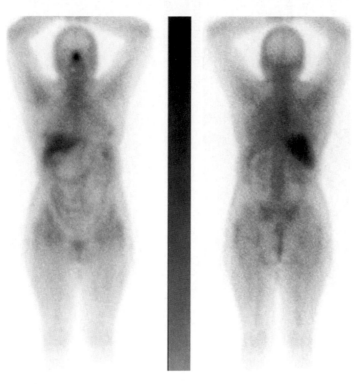

Fig. 105.1 Whole-body image, anterior, and posterior projections, ^{67}Ga.

Technique

- A 7.5 mCi dose of ^{67}Ga-citrate is injected intravenously 3 days before scan.
- Whole-body imaging in anterior and posterior projections
  - Dual-detector gamma camera
  - Medium-energy collimators
  - Energy peak at 93-, 185-, and 300-keV photopeaks

Image Interpretation

Whole-body images **(Fig. 105.1)** demonstrate a normal biodistribution pattern. Typically, ^{67}Ga localizes in the nose, salivary glands, lacrimal glands, breasts, liver, spleen, genitalia, and skeleton; it is not unusual to have varying degrees of large-bowel activity. No abnormal tracer localization is seen to suggest active inflammation/infection.

Table 105.1 Comparison of Radiopharmaceuticals for Inflammation/Infection Imaging

	67Ga-Citrate	111In-WBCs	99mTc-WBCs
Advantages	No preparation (readily available)	No excretion by GU and GI tracts	Photopeak of 140 keV ideal for imaging
	Localization is by: hyperemia/capillary permeability/iron-binding proteins/siderophores	Wait only 18–24 h prior to imaging	Wait only 2–4 h prior to imaging
	(Independent of WBCs)	—	Dose favorable for children
Disadvantages	Evaluation of abdomen limited by excretion into GU and GI tracts	In vitro labeling: draw blood, isolate WBCs, incubate with 111In-oxine; reinject labeled WBCs	In vitro labeling: draw blood, isolate WBCs, incubate with 99mTc-HMPAO; reinject labeled WBCs
	Wait 48–72 h prior to imaging	Localization dependent on migration of WBCs/chemotaxis	Localization dependent on migration of WBCs/chemotaxis
	Photopeaks: 93/185/300 keV are less ideal for imaging	Photopeaks: 173/247 keV less ideal for imaging, low photon flux	Evaluation of abdomen limited by excretion into GU and GI tracts
	—	Leukopenic patients are excluded	Leukopenic patients are excluded
Clinical indications	Chronic/nonpyogenic abscess (outside abdomen)	Acute/pyogenic abscess; abdominal or renal abscess	—
	—	Inflammatory bowel disease	Inflammatory bowel disease
	Pulmonary infection and lymphadenitis in HIV+	Nonpulmonary infection in HIV+	Nonpulmonary infection in HIV+
	Chronic bone and joint infection	Acute/complicated/prosthetic bone and joint infection	—
	—	Infected catheters/vascular grafts	—
	Granulomatous disease (sarcoidosis)	Occult sepsis	—

Abbreviations: GI, gastrointestinal; GU, genitourinary; HIV, human immunodeficiency virus; HMPAO, hexamethylpropylene amine oxime (exametazime); IV, intravenous; WBC, white blood cell.

Differential Diagnosis

- Normal ^{67}Ga scan

Diagnosis and Clinical Follow-Up

Normal. No active inflammation/infection identified. Diagnosis final, no clinical follow-up.

Discussion

The best-known and most widely used inflammation/infection–seeking radiopharmaceuticals are ^{67}Ga and autologous white blood cells (WBCs) radioactively labeled with either ^{111}In or ^{99m}Tc. Each agent has its advantages, disadvantages, and preferred clinical indications (**Table 105.1**). As a general principle, they have comparable sensitivity rates on the order of 90% for inflammation, but WBCs are generally more specific than ^{67}Ga for infection. The choice of radiotracer will depend on factors including availability of the radiopharmaceutical, familiarity and experience of the particular physician with the radiopharmaceutical, the patient's region-of-interest, and the chronicity of the process. Newer inflammation/infection–seeking agents are under investigation; for example, radiolabeled monoclonal antibodies, radiolabeled ciprofloxacin, and ^{18}F-FDG offer the potential to target inflammation/infection for a faster and more specific diagnosis.

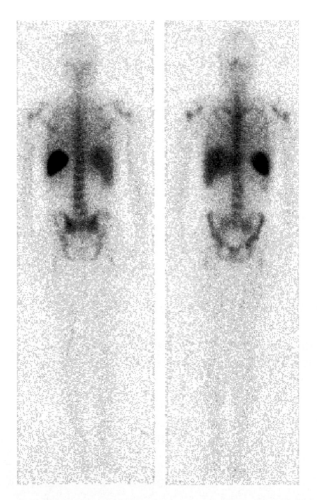

Fig. 105.2 Whole-body image, anterior and posterior projections, ^{111}In-WBCs.

By contrast, the normal biodistribution of radiolabeled WBCs is quite different from that of ^{67}Ga; ^{111}In- WBCs localize only to spleen, liver, and bone marrow (**Fig. 105.2**). The in vitro process of radiolabeling WBCs requires special in-house facilities or access to a nearby commercial nuclear pharmacy. Because of nonspecific cell labeling, WBCs must be separated from the red blood cells and platelets by differential centrifugation, then incubated with ^{111}In-oxine or ^{99m}Tc-HMPAO while their functional integrity is preserved so that they can later be injected into the patient. As with any blood products, universal precautions are in order for the personnel handling the blood. Care must be taken to ensure strict quality control of the whole blood and WBCs during each step so that the patient receives his or her own WBCs.

Despite advances in antimicrobial therapy, infection remains a major cause of morbidity and mortality, and clinically it can present a vexing problem in some patients. Radionuclide imaging provides whole-body surveillance and can be quite helpful in identifying and localizing sites of active inflammation/infection. In the postoperative patient, radionuclide imaging is complementary to CT and can differentiate postoperative changes from active infection. Currently, in immunocompetent patients, WBCs are the radiopharmaceutical of choice; in immunocompromised patients, it is ^{67}Ga.

PEARLS AND PITFALLS

- It is essential to be familiar with the variability of the normal skeletal biodistribution patterns of ^{67}Ga and radiolabeled WBCs to avoid misinterpretation. The skeleton can appear irregular and patchy.
- The liver should be the "hottest" organ on ^{67}Ga images; the spleen is so intense on ^{111}In-WBC images that the "blooming" effect limits the evaluation of spleen size.
- Delayed ^{67}Ga images may be useful to allow for bowel clearance; physiologic activity should clear with time, whereas pathologic localization persists.
- Radiolabeled WBCs should be handled gently and injected as soon as possible following labeling to preserve function.
- In children, ^{99m}Tc-WBCs are the radiopharmaceutical of choice because of relatively favorable dosimetry and imaging characteristics.
- Examining the patient for ostomy sites, drains, surgical scars, and ulcerations/open wounds can avoid misinterpretation because ^{67}Ga and WBCs can localize at these sites.
- On ^{111}In-WBC images, diffuse lung activity is expected on early images (< 4 hours) and will clear by 18 to 24 hours.

Suggested Reading

Boerman OC, Rennen H, Oyen WJ, Corstens FH. Radiopharmaceuticals to image infection and inflammation. Semin Nucl Med 2001;31(4):286–295

Hughes DK. Nuclear medicine and infection detection: the relative effectiveness of imaging with ^{111}In-oxine-, 99mTc-HMPAO-, and 99mTc-stannous fluoride colloid-labeled leukocytes and with 67Ga-citrate. J Nucl Med Technol 2003;31(4):196–201, quiz 203–204

Love C, Palestro CJ. Radionuclide imaging of infection. J Nucl Med Technol 2004;32(2):47–57, quiz 58–59

Rini JN, Bhargava KK, Tronco GG, et al. PET with FDG-labeled leukocytes versus scintigraphy with 111In-oxine-labeled leukocytes for detection of infection. Radiology 2006;238(3):978–987

Society of Nuclear Medicine Procedure Guideline for Gallium Scintigraphy in Inflammation Version 3.0, approved June 6, 2004. www.snm.org. Accessed April 21, 2010

Society of Nuclear Medicine Procedure Guideline for [111]In Leukocyte Scintigraphy for Suspected Infection/Inflammation Version 3.0, approved June 2, 2004. www.snm.org. Accessed April 21, 2010

Society of Nuclear Medicine Procedure Guideline for Tc-99m Exametazime (HMPAO)-Labeled Leukocyte Scintigraphy for Suspected Infection/Inflammation Version 3.0, approved June 2, 2004. www.snm.org

CASE 106

Clinical Presentation

A 48-year-old man with uveitis is referred by ophthalmology for suspected sarcoidosis.

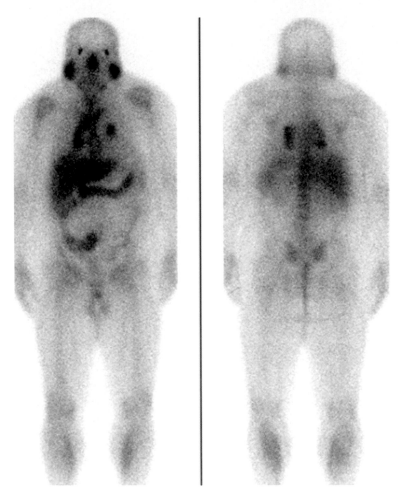

Fig. 106.1 Whole-body planar image, anterior and posterior projections, ^{67}Ga.

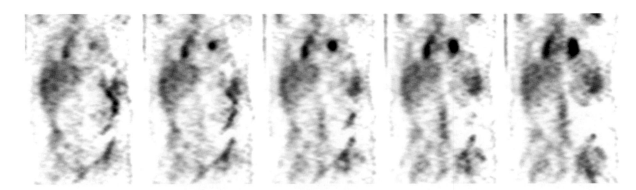

Fig. 106.2 Selected "whole-body" SPECT image, coronal projection, ^{67}Ga.

Technique

- A 7.5 mCi dose of ^{67}Ga-citrate is injected intravenously 3 days before scan.
- Whole-body imaging in anterior and posterior projections
  - Dual-detector gamma camera
  - Medium-energy collimators
  - Energy peak at 93-, 185-, and 300-keV photopeaks

Image Interpretation

Whole-body planar images (**Fig. 106.1**) and "whole-body" SPECT images (**Fig. 106.2**) demonstrate intense right paratracheal and symmetric bilateral hilar uptake; this pattern has been termed the *lambda sign* because it resembles the Greek letter. Coupled with intense, symmetric uptake in the parotid glands and lacrimal glands, this is a characteristic pattern of sarcoidosis. The colon activity is physiologic.

Differential Diagnosis

- Sarcoidosis
- Lymphoma
- Inflammatory/infectious lymphadenitis

Diagnosis and Clinical Follow-Up

Active sarcoidosis. No follow-up obtained.

Discussion

Sarcoidosis is a multisystem granulomatous disease of unknown etiology, characterized by noncaseating granulomas in involved tissues. The disease typically affects adults 20 to 40 years of age, is slightly more common in women than men, and is three to four times more prevalent in blacks than whites. It often presents with bilateral hilar adenopathy, pulmonary infiltrates, and skin or eye involvement (25–80%) but may also involve the skeletal and cardiac muscles, bones and joints.

Noninvasive imaging studies for the diagnosis of sarcoidosis include chest radiography, CT and gallium scintigraphy. Normally, the lacrimal glands, parotid glands, and submandibular glands show mild, symmetric gallium uptake. In sarcoidosis, increased uptake in these structures renders a characteristic pattern termed the *panda sign*; not all components need to be present for the scintigraphic diagnosis. **Figure 106.3** shows "hot" salivary glands, as can also be seen with sialadenitis of another etiology; the nose is also hot. **Figure 106.4** shows only hot lacrimal glands, with sparing of the salivary glands.

Scintigraphy with ^{67}Ga retains its value in patients with sarcoidosis because it can establish the diagnosis, assess the location and extent of disease, differentiate active disease from chronic scarring, guide biopsy, determine recurrence, and predict response to therapy. For example, a positive gallium scan can have prognostic significance in cardiac sarcoidosis because active granulomas may be associated with ventricular tachycardia.

Biopsy showing classic noncaseating granulomas is required for definitive diagnosis. Oral corticosteroids are the mainstay of treatment.

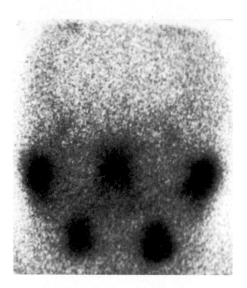

Fig. 106.3 Head and neck planar image, anterior view, ^{67}Ga.

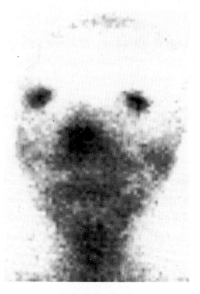

Fig. 106.4 Head and neck planar image, anterior view, ^{67}Ga.

PEARLS AND PITFALLS

- Head-to-toe imaging is indicated for this systemic disease process; images of the head and neck are particularly relevant to evaluate the lacrimal glands and salivary glands.
- A dose of 7.5 mCi of ^{67}Ga permits high-quality, "whole-body" SPECT imaging.
- "Whole-body" SPECT images better define involved structures than do planar images and facilitate correlation with anatomic imaging.
- Localization of ^{67}Ga is nonspecific; thus, correlation with the history, laboratory test results, and other imaging is essential to add specificity and to render an appropriate differential diagnosis.
- Sarcoidosis can involve intra-abdominal tissues; thus, delayed planar and SPECT imaging can distinguish physiologic from pathologic uptake, avoiding false-positive and false-negative interpretations.

Suggested Reading

Bonfioli AA, Orefice F. Sarcoidosis. Semin Ophthalmol 2005;20(3):177–182

Fayad F, Duet M, Orcel P, Lioté F. Systemic sarcoidosis: the "leopard-man" sign. Joint Bone Spine 2006;73(1):109–112

Futamatsu H, Suzuki J, Adachi S, et al. Utility of gallium-67 scintigraphy for evaluation of cardiac sarcoidosis with ventricular tachycardia. Int J Cardiovasc Imaging 2006;22(3-4):443–448

Kawamura S, Ishibashi M, Fukushima S, et al. Study on the usefulness of whole body SPECT coronal image, MIP image in 67Ga scintigraphy. Ann Nucl Med 2002;16(3):221–226

Kurdziel KA. The panda sign. Radiology 2000;215(3):884–885

Otake S, Ishigaki T. Muscular sarcoidosis. Semin Musculoskelet Radiol 2001;5(2):167–170

Schuster DM, Alazraki N. Gallium and other agents in diseases of the lung. Semin Nucl Med 2002;32(3):193–211

Sy WM, Seo IS, Homs CJ, et al. The evolutional stage changes in sarcoidosis on gallium-67 scintigraphy. Ann Nucl Med 1998;12(2):77–82

CASE 107

Clinical Presentation

A 36-year-old man with a history of intravenous drug abuse presents with right hip and flank pain radiating down his right leg.

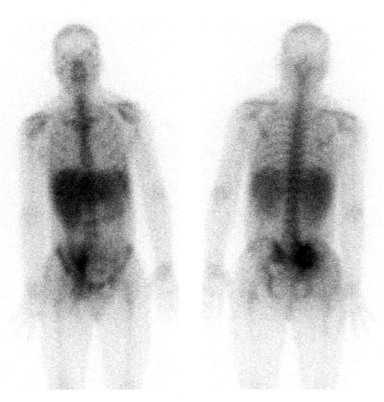

Fig. 107.1 Whole-body planar image, anterior and posterior projections, ⁶⁷Ga.

Technique

- A 7.5 mCi dose of ⁶⁷Ga-citrate is injected intravenously 3 days before scan.
- Whole-body imaging in anterior and posterior projections
  - Dual-detector gamma camera
  - Medium-energy collimators
  - Energy peak at 93-, 185-, and 300-keV photopeaks

Image Interpretation

Intense tracer uptake is noted in the region of the right sacroiliac joint (**Fig. 107.1**). Note the "cold" center on the posterior view; this suggests an advanced process with central devitalization (necrosis). Faint tracer uptake is apparent in the soft tissues of the right buttock.

Differential Diagnosis

- Osteomyelitis
- Sacroiliitis
- Soft tissue inflammation/infection
- Acute trauma
- Malignancy

Diagnosis and Clinical Follow-Up

Findings consistent with unilateral sacroiliitis (with osteomyelitis) and adjacent cellulitis. Correlative MRI demonstrates local sacroiliac bone destruction and edema of adjacent gluteus muscles.

Discussion

Three-phase bone scans have a high sensitivity and specificity for bone and joint disease when plain radiographic findings are normal and are generally a reasonable first-line imaging examination in patients whose skeleton has not been previously violated. When the three-phase bone scan results are equivocal or when the radiographic results are abnormal, ^{67}Ga scintigraphy can be useful in distinguishing bone remodeling related to trauma from underlying infection of the bone, joint, or adjacent soft tissues.

The spine and joints can be "seeded" from another source; intravenous drug users and immunocompromised patients (including those with diabetes) are at particular risk. A corollary case of disseminated infection in an intravenous drug user is shown in **Figs. 107.2** and **107.3**; the right sternoclavicular joint is moderately intense on the bone scan (**Fig. 107.2**), but markedly more intense and more extensive on the ^{67}Ga scan obtained 3 days later (**Fig. 107.3**). Patients with spondyloarthropathy and other conditions (eg, inflammatory bowel disease) can have unilateral or bilateral sacroiliitis.

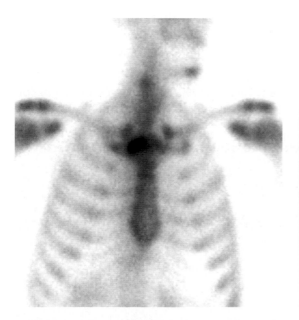

Fig. 107.2 Thoracic planar image, anterior projection, ^{99m}Tc-HDP.

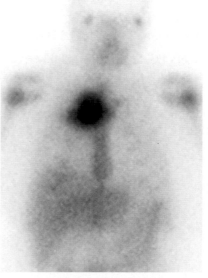

Fig. 107.3 Thoracic planar image, anterior projection, ^{67}Ga.

Gallium scintigraphy can identify one or multiple sites of bone and joint infection, symptomatic or asymptomatic. It is a highly sensitive approach compared with radiographs. MRI is complementary and can evaluate the soft tissues. No single complementary imaging technique has 100% specificity and sensitivity for every case of musculoskeletal infection. Thus, imaging must be tailored to the particular patient depending on his or her age, the presence of orthopedic hardware, location of the infection, and any underlying bone and other systemic conditions. In some patients, plain radiographs are performed first and may be diagnostic. In children, a bone scan can be highly accurate, whereas in adults, either radiolabeled white blood cells or ^{67}Ga may be required. MRI and CT are anatomic approaches, particularly useful in the spine and pelvis.

PEARLS AND PITFALLS

- In osteomyelitis, the gallium scan demonstrates more extensive and more intense uptake compared with the pattern of uptake seen with bone tracers. The value of the combined bone and gallium scans versus MRI for the diagnosis of osteomyelitis has been debated. In difficult cases, all three studies may be needed to make the most accurate diagnosis.
- Sequential bone/gallium scans are particularly useful in complicated cases of patients with limited venous access and chronic processes.
- Infectious deposits tend to accumulate in the sacroiliac joints and sternoclavicular joints. However, any bone and any joint can be involved; thus, whole-body imaging is essential.
- Gallium scans are often positive at sites of trauma; it is difficult to distinguish noninfectious from infectious causes of local inflammation by ^{67}Ga alone.

Suggested Reading

Doita M, Yoshiya S, Nabeshima Y, et al. Acute pyogenic sacroiliitis without predisposing conditions. Spine (Phila Pa 1976) 2003;28(18):E384–E389

Love C, Patel M, Lonner BS, Tomas MB, Palestro CJ. Diagnosing spinal osteomyelitis: a comparison of bone and Ga-67 scintigraphy and magnetic resonance imaging. Clin Nucl Med 2000;25(12):963–977

Nolla JM, Ariza J, Gómez-Vaquero C, et al. Spontaneous pyogenic vertebral osteomyelitis in nondrug users. Semin Arthritis Rheum 2002;31(4):271–278

Termaat MF, Raijmakers PG, Scholten HJ, Bakker FC, Patka P, Haarman HJ. The accuracy of diagnostic imaging for the assessment of chronic osteomyelitis: a systematic review and meta-analysis. J Bone Joint Surg Am 2005;87(11):2464–2471

Turpin S, Lambert R. Role of scintigraphy in musculoskeletal and spinal infections. Radiol Clin North Am 2001;39(2):169–189

CASE 108

Clinical Presentation

A 45-year-old man, a heroin user and HIV-positive, presents with headache and fever. CT of the head shows a low-attenuation lesion in the left frontal lobe (**Fig. 108.1**).

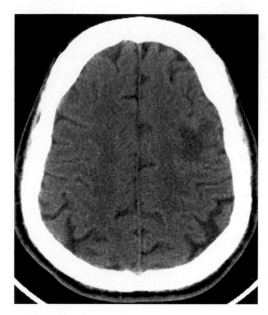

Fig. 108.1 CT, axial image.

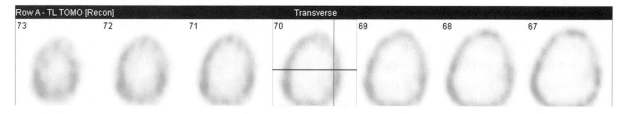

Fig. 108.2 Sequential ^{201}Tl SPECT, axial images.

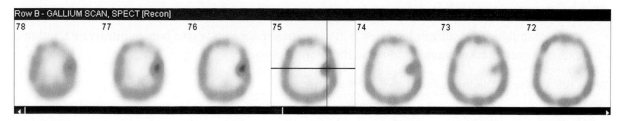

Fig. 108.3 ^{67}Ga SPECT.

Technique

- A 4.0 mCi dose of ^{201}Tl is injected intravenously for scan on day 1.
- A 7.5 mCi dose of ^{67}Ga is injected intravenously on day 1 (after ^{201}Tl scan) for scan on day 4.
- Sequential ^{201}Tl SPECT imaging of the brain on day 1 with a dual-detector gamma camera
  - Low-energy, high-resolution collimators peaked at 80 keV (**Fig. 108.2**)
  - ^{67}Ga SPECT imaging of brain on day 4 with same gamma camera
  - Medium-energy collimators
  - Triple-peaked at 93, 185, and 300 keV (**Fig. 108.3**)

Image Interpretation

CT scan reveals a mass lesion in the left frontal lobe of the brain. Normally, both ^{201}Tl and ^{67}Ga are excluded from the cerebrum. This lesion is thallium-negative (**Fig. 108.2**) but gallium-positive (**Fig. 108.3**). The two sets of images are coregistered; the crosshairs on both rows of images point to the same location in the brain.

Differential Diagnosis

- By CT scan alone, possible causes of the finding include tumor inflammation/infection and other processes (infarction, demyelination).
- Lesions avid for thallium include tumors, whereas lesions avid for gallium include tumors and inflammation/infection.

Diagnosis and Clinical Follow-Up

Biopsy-proven active inflammatory lesion without organism isolated. Diagnosis final, no clinical follow-up.

Discussion

Radiotracers that localize in neoplasms and/or inflammatory/infectious processes can be used in combination to characterize anatomic lesions detected by CT or MRI. As illustrated here, sequential ^{201}Tl/^{67}Ga scintigraphy differentiates cerebral inflammation/infection (eg, toxoplasmosis) from tumor (eg, lymphoma), particularly in the HIV-positive population (**Table 108.1**). Avidity for ^{201}Tl would also indicate viable tumor in patients who have undergone surgery and/or radiotherapy for brain neoplasms. The fusion of physiologic SPECT images with anatomic CT or MR images can facilitate a more confident diagnostic interpretation, guiding proper clinical management.

PEARLS AND PITFALLS

- ^{99m}Tc sestamibi can be substituted for ^{201}Tl in evaluating malignant versus benign intracranial lesions; note, however, that sestamibi localizes in the choroid plexus.

Table 108.1   Key to Diagnosis Based on ^{201}Tl/^{67}Ga Patterns

^{201}Tl	^{67}Ga	Diagnosis
Avid	Avid	Tumor (eg, lymphoma)
Avid	Not avid	Tumor
Not avid	Avid	Inflammation/infection
Not avid	Not avid	Other pathology

- Because of the low administered dose and low-energy imaging photon of ^{201}Tl, it is preferable to complete the thallium scan before dosing with ^{67}Ga. Imaging with ^{67}Ga can be performed as early as 2 days after injection because there is little soft tissue background activity in the brain.
- SPECT/CT and SPECT/MR fusion imaging can be of particular value for small, deep lesions with mild avidity; coregistering the image data sets allows lesions to be more accurately and confidently characterized.
- Motion and positioning artifacts can be problematic. Often, because of the underlying brain pathology, these patients cannot easily cooperate for the long duration of imaging; head holders/restraints can improve the imaging results. Processing software allows the physician or technologist to reorient the brain for direct correlation with anatomic images.

Suggested Reading

Bunyaviroch T, Aggarwal A, Oates ME. Optimized scintigraphic evaluation of infection and inflammation: role of single-photon emission computed tomography/computed tomography fusion imaging. Semin Nucl Med 2006;36(4):295–311

Goethals I, Dierckx R, Van Laere K, Van De Wiele C, Signore A. The role of nuclear medicine imaging in routine assessment of infectious brain pathology. Nucl Med Commun 2002;23(9):819–826

Lee VW, Antonacci V, Tilak S, Fuller JD, Cooley TP. Intracranial mass lesions: sequential thallium and gallium scintigraphy in patients with AIDS. Radiology 1999;211(2):507–512

Turoglu HT, Akisik MF, Naddaf SY, Omar WS, Kempf JS, Abdel-Dayem HM. Tumor and infection localization in AIDS patients: Ga-67 and Tl-201 findings. Clin Nucl Med 1998;23(7):446–459

CASE 109

Clinical Presentation

A 41-year-old man presents with persistent bacteremia and fevers despite antibiotic treatment.

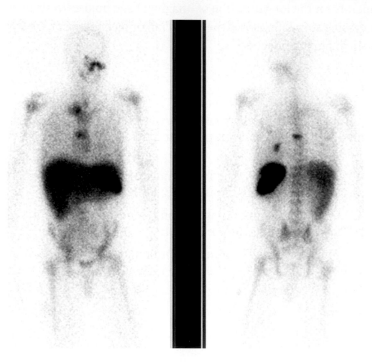

Fig. 109.1 Whole-body planar image, anterior and posterior projections, ^{111}In-WBCs on the posterior view. SPECT images (**Figs. 109.2** and **109.3**) localize the spine focus to the vertebral bodies.

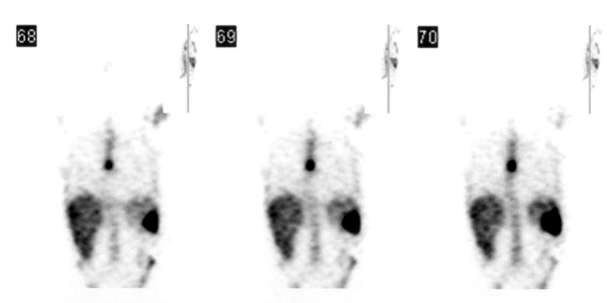

Fig. 109.2 Whole-body SPECT, coronal projection, ^{111}In-WBCs.

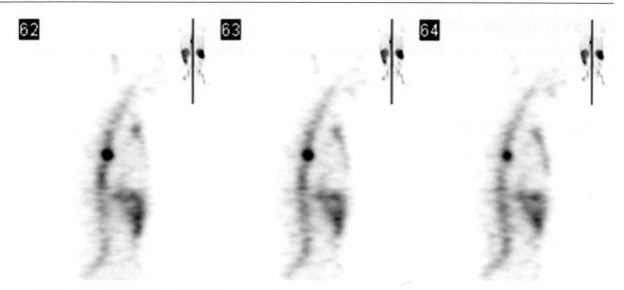

Fig. 109.3 Whole-body SPECT, sagittal projection, ¹¹¹In-WBCs.

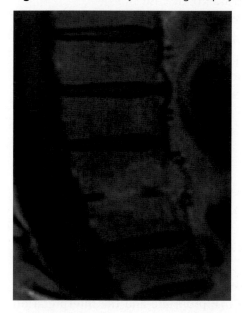

Fig. 109.4 Thoracic spine, sagittal projection, MRI.

Technique

- A 0.5 mCi dose of ¹¹¹In-WBCs is injected intravenously 24 hours before imaging.
- Whole-body planar imaging (**Fig. 109.1**) and whole-body SPECT imaging (**Figs. 109.2** and **109.3**) with a dual-detector gamma camera
  - Medium-energy collimators
  - Energy peaks: 173 and 247 keV

Image Interpretation

Multiple sites of abnormal WBC localization are seen, including in the maxillary sinuses and right sterno-clavicular joint on the anterior view, and in the left lung base and midthoracic spine on the posterior view.

Differential Diagnosis

- Multifocal inflammation/infection: septic joint, diskitis/osteomyelitis, sinusitis, and pneumonia
- Neoplastic metastases
- Active bleeding from multiple sites of trauma

Diagnosis and Clinical Follow-Up

Multifocal infection, including thoracic spine disk space infection and vertebral osteomyelitis. Diagnosis final, no clinical follow-up.

Discussion

For evaluating fever of unknown origin in immunocompetent patients, ^{111}In-WBCs are the radiopharmaceutical of choice. On injection, the radiolabeled WBCs seek out and localize in inflammatory/infected sites, just as unlabeled WBCs do. This is a relatively noninvasive approach for physiologically targeting the disease process. One of the most valuable aspects of WBC scintigraphy is the ability to survey the entire body and the potential to uncover unsuspected sites of disease.

In general, ^{111}In-WBCs are *not* considered the test of choice for vertebral infections, having up to a 40% false-negative rate. A bone scan and ^{67}Ga scan are more sensitive for infections at this site. Infections are usually hematogenously spread; in the spine, the end plate is affected first, with subsequent spread to the disk and adjacent vertebral bodies. MRI is highly sensitive and generally available for the immediate diagnosis of spine infection. In this case, MRI (**Fig. 109.4**) confirmed the disk space infection with involvement of adjacent vertebral bodies.

PEARLS AND PITFALLS

- "Whole-body" (multiple-bed) SPECT imaging permits the accurate localization of focal WBC collections and facilitates correlation with anatomic studies, which can be obtained either before or after scintigraphy.
- WBCs can localize in pneumonias before anatomic evidence is found by chest radiography or even CT.
- Without careful correlation with patient history, physical examination findings, laboratory test results, and other imaging studies, WBC scintigraphy can be inappropriate and the interpretation flawed.
- Focal concentration of WBCs can be seen at stoma sites, hematomas, neoplasms, and healing fractures. Inflammation at these sites may be present without infection.

Suggested Reading

Adams BK, Youssef I, El-Tom el-FA. Imaging in acute pyogenic spondylitis. Clin Nucl Med 2006;31(2):85–86

Becker W, Meller J. The role of nuclear medicine in infection and inflammation. Lancet Infect Dis 2001;1(5):326–333

Medina M, Viglietti AL, Gozzoli L, et al. Indium-111 labelled white blood cell scintigraphy in cranial and spinal septic lesions. Eur J Nucl Med 2000;27(10):1473–1480

CASE 110

Clinical Presentation

A 38-year-old man with poorly healing fractures of the left tibia that were previously repaired with orthopedic hardware now presents with pain and tenderness in his lower left leg. There is no erythema or draining sinus (**Figs. 110.1, 110.2, 110.3,** and **110.4**).

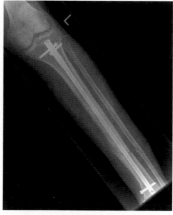

Fig. 110.1 Radiograph of left tibia (knee), anteroposterior projection.

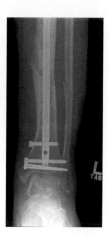

Fig. 110.2 Radiograph of left tibia (ankle), anteroposterior projection.

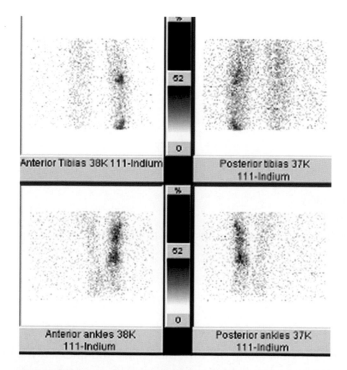

Fig. 110.3 Four views, tibiae (knee to ankle), anterior and posterior projections, ^{111}In-WBCs.

365

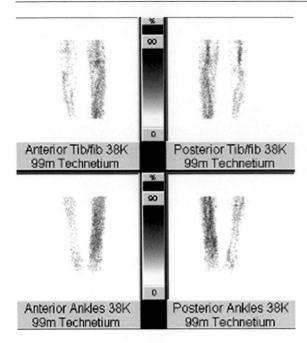

Fig. 110.4 Four matching views, tibiae (knee to ankle), anterior and posterior projections, 99mTc-SC.

Technique

111In-WBC Scan

- A 0.5 mCi dose of 111In-WBCs is injected intravenously.
- Images 24 hours following tracer injection
- Whole-body planar images (not shown) and spot views of the lower legs (**Fig. 110.3**) obtained with a dual-detector gamma camera
- Medium-energy collimators
- Energy peaks: 173 and 247 keV

99mTc-SC Scan

- A 12 mCi dose of 99mTc-SC is injected intravenously.
- Image at 20 minutes (bone marrow "mapping" scan)
- Dual-detector spot views of the lower legs in the same projections used to obtain the WBC spot views (**Fig. 110.4**)
- Low-energy, all-purpose (LEAP) collimators
- Energy peak of 140 keV

Image Interpretation

Intense WBC localization is seen throughout the left tibia along the intramedullary rod and screws, discordant with the SC bone marrow pattern, indicating extensive infection.

Table 110.1 **Diagnostic Patterns of White Blood Cells and Sulfur Colloid in Complicated Bones and Joints**

Localization of ^{111}In-WBCs	Localization of ^{99m}Tc-SC	WBC/SC Pattern	Combined Diagnosis
Negative	Negative or minimal	Concordant	No marrow or minimal marrow (no infection)
Positive	Positive	Concordant	Hyperplastic or displaced marrow (no infection)
Positive	Negative	Discordant	Infection

Abbreviations: SC, sulfur colloid; WBC, white blood cell.

Differential Diagnosis

- Infected hardware with osteomyelitis
- Hyperplastic, reactive, or displaced bone marrow
- Healing fractures; inflammatory response without superimposed infection

Diagnosis and Clinical Follow-Up

Tibial osteomyelitis. This diagnosis prompted surgical removal of the infected orthopedic hardware.

Discussion

Imaging with ^{111}In-WBCs is a sensitive, specific test for the diagnosis of soft tissue infections and osteomyelitis. When WBCs are used for the diagnosis of osteomyelitis in marrow-containing bone, it is often necessary to compare the pattern of WBC localization with that of labeled colloid. The colloid "maps" the red marrow distribution. Red marrow will also normally concentrate labeled WBCs, and the difference between the marrow concentration of WBCs and the concentration of WBCs at the site of inflammation may be subtle. If the WBCs are seen where there is no colloid uptake, it may be assumed that no red marrow is present at that site, and therefore the concentration of WBCs is suggestive of infection (**Table 110.1**).

Radiocolloid images significantly improve the overall scintigraphic specificity for osteomyelitis compared with WBC imaging alone without loss of sensitivity. However, complementary marrow imaging does add complexity and expense to the procedure and can be an inconvenience to patients if performed on separate days.

Besides ^{111}In-WBC scintigraphy, ^{99m}Tc-HMPAO–WBC scintigraphy can be useful in the diagnosis of acute or exacerbated bone infection. Given the higher administered dose, the photon flux is much more abundant, rendering a better-quality image. One of the potential advantages of ^{99m}Tc-WBCs is same-day imaging, although early imaging with ^{111}In-WBCs may be performed.

PEARLS AND PITFALLS

- Bone marrow images can be completed on the same day as ^{111}In-WBC imaging simply by re-peaking the gamma camera for the 140-keV photon of ^{99m}Tc. There is much more abundant photon flux of ^{99m}Tc than of ^{111}In because of substantial differences in the doses administered (eg, ~25 times greater).
- Marrow hyperplasia and marrow displacement are greatly variable and can be identified with confidence only by matching the WBC distribution pattern with that of SC (**Table 110.1**).

- Because of the relatively small percentage of administered activity to normal bone marrow, the dose of ^{99m}Tc-SC should be higher (doubled or tripled) than that administered for a standard liver/spleen scan.
- Same-day marrow mapping is not possible with ^{99m}Tc-WBCs because the ^{99m}Tc photons from ^{99m}Tc-SC cannot be differentiated from those of the WBCs. Marrow imaging has to be performed on another day.

Suggested Reading

Achong DM, Oates E. The computer-generated bone marrow subtraction image: a valuable adjunct to combined In-111 WBC/Tc-99m in sulfur colloid scintigraphy for musculoskeletal infection. Clin Nucl Med 1994;19(3):188–193

Dutton JA, Bird NJ, Skehan SJ, Peters AM. Evaluation of a 3-hour indium-111 leukocyte image as a surrogate for a technetium-99m nanocolloid marrow scan in the diagnosis of orthopedic infection. Clin Nucl Med 2004;29(8):469–474

El Espera I, Blondet C, Moullart V, et al. The usefulness of 99mTc sulfur colloid bone marrow scintigraphy combined with 111In leucocyte scintigraphy in prosthetic joint infection. Nucl Med Commun 2004;25(2):171–175

Seabold JE, Nepola JV, Marsh JL, et al. Postoperative bone marrow alterations: potential pitfalls in the diagnosis of osteomyelitis with In-111-labeled leukocyte scintigraphy. Radiology 1991;180(3):741–747

Wolf G, Aigner RM, Schwarz T. Diagnosis of bone infection using ^{99m}Tc-HMPAO labelled leukocytes. Nucl Med Commun 2001;22(11):1201–1206

CASE 111

Clinical Presentation

A 72-year-old man develops fever and leukocytosis several weeks after placement of an aortoiliac arterial endograft.

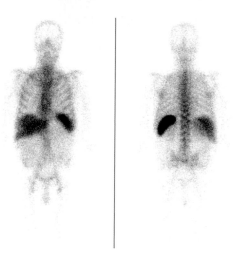

Fig. 111.1 Whole-body planar image, anterior and posterior projections, ^{111}In-WBCs.

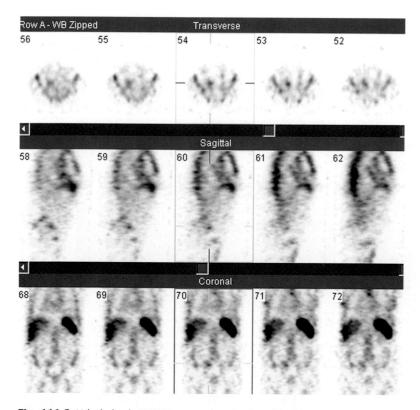

Fig. 111.2 Whole-body SPECT, coronal projection, ^{111}In-WBCs.

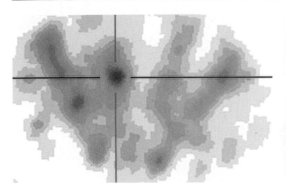

Fig. 111.3 Abdominal SPECT, axial projection, ^{111}In-WBCs.

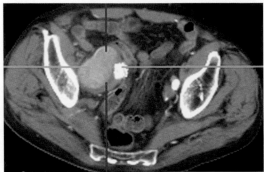

Fig. 111.4 Abdominal CT, axial projection.

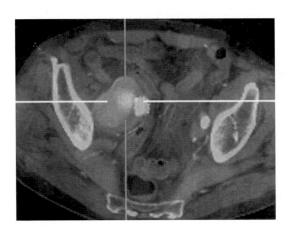

Fig. 111.5 Fused SPECT/CT (**Figs. 111.3** and **111.4**), axial projection.

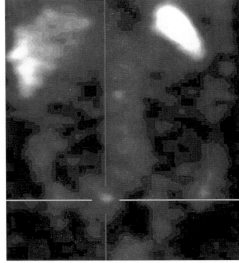

Fig. 111.6 Abdominal SPECT, coronal projection, ^{111}In-WBCs.

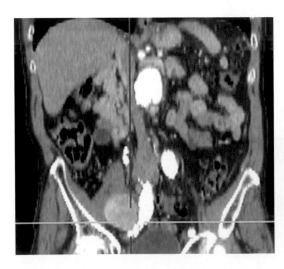

Fig. 111.7 Abdominal CT, coronal projection.

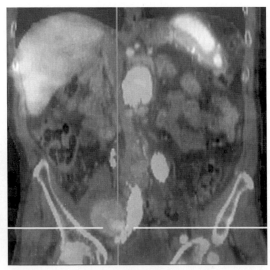

Fig. 111.8 Fused SPECT/CT (**Figs. 111.6** and **111.7**), coronal projection.

Technique

- A 0.5 mCi dose of white blood cells labeled with ^{111}In-WBCs is injected intravenously.
- Images are obtained 24 hours following tracer injection.
- Whole-body planar imaging (**Fig. 111.1**) and whole-body SPECT imaging (**Fig. 111.2**) with a dual-detector gamma camera
- Medium-energy collimators
- Energy peaks: 173 and 247 keV
- Use of software to fuse SPECT and CT images in axial and coronal projections (**Figs. 111.3, 111.4, 111.5, 111.6, 111.7,** and **111.8**)

Image Interpretation

Intense, focal WBC localization in the right pelvis is clearly apparent only on SPECT images. This focus corresponds exactly to the postoperative fluid collection (pseudoaneurysm) adjacent to the right iliac artery endograft. No abnormal localization is seen in the other vascular grafts.

Differential Diagnosis

- By WBC SPECT alone, the following are possible:
  - Soft tissue abscess
  - Inflammatory bowel disease
  - Diverticulitis
  - Appendicitis
  - Infarcted bowel
  - Neoplasm
  - Gastrointestinal bleeding while WBCs circulating (6- to 8-hour half-time in blood)
  - Migration of swallowed WBCs into small or large bowel.
- With CT correlation, the differential diagnosis is greatly refined to vascular graft infection.

Diagnosis and Clinical Follow-Up

Infected pseudoaneurym of right iliac artery endograft. Diagnosis final, no clinical follow-up.

Discussion

Post-operative infections are a serious cause of morbidity and mortality and can be difficult to diagnose clinically with certainty. Signs and symptoms may be confounded by expected post-operative changes. CT provides excellent anatomic detail and is generally the procedure of choice for initial evaluation. CT is readily available, easy to perform, and accurate. However, negative or nondiagnostic anatomic studies in some patients prompt further evaluation with radionuclide studies. It is well recognized that physiologic processes can precede anatomic changes, and nuclear medicine can help differentiate expected postoperative inflammation from serious infection.

In general, ^{111}In-WBCs are preferred for the evaluation of abdominal processes, because unlike ^{67}Ga or WBCs labeled with ^{99m}Tc, they normally are not excreted through the gastrointestinal or urinary tract. Thus, localization of ^{111}In-WBCs in the abdomen is always abnormal and requires further investigation. Given the sensitivity and specificity in the appropriate clinical setting, ^{111}In-WBCs are the first-line investigation for vascular graft infections, as shown here.

SPECT imaging is important to precisely locate the site of obvious abnormal WBC accumulation on planar imaging for a better diagnosis; furthermore, it may be the only means to detect the abnormality, as shown here. Correlation with CT scan is essential for proper diagnosis, and SPECT imaging facilitates this correlation. SPECT/CT fusion imaging is possible today with the use either of software programs or of a dual-modality SPECT/CT device. SPECT/CT fusion has been shown to be of value in patients with suspected infections because it improves the diagnosis, localization, and definition of the extent of disease and adds considerable confidence to the diagnosis, either excluding or confirming disease. SPECT/CT has an important role with highly specific, low-background, infection-seeking tracers such as ^{111}In-WBCs.

PEARLS AND PITFALLS

- Cardiac valvular abscesses can be positive on WBC scans, but endocarditis itself does not recruit many WBCs; thus, it is more likely to be negative scintigraphically.
- Follow-up WBC scintigraphy after a course of antibiotics can confirm resolution of the inflammatory/infectious process.
- Check for cardiac blood pool activity; if present, this suggests incomplete separation of the WBCs from the red blood cells and/or platelets during the labeling process. Because ^{111}In labels cells non-specifically, activity localizing to vascular structures can reflect stasis of red blood cells or adherence of platelets, not WBCs responding to inflammation or infection.
- If evaluating possible central venous catheter infection, do not use that line to inject the radiolabeled WBCs because a finding of activity there will be of unclear significance.

Suggested Reading

Bar-Shalom R, Yefremov N, Guralnik L, et al. SPECT/CT using 67Ga and 111In-labeled leukocyte scintigraphy for diagnosis of infection. J Nucl Med 2006;47(4):587–594

Bunyaviroch T, Aggarwal A, Oates ME. Optimized scintigraphic evaluation of infection and inflammation: role of single-photon emission computed tomography/computed tomography fusion imaging. Semin Nucl Med 2006;36(4):295–311

Ingui CJ, Shah NP, Oates ME. Infection scintigraphy: added value of single-photon emission computed tomography/computed tomography fusion compared with traditional analysis. J Comput Assist Tomogr 2007;31(3):375–380

Palestro CJ, Love C, Tronco GG, Tomas MB. Role of radionuclide imaging in the diagnosis of postoperative infection. Radiographics 2000;20(6):1649–1660, discussion 1660–1663

Sirinek KR. Diagnosis and treatment of intra-abdominal abscesses. Surg Infect (Larchmt) 2000;1(1):31–38

CASE 112

Clinical Presentation

A 77-year-old woman on peritoneal dialysis has fever and abdominal pain.

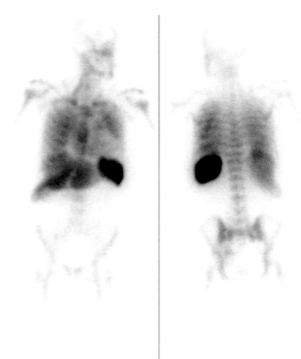

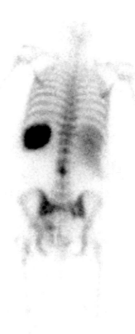

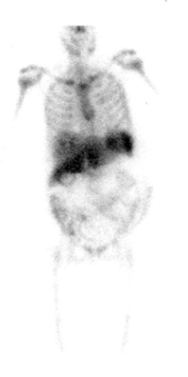

Fig. 112.1 Whole-body 4-hour planar image, anterior and posterior projections, ^{99m}Tc-WBCs.

Fig. 112.2 Whole-body 24-hour planar image, anterior and posterior projections, ^{99m}Tc-WBCs.

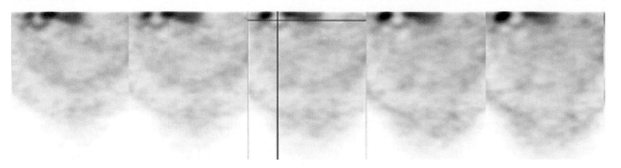

Fig. 112.3 Abdominal 24-hour SPECT, coronal projection, ⁹⁹ᵐTc-WBCs.

Technique

- A 20 mCi dose of white blood cells labeled with ⁹⁹ᵐTc-WBCs is injected intravenously.
- Whole-body planar imaging in anterior and posterior projections at 4 hours and 24 hours
- Abdominal SPECT at 24 hours
- Dual-detector gamma camera
- Low-energy, high-resolution collimators
- Energy peak of 140 keV

Image Interpretation

At 4 hours, blood pool activity and early localization in the gallbladder fossa and left posterior pelvis are subtle findings (**Fig. 112.1**). At 24 hours, blood pool activity has cleared; a rim of WBC localization in the subhepatic region is clearly defined and suggests activity in the gallbladder wall (**Figs. 112.2** and **112.3**); diffuse, moderately intense activity throughout the abdomen suggests peritoneal activity, and linear activity in the anterior right lower pelvis conforms to the peritoneal dialysis catheter. The abdominal activity does not conform to the bowel lumen, as would be seen with excreted activity.

Differential Diagnosis

- Subhepatic abscess or inflammatory mass
- Peritonitis related to gallbladder perforation and/or peritoneal dialysis catheter infection
- Peritoneal tumor implants
- Gastrointestinal tract inflammation

Diagnosis and Clinical Follow-Up

Peritonitis related to infected peritoneal dialysis catheter. Diagnosis final, no clinical follow-up.

Discussion

⁹⁹ᵐTc as a radiolabel has advantages over ¹¹¹In, including a higher administered dose, which results in greater photon flux and count-rich images. Imaging can be performed soon after administration, but repeated imaging at 24 hours is possible by increasing the imaging time to compensate for decay. The improved target-to-background ratio on delayed images may facilitate the detection of disease, as in this case.

Acute cholecystitis is generally diagnosed by ultrasonography or hepatobiliary scintigraphy. Some patients, such as those who are on steroids, have diabetes, or are in renal failure, may not manifest overt signs or symptoms of this serious, potentially life-threatening condition. At times, inflammation/infection scintigraphy may uncover cholecystitis, as in this case.

PEARLS AND PITFALLS

- Logistically, it is necessary to draw the patient's blood early in the morning and return the cells to the patient by noon to acquire images on the same day at 2 to 4 hours after injection.
- SPECT imaging can be performed (as shown here) and has two advantages over planar imaging: removing superimposed activity and localizing tracer collection more accurately.
- When ^{111}In (cyclotron-produced) is unavailable, ^{99m}Tc is an alternative radiolabel.
- Bowel activity will be apparent because a breakdown product with the ^{99m}Tc label is excreted via the biliary system.
- Urinary activity is a normal finding, making the diagnosis of urinary tract disease more difficult.

Suggested Reading

Gratz S, Rennen HJ, Boerman OC, et al. 99mTc-HMPAO-labeled autologous versus heterologous leukocytes for imaging infection. J Nucl Med 2002;43(7):918–924

Moreno AJ, Rampy RJ, Ward DL. Dramatic example of peritonitis revealed by In-111-labeled leukocyte scintigraphy. Clin Nucl Med 2000;25(11):911–912

Mountford PJ, Kettle AG, O'Doherty MJ, Coakley AJ. Comparison of technetium-99m-HM-PAO leukocytes with indium-111-oxine leukocytes for localizing intraabdominal sepsis. J Nucl Med 1990;31(3):311–315

Ruiz Solís S, García Vicente A, Rodado Marina S, et al. [Diagnosis of the infectious complications of continuous ambulatory peritoneal dialysis by 99mTc-HMPAO labelled leukocytes]. Rev Esp Med Nucl 2004;23(6):403–413

Section VIII

Renal Scintigraphy

Scott H. Britz-Cunningham

CASE 113

Clinical Presentation

A 53-year-old woman with diabetes mellitus and end-stage renal disease presents with rising serum creatinine 2 months after receiving a cadaveric renal transplant. (A living related donor transplant had failed 8 years previously.) The postoperative course was complicated by febrile neutropenia. Multiple biopsies of the transplant kidney showed moderate-severe acute tubular necrosis but no evidence of rejection. Multiple CT examinations of the pelvis showed a stable 8.1 × 3.4-cm accumulation of fluid adjacent to the transplant kidney.

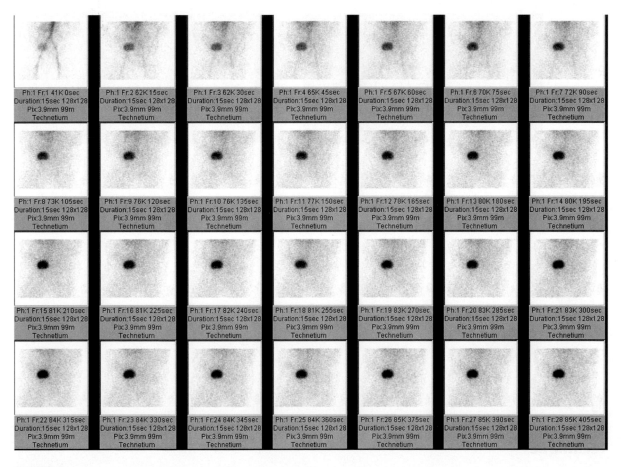

Fig 113.1

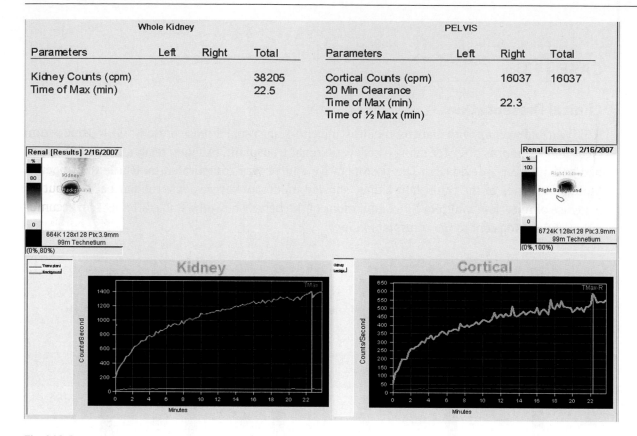

Fig 113.2

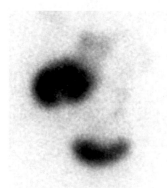

Fig 113.3

Technique

- ⁹⁹ᵐTc-MAG-3 (5-10mCi) is the radiopharmaceutical of choice because of its higher extraction fraction, although ⁹⁹ᵐTc-DTPA (10-20mCi) is an acceptable substitute.
- Dynamic imaging of the pelvis for 20 or 30 minutes is followed by 10-minute static views, repeated as necessary for up to 2 hours.
- For transplants located in the pelvis, imaging should be performed in the anterior view to avoid attenuation from the sacrum and pelvic bones.
- When possible, correlation should be made with anatomic imaging (CT, MRI, or ultrasound) to evaluate any grossly evident fluid collections.

Image Interpretation

Dynamic images (**Fig. 113.1**) show the transplant kidney in the left hemipelvis. Homogeneous perfusion is seen in the first frame, immediately after arrival of the injection bolus in the internal and external iliac arteries. There is slightly delayed tracer uptake in the renal cortex; however, no activity is seen in the renal pelvis, ureter, or bladder.

The time-activity curves (**Fig. 113.2**) show that tracer activity in the cortex continues to rise slowly until the termination of imaging after 24 minutes. The whole-kidney and cortical curves are identical in shape, reflecting the absence of excretion into the collecting system.

On an anterior 10-minute static view taken after 1 hour, tracer activity is finally seen in the bladder, although most of the activity is still in the renal cortex. The renal pelvis and ureter are not visualized (**Fig. 113.3**). This pattern is typical of acute tubular necrosis, which was biopsy-proven in this case. In addition, an ill-defined collection of tracer is seen superomedial to the transplant kidney, reflecting extravasation of tracer due to a small urinary leak.

Differential Diagnosis

- Perirenal seroma/hematoma
- Urinary leak (urinoma)
- Acute tubular necrosis (vasomotor nephropathy)
- Acute rejection

Diagnosis and Clinical Follow-Up

The diagnosis was urinary leak and acute tubular necrosis. The patient's creatinine continued to rise to pre-transplant levels, and she became dependent on hemodialysis once more. No surgical repair of the urinary leak was attempted.

Discussion

Urinary leaks may occur at the site of an anastomosis (typically ureteroneocystostomy or pelvineoureterostomy) or from the ureter itself as a result of operative injury or rejection. Urinary leaks may be treated by conservative medical management or may require surgical intervention, depending on their severity.

Other common complications of a renal transplant include the following:
- Vascular occlusion/thrombosis: In this condition, the entire transplant kidney appears photopenic.
- Infarct: This appears as a focal area of photopenia, sometimes with a hyperemic rim.
- Hyperacute rejection: This has the same appearance as vascular occlusion.
- Acute rejection: This appears similar to acute tubular necrosis, but uptake may be less and may appear patchy. The most specific diagnostic finding is a scan that deteriorates if repeated after 1 to 2 days.
- Chronic rejection: This is characterized by decreased uptake that worsens over a prolonged time course. The pattern is indistinguishable from that of cyclosporine toxicity or recurrence of the patient's original kidney disease (eg, glomerulonephritis), and chronic rejection can be confirmed only by biopsy.
- Renal arterial stenosis, typically at the anastomosis site: This can be evaluated with a captopril scan.
- Urinary obstruction: Tracer is retained in the renal pelvis and calyces but is slow to appear in the bladder. A post-furosemide renogram shows an abnormally prolonged half-time of clearance.

A prominent renal pelvis may be a late manifestation and is not required for the diagnosis. Perfusion and cortical uptake are usually normal unless the disease has persisted for some time.

PEARLS AND PITFALLS

- A lateral decubitus anterior static image may help to identify a urinary leak that pools around the bladder.
- A large, loculated urinoma will appear photopenic on dynamic and early static images, when it is indistinguishable from a postoperative perinephric fluid collection, seroma, or hematoma. The differential is resolved on later images as tracer slowly begins to appear outside the urinary tract.
- Because of a dilution effect, activity within a urinoma may be faint and is generally less intense than that seen in the bladder or renal pelvis. However, any amount of tracer accumulating outside the urinary tract should be considered abnormal.
- Occasionally, reflux into the native ureter can be seen. Unlike a urinary leak, this activity remains confined to the ureteral lumen over time.

Suggested Reading

Maaloul M, Krivochiev M, Evangelista E, Itti E, Hoznek A, Meignan M. Diagnosis of urinoma complicating a renal graft using 99mTc-DTPA scintigraphy and factor analysis. Eur J Nucl Med Mol Imaging 2005;32(7):854

Nicoletti R. Evaluation of renal transplant perfusion by functional imaging. Eur J Nucl Med 1990;16 (8–10):733–739

Padhy AK, Gopinath PG, Mehta SN, Tiwari DC, Dhawan IK. Technetium-99m DTPA renal transplant imaging in the diagnosis of urinoma. Clin Nucl Med 1989;14(10):769–771

Titton RL, Gervais DA, Hahn PF, Harisinghani MG, Arellano RS, Mueller PR. Urine leaks and urinomas: diagnosis and imaging-guided intervention. Radiographics 2003;23(5):1133–1147

CASE 114

Clinical Presentation

A 37-year-old woman is incidentally noted to have a 2.5-cm mass-like structure in the interpolar region of the right kidney on a gynecologic ultrasound examination. Follow-up MRI shows a 2.6 × 2.0-cm prominence in the right interpolar region that is equivocal for renal tumor versus hypertrophic columns of Bertin.

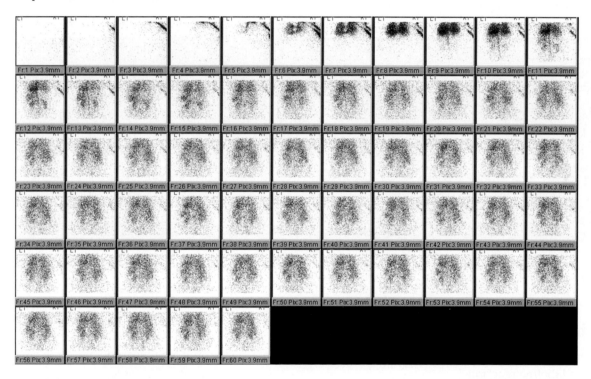

Fig. 114.1

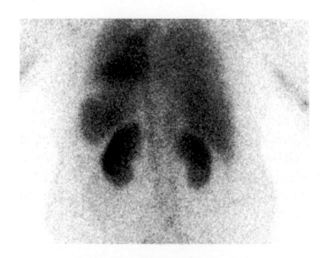

Posterior 498K Duration:227sec 256x256 Pix:1.9mm 99m
Technetium

Fig. 114.2

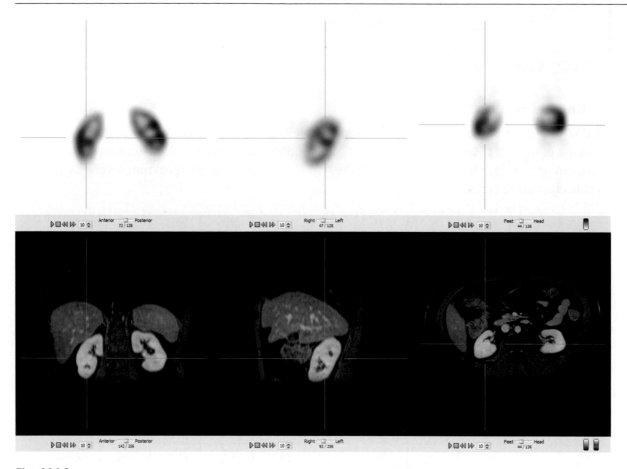

Fig. 114.3

Technique

- Inject 1 to 5 mCi of ^{99m}Tc-DMSA. Use within 30 minutes of labeling, and avoid introducing air during the labeling reaction.
- Use a low-energy, high-resolution collimator.
- Image 2 to 3 hours after injection.
- For infants, pinhole collimators may be used for better anatomic definition. For adults, SPECT is preferable, given the greater depth of the kidney.

Image Interpretation

Dynamic images (**Fig. 114.1**) show prompt perfusion of both kidneys, which appear similar in size. On the 4-minute static image (**Fig. 114.2**), both kidneys show homogeneous uptake. Note that the blood pool activity persists longer than on ^{99m}Tc-DTPA or ^{99m}Tc-MAG-3 imaging because of slower cortical uptake. **Figure 114.3** shows SPECT images (top) obtained at 3 hours after injection. Fusion with MR image (bottom) indicates that the mass-like feature adjacent to the right renal pelvis at the crossline intersection has ^{99m}Tc-DMSA uptake similar to that of the remainder of the renal cortex, confirming that it consists of functional renal tissue.

Differential Diagnosis

- Hypertrophic columns of Bertin
- Renal cell carcinoma or other neoplasm

Diagnosis and Clinical Follow-Up

The diagnosis was hypertrophic columns of Bertin. A planned renal biopsy was cancelled. No further management was required.

Discussion

^{99m}Tc-DMSA provides a useful method for estimating the amount of functional renal cortex and evaluating focal renal parenchymal lesions. It can be particularly helpful in the setting of renal trauma, pyelonephritis, pediatric vesico-ureteral reflux, chronic ureteropelvic junction obstruction, renal infarcts, and renal mass lesions.

Although the functional information obtained from ^{99m}Tc-DMSA imaging is often best employed as an adjunct to CT imaging, the use of radioiodinated contrast may be contraindicated in patients with compromised renal function. In such patients, SPECT imaging with ^{99m}Tc-DMSA may provide enough anatomic information to effectively substitute for CT.

Most benign and malignant neoplasms appear as photopenic defects as seen in ^{99m}Tc-DMSA imaging. Oncocytomas and mesoblastic nephromas have been reported to concentrate renal imaging agents; however, these are relatively rare.

Hypertrophic columns of Bertin are a normal anatomic variant in which the renal cortex extends deeply into the medulla, often forming a masslike structure. The columns are not neoplastic and are functionally and histologically similar to renal cortex elsewhere in the same kidney. Thus, on ultrasound, they appear isoechoic to cortex; on CT, they are isodense to cortex, with homogeneous contrast enhancement; and on MR, they are isointense to cortex. They will show positive uptake, similar to that of cortex, on ^{99m}Tc-DTPA, ^{99m}Tc-MAG-3, and ^{99m}Tc-DMSA scans. However, only ^{99m}Tc-DMSA persists long enough to allow detailed tomographic correlation with CT or MR images.

PEARLS AND PITFALLS

- ^{99m}Tc-DMSA binds tubular cells in the renal cortex. At 3 hours after injection, approximately 40% of the injected dose remains within the cortex.
- Because of protein binding, clearance of ^{99m}Tc-DMSA from the blood pool is slow. Consequently, imaging should be performed 2 to 3 hours after injection.
- Extrarenal excretion is normally seen in the liver, gallbladder, and bowel. This can be increased if air or oxygen is inadvertently introduced into the labeling mixture.
- The slow clearance of ^{99m}Tc-DMSA from the renal cortex permits SPECT imaging, which should be routinely employed in older children and adults because it provides detailed anatomic information.
- Correct interpretation of ^{99m}Tc-DMSA SPECT images requires accurate knowledge of the appearance of normal scans so that anatomic features, such as cortical thinning toward the upper poles, are not misinterpreted as lesions.
- Because of the very slow excretion of ^{99m}Tc-DMSA, imaging with this agent cannot be used to evaluate cortical transit time, obstruction of the renal excretory apparatus, or urinary leaks.

Suggested Reading

Piepsz A, Blaufox MD, Gordon I, Granerus G, Majd M, O'Reilly P, Rosenberg AR, Rossleigh MA, Sixt R. Scientific Committee of Radionuclides in Nephrourology. Consensus on renal cortical scintigraphy in children with urinary tract infection. Semin Nucl Med 1999;29(2):160–174

Rossleigh MA. Renal infection and vesico-ureteric reflux. Semin Nucl Med 2007;37(4):261–268

Rushton HG, Majd M. Dimercaptosuccinic acid renal scintigraphy for the evaluation of pyelonephritis and scarring: a review of experimental and clinical studies. J Urol 1992;148(5 Pt 2):1726–1732

Tondeur MC, De Palma D, Roca I, Piepsz A, Ham HH. Interobserver reproducibility in reporting on renal cortical scintigraphy in children: a large collaborative study. Nucl Med Commun 2009;30(4):258–262

Vitti RA, Maurer AH. Single photon emission computed tomography and renal pseudotumor. Clin Nucl Med 1985;10(7):501–503

CASE 115

Clinical Presentation

A 39-year-old woman with a history of congenital bladder exstrophy, repaired with an ileal loop and Indiana pouch, presents with recurrent pyelonephritis and severe right-sided flank pain.

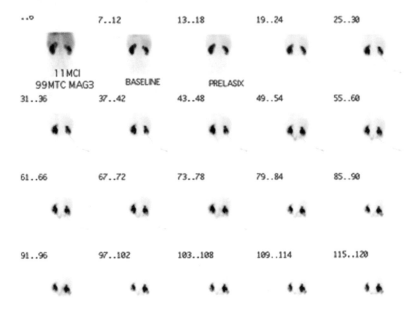

Fig. 115.1

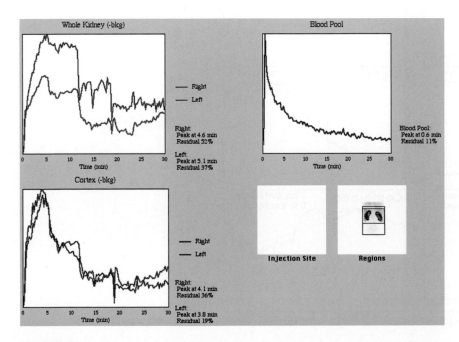

Fig. 115.2

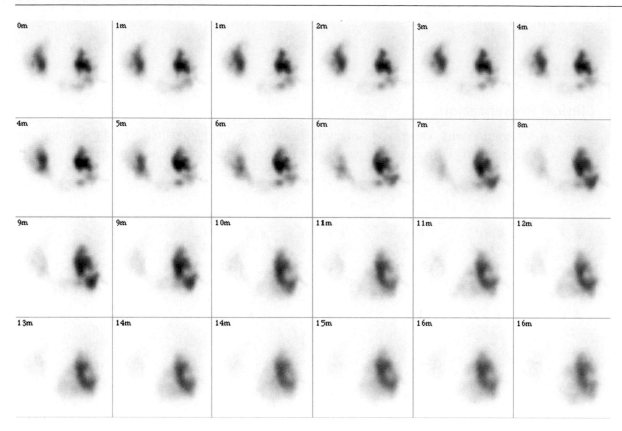

Fig. 115.3

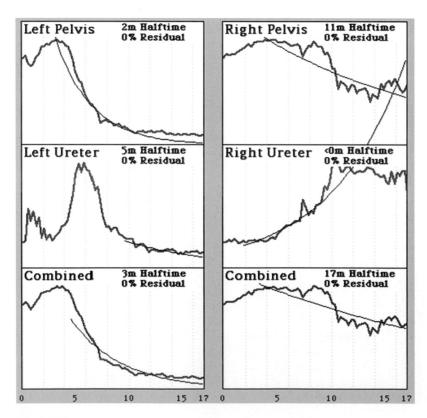

Fig. 115.4

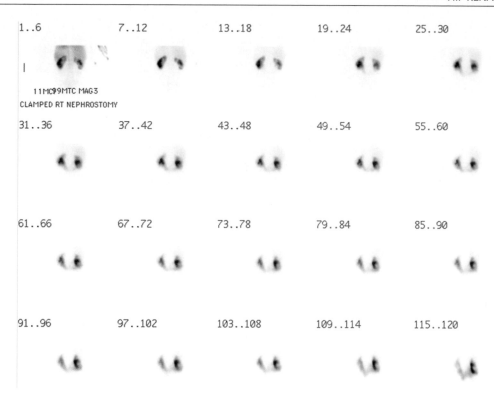

Fig. 115.5

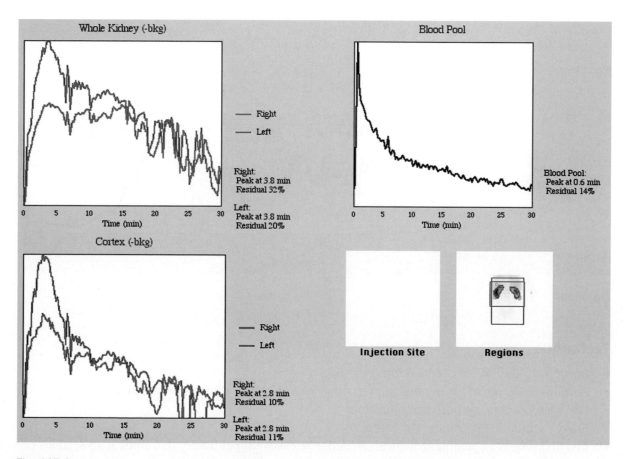

Fig. 115.6

0m 11M99MTC MAG3	1m	3m	4m	5m	6m
RIGHT NEPHROSTOMY UNCLAMPED					
8m	9m	10m	11m	13m	14m
15m	16m	18m	19m	20m	21m
23m	24m	25m	26m	28m	29m

Fig. 115.7

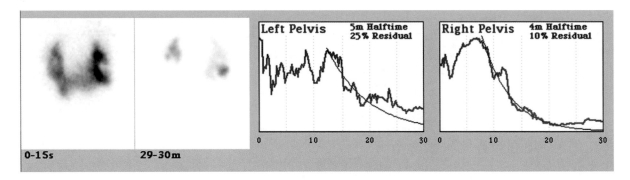

| 0-15s | 29-30m | Left Pelvis 5m Halftime 25% Residual | Right Pelvis 4m Halftime 10% Residual |

Fig. 115.8

Technique

- Inject 5–10 mCi of ^{99m}Tc-MAG-3 intravenously.
- Administer 20 mg of furosemide intravenously at 20 minutes after tracer injection.
- Use a low-energy, all-purpose collimator.
- Energy window 20% centered at 140 keV.
- Imaging time is a dynamic sequence: 24 frames at 2 seconds per frame, 16 frames at 15 seconds per frame, and 60 frames at 30 seconds per frame.

Image Interpretation

The patient had a right nephrostomy tube. Dynamic images (**Fig. 115.1**) obtained in the posterior position with the tube unclamped show that excretion from the right kidney is primarily through the tube. The time–activity curves (**Fig. 115.2**) show a split function: left 56% and right 44%. Tracer accumulation was seen in the right renal pelvis; however, this cleared substantially following the administration of 40 mg of furosemide (**Figs. 115.3** and **115.4**).

Two days later, the study was repeated with the nephrostomy tube clamped. Right-sided urinary collecting system activity can be seen on dynamic images (**Fig. 115.5**). The right kidney appears slightly worse on split function: left 60% and right 40% (**Fig. 115.6**). At the end of the baseline part of the study, the patient experienced severe right flank pain, which precluded the administration of furosemide. Instead, the nephrostomy tube was unclamped. The residual activity in the right renal pelvis cleared rapidly (**Figs. 115.7** and **115.8**).

Differential Diagnosis

- Right-sided urinary obstruction, likely at the junction of the right ureter and the diversion pouch.

Diagnosis and Clinical Follow-Up

The imaging diagnosis was high-grade obstruction of the right ureter at the level of the diversion. A kidney biopsy showed focal subcapsular vascular scarring with moderate arterial and arteriolar sclerosis, but no evidence of acute or chronic obstructive uropathic changes. The patient continued to have severe flank pain and elected to have a right nephrectomy a year after the study.

Discussion

As a rule of thumb, the emptying half-time of the pelvis after furosemide (the time it takes for half of the tracer activity to leave the pelvis) should be less than 10 minutes. If the emptying half-time is 10 to 20 minutes, mild obstruction or dilatation is suggested, or both. An emptying half-time of more than 20 minutes is consistent with moderate to high-grade or total obstruction.

With diminished renal function, a less vigorous response to diuretics should be expected. Where cortical function is very poor, furosemide may be ineffective, and the half-time of clearance will reflect the poor cortical function rather than mechanical obstruction. In such cases, it may be better to consider the study nondiagnostic, and not to report half-times that may be little more than misleading.

PEARLS AND PITFALLS

- Quantitative analysis of excretory function requires that renal pelvic and ureteral regions-of-interest be carefully drawn. Frame-by-frame inspection of the study will identify when the pelvis of each kidney is optimally visualized. The region-of-interest can then be drawn by using the most appropriate frames.
- When high-grade obstruction leads to marked reduction in function, the time–activity curve often has very low amplitude when it is displayed alongside the curve of a well-functioning contralateral kidney. If the curves are displayed and scaled individually, the details of the lower-count curve can be made more apparent.
- Optimally, furosemide should be given when the cortex has cleared and the renal pelvis has filled. The images should therefore be monitored as they are acquired. When cortical function is poor,

tracer may be slow to reach the renal pelvis. In such cases, monitoring may have to be continued beyond the typical 20- to 30-minute sequence before furosemide is given.

- Furosemide is unnecessary when the clearance of both kidneys is normal on the baseline images, as evidenced by rapid diminution of activity from the renal pelves and good visualization of the ureters over their full length. In such cases, obstruction can be ruled out by simple inspection.

- The half-time of clearance after furosemide should be reported only if there is a significant amount of activity in the renal pelvis at the time that furosemide is given. Paradoxically, a normal kidney may have a spuriously abnormal half-time of clearance because there is little relative change when the activity is already at a minimal level. Therefore, clearance half-times should not be reported for kidneys that are obviously normal.

- A full bladder will inhibit clearance from the renal pelves. If possible, the bladder should be emptied before the administration of furosemide. Consider catheterizing patients with neurogenic bladders or obvious large residuals after voiding.

- Proper hydration is essential for quantitative radionuclide renography. On the day of the study, eating and drinking are permitted as usual, with an additional intake of 500 to 750 mL of water (10 mL/kg) encouraged in the hour before imaging. When in doubt, or when the patient cannot drink normally, consider administering fluids intravenously before and during the study.

- When furosemide cannot be administered, alternative protocols include imaging the patient in an upright sitting position, or simply acquiring delayed images at longer intervals. Occasionally, the kidneys will clear completely after these maneuvers, allowing a high-grade obstruction to be ruled out. Note, however, that partial obstruction is often position-dependent.

Suggested Reading

Conway JJ. "Well-tempered" diuresis renography: its historical development, physiological and technical pitfalls, and standardized technique protocol. Semin Nucl Med 1992;22(2):74–84

O'Reilly PH. Diuresis renography: recent advances and recommended protocols. Br J Urol 1992;69(2): 113–120

Sarkar SD. Diuretic renography: concepts and controversies. Urol Radiol 1992;14(2):79–84

Yung BCK, Sostre S, Gearhart JP. Normalized clearance-to-uptake slope ratio: a method to minimize false-positive diuretic renograms. J Nucl Med 1993;34(5):762–768

CASE 116

Clinical Presentation

A 54-year-old woman is anuric for 2 days after receiving a renal transplant.

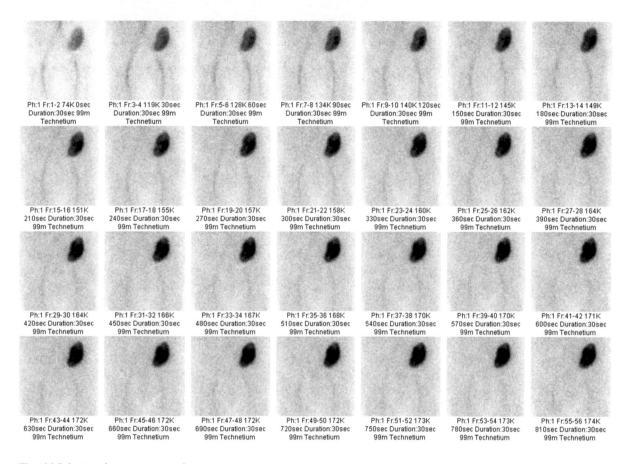

Ph:1 Fr:1-2 74K 0sec Duration:30sec 99m Technetium

Ph:1 Fr:3-4 119K 30sec Duration:30sec 99m Technetium

Ph:1 Fr:5-6 128K 60sec Duration:30sec 99m Technetium

Ph:1 Fr:7-8 134K 90sec Duration:30sec 99m Technetium

Ph:1 Fr:9-10 140K 120sec Duration:30sec 99m Technetium

Ph:1 Fr:11-12 145K 150sec Duration:30sec 99m Technetium

Ph:1 Fr:13-14 149K 180sec Duration:30sec 99m Technetium

Ph:1 Fr:15-16 151K 210sec Duration:30sec 99m Technetium

Ph:1 Fr:17-18 155K 240sec Duration:30sec 99m Technetium

Ph:1 Fr:19-20 157K 270sec Duration:30sec 99m Technetium

Ph:1 Fr:21-22 158K 300sec Duration:30sec 99m Technetium

Ph:1 Fr:23-24 160K 330sec Duration:30sec 99m Technetium

Ph:1 Fr:25-26 162K 360sec Duration:30sec 99m Technetium

Ph:1 Fr:27-28 164K 390sec Duration:30sec 99m Technetium

Ph:1 Fr:29-30 164K 420sec Duration:30sec 99m Technetium

Ph:1 Fr:31-32 166K 450sec Duration:30sec 99m Technetium

Ph:1 Fr:33-34 167K 480sec Duration:30sec 99m Technetium

Ph:1 Fr:35-36 168K 510sec Duration:30sec 99m Technetium

Ph:1 Fr:37-38 170K 540sec Duration:30sec 99m Technetium

Ph:1 Fr:39-40 170K 570sec Duration:30sec 99m Technetium

Ph:1 Fr:41-42 171K 600sec Duration:30sec 99m Technetium

Ph:1 Fr:43-44 172K 630sec Duration:30sec 99m Technetium

Ph:1 Fr:45-46 172K 660sec Duration:30sec 99m Technetium

Ph:1 Fr:47-48 172K 690sec Duration:30sec 99m Technetium

Ph:1 Fr:49-50 172K 720sec Duration:30sec 99m Technetium

Ph:1 Fr:51-52 173K 750sec Duration:30sec 99m Technetium

Ph:1 Fr:53-54 173K 780sec Duration:30sec 99m Technetium

Ph:1 Fr:55-56 174K 810sec Duration:30sec 99m Technetium

Fig. 116.1 Two days post-transplant.

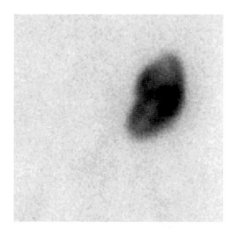

Fig. 116.2 Two days post-transplant.

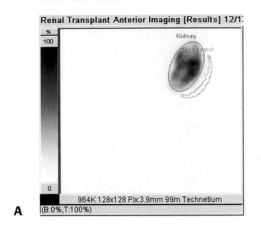

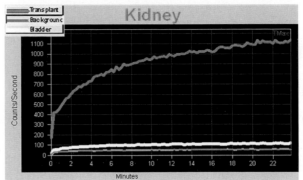

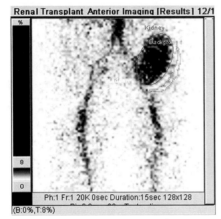

Fig. 116.3 Two days post-transplant.

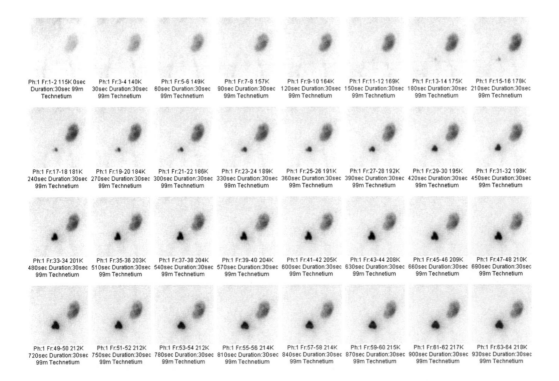

Fig. 116.4 Three weeks post-transplant.

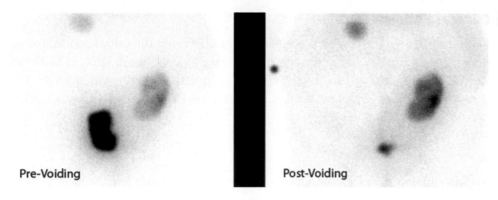

Pre-Voiding Post-Voiding

Fig. 116.5 Three weeks post-transplant.

Technique

- Inject 10 mCi of ^{99m}Tc-MAG-3 with a tight intravenous bolus. ^{99m}Tc-DTPA (10–20mCi) can also be used.
- Use a low-energy, medium-resolution collimator.
- Image native kidneys in the posterior view and pelvic transplant kidneys in the anterior view.
- Image for the first minute with 1- to 2-second frames. Then image for 2 to 30 minutes with 30- to 60-second frames. A 5-minute static image at the end may help to demonstrate ureteral uptake.
- A 1mg/kg (max 40 mg) dose of furosemide can be administered if the initial set of images suggests obstruction. Image another 20 to 30 minutes after the furosemide injection, and compute the final residual activity in the collecting system (renal pelvis ± ureter) plus the half-time of emptying (see Case 115).

Image Interpretation

Anterior dynamic images (**Fig. 116.1**) obtained on postoperative day 2 show prompt perfusion of the transplant kidney in the left iliac fossa. This key finding excludes arterial thrombosis as a cause of the patient's anuria. There is good cortical uptake, with at most a slight lack of homogeneity, and blood pool activity visibly decreases as tracer is concentrated in the kidney. However, no activity is seen in the renal pelvis, ureter, or bladder, either on the dynamic images or on a 5-minute static image taken after 30 minutes (**Fig. 116.2**). The time–activity curve (**Fig. 116.3**) shows steadily increasing uptake, which does not maximize until the end of the study.

Anterior dynamic images taken from a repeated study 3 weeks later (**Fig. 116.4**) show good cortical uptake, with only slight clearance from the transplant kidney toward the end of the study. A modest amount of activity is seen in the bladder, indicating that urinary excretion is now taking place. This is confirmed on pre- and post-voiding 5-minute static images taken after 30 minutes (**Fig. 116.5**). Note the presence of a small amount of uptake in a remaining native kidney in the right upper quadrant.

Differential Diagnosis

- Acute tubular necrosis
- Acute rejection
- Cyclosporin A toxicity
- Acute interstitial nephritis

Diagnosis and Clinical Follow-Up

The diagnosis was acute tubular necrosis, with partial resolution between the initial and follow-up studies. The serum creatinine was 3.97 mg/dL on the day of imaging. One week later, it had risen to 9.71 mg/dL. Three weeks later, at the time of the second renogram, it had normalized to 1.58 mg/dL. No hemodialysis or renal biopsy was performed. Only routine clinical follow-up was needed afterward.

Discussion

Acute tubular necrosis, also known as vasomotor nephropathy, is a form of acute renal failure. It can be seen (1) in the setting of ischemia or hypovolemia caused by cardiac arrest, major surgery, trauma, or burns; (2) as the consequence of intrarenal vasoconstriction induced by radiographic contrast agents or cyclosporin A; and (3) as a direct toxic effect of drugs such as aminoglycosides, amphotericin B, cisplatin, carboplatin, and ifosfamide, as well as endogenous toxins such as myoglobin, hemoglobin, and myeloma light chains. Once the inciting cause is corrected, renal function will typically remain low for 1 to 2 weeks, followed by a gradual spontaneous recovery. Treatment is therefore mainly supportive. However, it is essential to accurately distinguish acute tubular necrosis from other causes of acute failure, such as transplant rejection, glomerulonephritis, and vascular thrombosis, which may require more aggressive therapy.

In a transplanted kidney, acute tubular necrosis can be impossible to distinguish from acute rejection or cyclosporin A toxicity on scintigraphic appearance alone. All of these show delayed uptake and markedly delayed clearance from the renal cortex. Various indices have been proposed to aid in making the differential diagnosis, such as the effective renal plasma flow (ERPF) and excretory index (**Table 116.1**).

However, none of these indices is in wide use, and the differential diagnosis ultimately rests on clinical criteria. Acute tubular necrosis and acute rejection both commonly occur in the early postoperative period. Acute tubular necrosis will typically show a stable or improving pattern on repeated scans, correlating with a rise in urinary volume. Acute rejection may show a worsening pattern if inadequately treated. Cyclosporin A toxicity is usually manifested several months after surgery.

Table 116.1   Effective Renal Plasma Flow and Excretory Index

	ERPF, mL/min	Excretory Index*
Normal post-transplant	270–450	0.8–1.2
Acute rejection	100–270	0.2–0.7
Chronic rejection	30–270	Normal; decreased if severe
ATN	50–300	< 0.2
Partial obstruction	Normal	0.5–0.7

Abbreviations: ATN, acute tubular necrosis; ERPF, effective renal plasma flow.
*Excretory index = ratio of the actual percentage of the dose excreted to the predicted excretion for the patient's ERPF.

PEARLS AND PITFALLS_____

- Even in the absence of detectable excretory function, a high rate of uptake in a kidney with acute tubular necrosis suggests a favorable prognosis. Conversely, poor uptake indicates a low likelihood of functional recovery.

- In acute tubular necrosis and acute rejection, renal tracer activity is confined to the renal cortex, and little or no accumulation is seen in the renal pelvis. If significant tracer retention is seen in the renal pelvis, consider acute obstruction in the differential diagnosis.

- In acute tubular necrosis, the scan images will become abnormal before the serum creatinine begins to rise. Similarly, normalization of the serum creatinine may lag for several days after images begin to show normal function.

Suggested Reading

Dubovsky EV, Russell CD, Bischof-Delaloye A, Bubeck B, Chaiwatanarat T, Hilson AJ, Rutland M, Oei HY, Sfakianakis GN, Taylor A Jr. Report of the Radionuclides in Nephrourology Committee for evaluation of transplanted kidney (review of techniques). Semin Nucl Med 1999;29(2): 175–188

Dunn EK. Radioisotopic evaluation of renal transplants. Urol Radiol 1992;14(2):115–126

El-Maghraby TA, de Fijter JW, van Eck-Smit BL, Zwinderman AH, El-Haddad SI, Pauwels EK. Renographic indices for evaluation of changes in graft function. Eur J Nucl Med 1998;25(11):1575–1586

Eva Dubovsky. Renal transplantation. In: Tauxe WN, Dubovsky EV. Nuclear Medicine in Clinical Urology and Nephrology. Norwalk, CT: Appleton-Century-Crofts; 1985:233–278

CASE 117

Clinical Presentation

A 48-year-old woman in generally good health presents for evaluation as a prospective renal transplant donor.

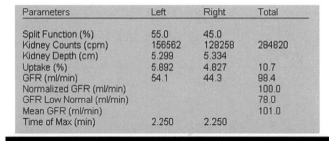

Fig. 117.1

Parameters	Left	Right	Total
Split Function (%)	55.0	45.0	
Kidney Counts (cpm)	156562	128258	284820
Kidney Depth (cm)	5.299	5.334	
Uptake (%)	5.892	4.827	10.7
GFR (ml/min)	54.1	44.3	98.4
Normalized GFR (ml/min)			100.0
GFR Low Normal (ml/min)			78.0
Mean GFR (ml/min)			101.0
Time of Max (min)	2.250	2.250	

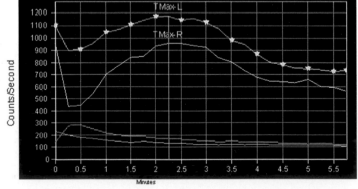

Fig. 117.2

Technique

- Best results are obtained with a medium-energy collimator, although a low-energy, all-purpose collimator can also be used.
- Administer 15 mCi of ^{99m}Tc-DTPA in a compact bolus injection.
- Obtain initial and post-injection syringe counts for 1 minute.
- Acquire twenty-four 15-second frames using a 128×128 matrix. Draw regions-of-interest for the whole kidney, cortex, and background.

Image Interpretation

Posterior dynamic images (**Fig. 117.1**) fail to show the aortic tracer bolus, indicating that imaging was started several seconds late. However, some cardiac and aortic blood pool activity is still seen in the first frame. The venous phase of blood pool activity persists for 2 to 3 minutes in the liver and spleen. This overlaps the renal regions-of-interest and adds to the measured counts in the earliest phase of the study. Both kidneys appear similar in size, with homogeneous cortical uptake. After a cortical transit time of about 2 minutes, tracer can be seen in the collecting systems of both kidneys. At the end of 6.5 minutes of imaging, nearly half of the maximal tracer activity has cleared from both renal cortices.

The shape of the time–activity curve differs from those of the other cases in this section because of the shorter imaging time: 6 minutes versus 20 or 30 minutes (**Fig. 117.2**). There is a transient, steeply dropping peak during the first 15 seconds of the study, which is due to the superimposed blood pool activity from the liver and spleen.

Differential Diagnosis

- Normal glomerular filtration rate (GFR)

Diagnosis and Clinical Follow-Up

Normal renal function, with a normalized total GFR of 100 mL/min per 1.73 m^2. The serum creatinine at the time of the study was 0.74 mg/dL. The estimated GFR, based on this serum creatinine level, was calculated to be 84 mL/min per 1.73 m^2. Abdominal CT showed normal kidneys bilaterally. No further clinical evaluation was performed. To date, no renal transplant has been performed.

Discussion

The GFR is the most useful and widely used measure of renal function, with renal insufficiency and renal failure defined directly in terms of reductions in the GFR. Changes in the effective renal plasma flow (ERPF) usually occur in concert with changes in the GFR; however, the two are not always proportional. In renal arterial stenosis/thrombosis or acute rejection, or under the influence of angiotensin-converting enzyme (ACE) inhibitors (including in captopril renography), the GFR will be affected more than the ERPF because of a decrease in the filtration fraction. In acute tubular necrosis and contrast nephropathy, the ERPF shows the greater decline. In obstructive uropathy, reductions in the GFR and ERPF are usually proportional.

The GFR can be estimated indirectly from the serum creatinine level by using one of several empiric formulas. However, this is an approximation that is affected by numerous factors, including the age and sex of the patient. The kidneys have a large functional reserve; therefore, the GFR needs to decrease by more than 50% before the serum creatinine levels rise. Furthermore, creatinine accumulates slowly as it is added to a preexisting reservoir in the blood. Accordingly, the serum levels will lag several days behind changes in the GFR itself.

For research applications, the most accurate GFR measurements are made from in vitro determinations of ^{99m}Tc-DTPA in serum samples collected at multiple (typically six to eight) time points. However, single serum activity measurements at 180 minutes (in adults) or 91 minutes (in children) have been shown to be nearly as accurate. Purely graphic methods are less accurate but still useful for most clinical applications. In addition to being simpler to perform, they permit separate GFR determinations for each kidney.

The GFR measurement is important in several clinical settings, including the following: (1) assessment of potential transplant donors; (2) serial monitoring of patients with chronic renal failure; (3) evaluation of patients at risk for renal failure (children with urinary obstruction or severe vesicoureteral reflux, or adults with spinal cord injury); and pre-treatment evaluation of patients scheduled for nephrectomy or irradiation of a kidney.

PEARLS AND PITFALLS

- Estimation of renal function by "eyeballing" the cinematic images is unreliable. However, persistent activity in the cardiac blood pool or soft tissues (interstitial fluid) can be suggestive of impaired function.
- True GFR measurement requires the use of a filtered agent, such as ^{99m}Tc-DTPA. ^{99m}Tc-MAG-3 is both filtered and secreted; consequently, this agent can be used to measure the ERPF, but not the GFR. ERPF measurements are typically approximately five times higher than the GFR.
- Although proprietary software analysis programs may vary, in the original Gates method the critical data are collected during the cortical uptake phase between 2 and 3 minutes after injection. If the camera is turned on too early or too late, this phase may be artifactually shifted to the left or to the right, leading to an erroneous GFR value. In such cases, the start and end points for data collection should be adjusted manually to correct for the error.
- In patients with chronic renal failure, the cortical uptake phase will be shifted to the right, sometimes markedly so. Again, the start and end points should be manually adjusted to compensate.
- A good injection bolus is essential for accurate results. A poor injection bolus or tracer infiltration at the injection site will tend to flatten the cortical uptake peak and shift it to the right. Manual correction may improve the results, but some loss of accuracy (usually consisting of a slight underestimation of the GFR) is unavoidable.
- As in all quantitative renal studies, good hydration is essential. Patients should be off diuretics for four to five drug half-lives before the study. They should be encouraged to drink 5 to 10 mL of water per kilogram of their weight for half an hour to an hour before the injection. In problematic cases, it may be necessary to run intravenous fluids before and during the study.
- The measured activity is critically dependent on the distance of the kidneys from the camera face. An increase in kidney depth of 1 cm can lead to an underestimation of the GFR by 14%, and an increase of 2 cm by as much as 26%. The Gates protocol estimates kidney depth as a function of weight and height with the Tonnesen equations:
  - Right Kidney Depth (cm) = 13.3 × (Weight [kg]/Height [cm])
  - Left Kidney Depth (cm) = 13.2 × (Weight [kg]/Height [cm])
- For patients with malrotated or ectopic kidneys (including transplant kidneys) or for very obese patients, the kidney depth should be measured directly by ultrasound or CT.

- If the renal regions-of-interest are drawn too tightly, the measured GFR will be artifactually reduced. Correct placement of background regions-of-interest is also critical and should follow directions on the specific software package being used.

Suggested Reading

Dubovsky EV, Russell CD. Quantitation of renal function with glomerular and tubular agents. Semin Nucl Med 1982;12(4):308–329

Filler G, Sharma AP. How to monitor renal function in pediatric solid organ transplant recipients. Pediatr Transplant 2008;12(4):393–401

Gaspari F, Perico N, Remuzzi G. Measurement of glomerular filtration rate. Kidney Int Suppl 1997;63: S151–S154

Gates GF. Split renal function testing using Tc-99m DTPA: a rapid technique for determining differential glomerular filtration. Clin Nucl Med 1983;8(9):400–407

Peters AM. Quantification of renal haemodynamics with radionuclides. Eur J Nucl Med 1991;18(4): 274–286

Tonnesen KH, Munck O, Hald T, Mogensen P, Wolf H. Influence on the renogram of variation in skin to kidney distance and the clinical importance thereof. In: Zum Winkel K, Blaufox MD, Funck-Brentano J-K, et al. *Radionuclides in Nephrology*. Acton, MA: Publishing Sciences Group; 1975:79–86

CASE 118

Clinical Presentation

A 34-year-old woman with a history of upper respiratory infection/sore throat presents with abnormally elevated serum creatinine.

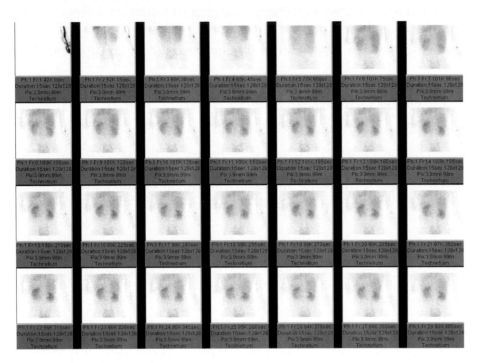

Fig. 118.1

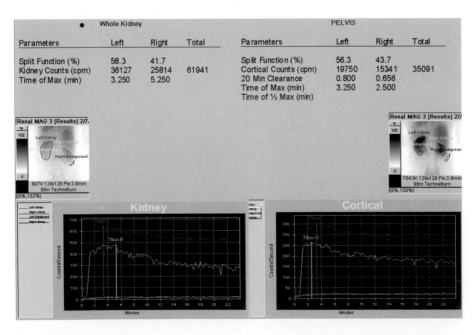

Fig. 118.2

Technique

- Inject 10 mCi of ^{99m}Tc-MAG-3 with a tight intravenous bolus. ^{99m}Tc-DTPA (10–20 mCi) can also be used.
- Use a low-energy, medium-resolution collimator.
- Image native kidneys in the posterior view.
- Image for the first minute with 1- to 2-second frames. Then image for 2 to 30 minutes with 30- to 60-second frames. A 5-minute static image at the end may help to demonstrate ureteral uptake.

Image Interpretation

Posterior dynamic images (**Fig. 118.1**) show a right kidney slightly smaller than the left, without focal abnormalities. The split function is 58% left and 42% right, likely reflecting this anatomic asymmetry. On the time–activity curves (**Fig. 118.2**), cortical uptake is relatively brisk, with maxima at 3.2 minutes on the left and 2.5 minutes on the right. Clearance is moderately delayed, however, and at the end of the study, residuals of 80% and 66% are seen on the left and right, respectively.

Differential Diagnosis

- Glomerulonephritis, probably post-infectious by history
- Acute tubular necrosis (mild)
- Lupus nephritis
- Drug-induced nephropathy
- Diabetic nephropathy
- Hypertensive nephropathy

Diagnosis and Clinical Follow-Up

A kidney biopsy was performed. The diagnosis was immune complex–mediated glomerulonephritis, probably post-infectious. The serum creatinine was mildly elevated at 1.9 mg/dL at the time of the renogram. Two months later, it had normalized to 1.2 mg/dL, indicating resolution of the glomerulonephritis. No further clinical intervention was required.

Discussion

Post-infectious glomerulonephritis is an immune complex–mediated disorder that typically presents with acute nephritic syndrome (often including oliguric renal failure, hematuria, flank pain, and systemic symptoms). It is most commonly seen beginning 10 to 14 days after pharyngeal or cutaneous infection by nephritogenic strains of β-hemolytic streptococci. It is usually self-limited, with complete spontaneous resolution within 6 to 8 weeks in children, although in adults changes may persist for a year or more after the initial infection. Hemodialysis is rarely necessary. Treatment consists of antibiotics, with the supportive use of diuretics and antihypertensives to manage fluid volume and blood pressure.

In acute interstitial nephritis of any cause (including drug-induced and immune complex–mediated disease), both the glomerular filtration rate (GFR) and the effective renal plasma flow (ERPF) are reduced, although the GFR is usually more affected because of a decrease in the filtration fraction. Consequently, a ^{99m}Tc-DTPA scan will tend to show more markedly decreased uptake than does a ^{99m}Tc-MAG-3 scan. A prolonged transit time may be seen with ^{99m}Tc-MAG-3 scanning, which can often resemble that of acute tubular necrosis. Uptake of ^{99m}Tc-DMSA is characteristically markedly decreased, but without focal abnormalities. A ^{67}Ga scan will show abnormally increased renal uptake, usually in a diffuse bilateral pattern.

- Split function should be calculated from whole-kidney regions-of-interest only. Although many automated programs provide split functions from cortical regions-of-interest as well, these are wholly inaccurate because they reflect the areas of the hand-drawn regions-of-interest rather than true differences in kidney function.

- The most useful indicators of cortical function that can be obtained directly from ^{99m}Tc-MAG-3 time-activity curves are the time-to-maximum activity, which reflects cortical uptake, and the residual activity at 20 minutes, which reflects cortical clearance. Both of these are derived from cortical regions-of-interest that are drawn to exclude the renal pelvis and calyces. For ^{99m}Tc-MAG-3, the 20-minute residual will normally be less than 35%. The time-to-maximum should be between 3 and 5 minutes; however, if there is a delay between injection and starting the camera, a shorter time will result.

- The cortical transit time is another useful indicator of cortical function that requires deconvolution analysis for precise calculation. However, it can be roughly estimated by moving frame by frame through the early cine sequence and simply noting the time interval between the first appearance of activity in the kidney and the first frame at which activity is seen in the collecting system. This appears as a slight heterogeneity within the previously homogeneous cortical background.

- The ^{99m}Tc-MAG-3 renogram is of little value in the initial diagnosis of nephritis because the abnormalities seen are common in a wide variety of conditions. However, it can be very useful in assessing the severity of disease. In particular, serial follow-up scans can be very helpful for monitoring disease progression or response to therapy.

Suggested Reading

Aperia A, Bergstrand A, Broberger O, Linné T, Wasserman J. Renal functional changes in acute glomerulonephritis in children: a one-year follow-up. Acta Paediatr Scand 1979;68(2):173–180

Herthelius M, Berg U. Renal function during and after childhood acute poststreptococcal glomerulonephritis. Pediatr Nephrol 1999;13(9):907–911

Sherman RA, Byun KJ. Nuclear medicine in acute and chronic renal failure. Semin Nucl Med 1982;12(3):265–279

CASE 119

Clinical Presentation

A 65-year-old woman presents with a history of peripheral vascular disease and hypertension. During the last year, her blood pressure has been increasingly difficult to control. She is now taking three antihypertensive drugs in high doses.

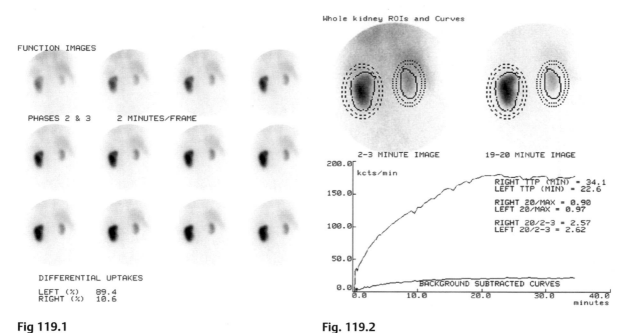

FUNCTION IMAGES

PHASES 2 & 3   2 MINUTES/FRAME

DIFFERENTIAL UPTAKES

LEFT (%)   89.4
RIGHT (%)   10.6

Fig 119.1

Whole kidney ROIs and Curves

2-3 MINUTE IMAGE   19-20 MINUTE IMAGE

200.0 ┐ kcts/min

RIGHT TTP (MIN) = 34.1
LEFT TTP (MIN) = 22.6

RIGHT 20/MAX = 0.90
LEFT 20/MAX = 0.97

RIGHT 20/2-3 = 2.57
LEFT 20/2-3 = 2.62

BACKGROUND SUBTRACTED CURVES

Fig. 119.2

Cortical ROIs and Curves

2-3 MINUTE IMAGE   19-20 MINUTE IMAGE

60.0 ┐ kcts/min

RIGHT TTP (MIN) = 24.1
LEFT TTP (MIN) = 24.1

RIGHT 20/MAX = 0.77
LEFT 20/MAX = 0.97

RIGHT 20/2-3 = 2.44
LEFT 20/2-3 = 2.57

BACKGROUND SUBTRACTED CURVES

Fig. 119.3

CAMERA BASED CLEARANCE

2-3 MINUTE IMAGE

200.0 ┐ kcts/min

BKGND SUBT'D CURVES

PATIENT INFORMATION

HEIGHT (CM) = 160   WEIGHT (KG) = 68.1
AGE = 64 BSA = 1.71 SQ M   % INFILTRATED DOSE = 0.28
DOSE INJ (mCi) = 10.30   DOSE COUNTED (mCi) = 1.15
L KID DEPTH (CM) = 7.7   R KID DEPTH (CM) = 7.8

	LEFT	RIGHT	TOTAL
% RELATIVE UPTAKE	89.2	10.8	
MAG3 CLEARANCE (ML/MIN)	81	10	91
EXPECTED MAG3 CL (ML/MIN)			223
OIH EQUIVALENT (ML/MIN)			154

Fig. 119.4

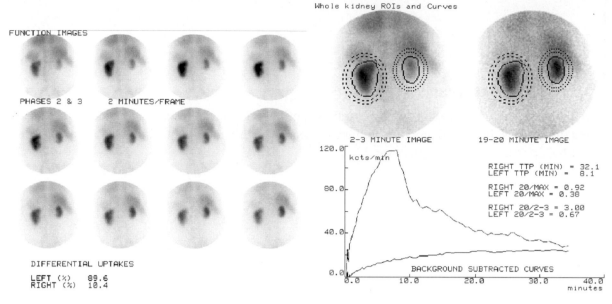

FUNCTION IMAGES

PHASES 2 & 3   2 MINUTES/FRAME

DIFFERENTIAL UPTAKES

LEFT (%)   89.6
RIGHT (%)   10.4

Fig. 119.5

Whole kidney ROIs and Curves

2-3 MINUTE IMAGE   19-20 MINUTE IMAGE

RIGHT TTP (MIN) = 32.1
LEFT TTP (MIN) = 8.1

RIGHT 20/MAX = 0.92
LEFT 20/MAX = 0.38

RIGHT 20/2-3 = 3.00
LEFT 20/2-3 = 0.67

BACKGROUND SUBTRACTED CURVES

Fig. 119.6

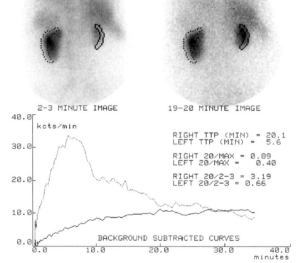

Cortical ROIs and Curves

2-3 MINUTE IMAGE   19-20 MINUTE IMAGE

RIGHT TTP (MIN) = 20.1
LEFT TTP (MIN) = 5.6

RIGHT 20/MAX = 0.89
LEFT 20/MAX = 0.40

RIGHT 20/2-3 = 3.19
LEFT 20/2-3 = 0.66

BACKGROUND SUBTRACTED CURVES

Fig. 119.7

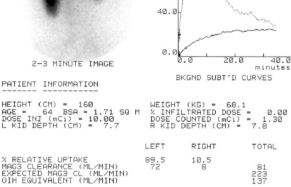

CAMERA BASED CLEARANCE

2-3 MINUTE IMAGE

BKGND SUBT'D CURVES

PATIENT INFORMATION

HEIGHT (CM) =   160   WEIGHT (KG) = 68.1
AGE =   64 BSA = 1.71 SQ M   % INFILTRATED DOSE =   0.00
DOSE INJ (mCi) = 10.00   DOSE COUNTED (mCi) =   1.30
L KID DEPTH (CM) = 7.7   R KID DEPTH (CM) = 7.8

	LEFT	RIGHT	TOTAL
% RELATIVE UPTAKE	89.5	10.5	
MAG3 CLEARANCE (ML/MIN)	72	8	81
EXPECTED MAG3 CL (ML/MIN)			223
OIH EQUIVALENT (ML/MIN)			137

Fig. 119.8

Technique

- A 4 to 12 mCi dose of ^{99m}Tc-MAG-3 is administered intravenously 1 hour after 50 mg of captopril (**Figs. 119.1, 119.2, 119.3,** and **119.4**).
- A baseline study is done 5 days later (**Figs. 119.5, 119.6, 119.7,** and **119.8**).
- The patient should be hydrated before imaging for both studies.
- Administer 25 to 50 mg of crushed (to ensure absorption) captopril 1 hour before imaging.
- Blood pressure measurements should be taken at 15- to 30-minute intervals between the administration of captopril and the start of imaging.
- Use a low-energy, general-purpose collimator.

- Energy window 20%.
- Centered at 140 keV.
- Imaging time is a dynamic sequence: 24 frames at 2 seconds per frame, 16 frames at 15 seconds per frame, and 60 frames at 30 seconds per frame.

Image Interpretation

Functional images from the captopril study (**Fig. 119.1**) show that the left kidney is of normal size with an inhomogeneous parenchymal distribution in the form of reduced tracer in the upper third. The renal collecting system is not visualized. The right kidney appears very small, but homogeneously functioning parenchyma is present. No collecting system details are identifiable.

The functional whole-kidney and cortex curves (**Figs. 119.2** and **119.3**) are very abnormal. The left-kidney curves are of continuous accumulation type; the right-kidney curves have very low amplitude and appear flat. Total function is markedly reduced (**Fig. 119.4**), and ^{99m}Tc-MAG-3 clearance is 91 mL/min, or 34% of expected (**Table 119.1**).

Functional images of the left kidney in the baseline study (**Fig. 119.5**) are similar to the images with captopril, but the collecting system is now visualized (from frame 4 forward). The functional whole-kidney and cortex curves (**Figs. 119.6** and **119.7**) for the left kidney now show a distinct peak and clear elimination.

The right-kidney curves are very similar to the curves seen during captopril challenge. Total function is markedly reduced (**Fig. 119.8**), and ^{99m}Tc-MAG-3 clearance is 81 mL/min (**Table 119.2**).

The marked increase in time to maximum and the increase in cortical retention during captopril challenge compared with baseline are diagnostic for functionally significant renal artery stenosis or renovascular hypertension on the left side.

The atrophic right kidney, with no appreciable change in time to maximum or cortical retention, may represent end-stage renal artery stenosis, but other conditions can also lead to this pattern.

Table 119.1   Captopril Study

Captopril	Left	Right
Split function, %	89	11
Residual cortical activity at 20 min	> 90	90
Time to peak, min	23	> 30

Table 119.2 Baseline Study

Baseline	Left	Right
Split function, %	90	10
Residual cortical activity at 20 min	38	92
Time to peak, min	8.1	> 30

Differential Diagnosis

- Left renal artery stenosis with atrophic right kidney
- Bilateral renal artery stenosis

Diagnosis and Clinical Follow-Up

Renal angiography was performed shortly after the second renogram, revealing (1) an occluded right main renal artery and (2) a 70% stenosis proximally in the left renal artery. Left renal artery angioplasty was performed successfully. The blood pressure was subsequently responsive to a single-drug regimen.

Discussion

An estimated 5% of cases of systemic hypertension are due to surgically correctable renal arterial stenosis. However, renal arterial stenosis is fairly common, and only a small percentage of patients who have it fall within this surgically correctable subgroup. The captopril renogram complements anatomic imaging (angiography) by providing information about the physiologic significance of the renal arterial stenosis. A positive captopril study predicts a good clinical response to renal artery dilation or surgical intervention.

Functionally significant renal arterial stenosis leads to reduced filtration pressure, which activates the intrarenal renin-angiotensin-aldosterone system locally. This constricts the efferent arterioles, ensuring a sufficient filtration pressure. Angiotensin-converting enzyme (ACE) inhibitors block this compensatory mechanism, resulting in an abrupt drop in filtration pressure. Along with the drop in filtration pressure, there is a decrease in tubular luminal transport, which results in the cortical retention of tubular agents like MAG-3.

A positive captopril study is defined by one or more of the following key findings compared with a baseline study:

* Decreased cortical uptake (> 10% change in split function difference between the two kidneys)
* Increased cortical transit time
* Increase of more than 11 minutes in time to peak activity
* Drop in absolute glomerular filtration rate (GFR) or effective renal plasma flow (ERPF) of more than 20%

When one or more of these criteria are present in a single kidney, the specificity and sensitivity of the study for identifying surgically correctable renal arterial stenosis approach 90%. The interpretation of similar changes in both kidneys becomes more problematic because this can reflect either bilateral renal arterial stenosis or chronic renal parenchymal disease in general.

Both 2-day and 1-day protocols are widely used; in the 2-day protocol, the captopril study is performed first. If the result is normal, functionally significant renal arterial stenosis is excluded, and the baseline study can be skipped. If the result is abnormal, the patient must return on a second day for the baseline study.

In the 1-day protocol, the baseline study is performed first. After the first dose of radiotracer has cleared from the kidneys, captopril is given, and a second round of imaging (with injection of a second dose of radiotracer) is performed 1 hour later.

Results of the 2-day and 1-day protocols are equivalent, and the rationale for choosing one or the other is the convenience to the patient of a 1-day study versus the slight cost savings that can be achieved by occasionally foregoing unnecessary baseline imaging.

PEARLS AND PITFALLS

* In captopril imaging, each kidney serves as its own control. The basis for diagnosis is the change in each kidney, captopril phase versus baseline. The same principle applies to patients with only one kidney.
* The whole-kidney time–activity curves are similar in renal obstruction and renal arterial stenosis. However, these can usually be distinguished by the relative degree of activity in the cortex and renal pelvis.

- Kidneys with very low function are difficult to evaluate. Such kidneys may have renal arterial stenosis but too little function to generate a measurable response to captopril. Equivocal results (intermediate probability for renal arterial stenosis) are typical.

- ACE inhibitors should be withheld for 24 to 72 hours before the test. Diuretics should also be discontinued for 24 to 48 hours.

- Standard hydration of all patients before both studies is important to avoid false-positive results, especially when tubular agents are used and cortical retention is a major diagnostic variable.

- Crushing the captopril tablet will facilitate rapid absorption of the medication.

- Blood pressure should be monitored and recorded just before the administration of captopril and every 15 to 30 minutes thereafter until imaging begins. A fall in systemic systolic pressure below 90 mm Hg will compromise kidney function and invalidate the examination. If this occurs, stop the study and expand the blood volume, elevating the extremities (the legs contain about 0.5 L of blood) while intravenous fluids are given. It may be prudent, particularly in older patients, to place an intravenous line before captopril is given because venous access may be difficult once the blood pressure drops.

- ACE inhibitor therapy should be withheld 48 to 72 hours before the study. If this is considered risky, a captopril-equivalent study can be performed by using the patient's regular morning dose of ACE inhibitor in place of captopril. If the captopril-equivalent renogram is normal, this excludes renal arterial stenosis, and no further imaging is required. If the captopril-equivalent renogram is abnormal, a baseline scan will be necessary. It may be sufficient to withhold an evening dose of ACE inhibitor the night before the baseline study and delay the morning dose until after imaging is complete.

- Both filtered agents (diethylenetriamine pentaacetic acid [DTPA]) and tubular agents (MAG-3) can be used. The tubular agents are more reliable because of a better target-to-background ratio, which allows for functional curves with less noise.

- If significant hydronephrosis is known or suspected, a small dose of furosemide (1 mg/Kg, maximum 40 mg) just before or early into imaging can minimize interference from tracer accumulating in the renal pelvis.

- Reduce the captopril dose (eg, to 25 mg) in older patients with arteriosclerosis. In these patients, compensation by means of peripheral vasoconstriction is more difficult.

Suggested Reading

Davidson R, Wilcox CS. Diagnostic usefulness of renal scanning after angiotensin converting enzyme inhibitors. Hypertension 1991;18(3):299–303

Dondi M, Fanti S, De Fabritiis A, Zuccala A, Gaggi R, Mirelli M, Stella A, Marengo M, Losinno F, Monetti N. Prognostic value of captopril renal scintigraphy in renovascular hypertension. J Nucl Med 1992;33(11):2040–2044

Erbslöh-Möller B, Dumas A, Roth D, Sfakianakis GN, Bourgoignie JJ. Furosemide-131I-hippuran renography after angiotensin-converting enzyme inhibition for the diagnosis of renovascular hypertension. Am J Med 1991;90(1):23–29

Nally JV Jr, Black HRS. State-of-the-art review: captopril renography—pathophysiological considerations and clinical observations. Semin Nucl Med 1992;22(2):85–97

Setaro JF, Saddler MC, Chen CC, Hoffer PB, Roer DA, Markowitz DM, Meier GH, Gosberg RJ, Black HR. Simplified captopril renography in diagnosis and treatment of renal artery stenosis. Hypertension 1991;18(3):289–298

Section IX

Biliary Scintigraphy

Kevin J. Donohoe

CASE 120

Clinical Presentation

A 45-year-old man presents with right upper quadrant pain (**Fig. 120.1**).

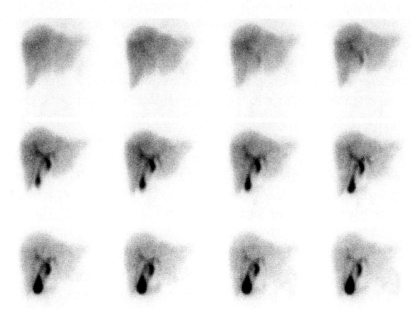

Fig. 120.1

Technique

- The patient should take nothing by mouth between less than 24 hours and more than 4 hours before the test.
- Immediately following the injection of 1.5 mCi of ^{99m}Tc-DISIDA, the patient is placed in a supine position beneath the gamma camera.
- Continuous images acquired in a 256 × 256 matrix are divided into 1-minute frames.
- Straight anterior views are obtained with a high-resolution, parallel-hole collimator.
- Delayed static images may be acquired as necessary.

Image Interpretation

Selected dynamic images show rapid uptake of tracer into the liver and subsequent excretion into the biliary tract and small bowel (**Fig. 120.1**). The gallbladder is seen within 10 minutes.

Differential Diagnosis

- Normal study
- False-negative study secondary to tracer in duodenum overlying gallbladder fossa (although this would be expected to vary over time)
- Bile leak into gallbladder fossa
- Acalculous cholecystitis
- Choledochal cyst overlying gallbladder fossa

Diagnosis and Clinical Follow-Up

Peptic ulcer disease was diagnosed. No evidence of biliary disease was noted.

Discussion

The biliary imaging study is a very sensitive and specific test for cystic duct obstruction in patients with the acute onset of right upper quadrant pain. The study has decreased in popularity in recent years, however, because alternative imaging modalities, such as ultrasonography, CT, and MRI, are more readily available. The anatomic imaging tests provide information not only about the liver and biliary tract but also about the adjacent structures in the abdomen, so that the anatomic imaging tests are better suited for the screening of abdominal pain. The scintigraphic study, on the other hand, provides information only about the liver and biliary tract, so that it is less valuable as a screening test. The study is therefore used more often in patients with equivocal findings on other tests. The patients have frequently been in the hospital for a period of time and may have taken nothing by mouth for more than 24 hours, making interpretation of the biliary study more difficult.

The normal sequence in which tracer appears in the biliary collecting system and gastrointestinal tract has been debated. Some believe that tracer should normally appear in the gallbladder before it appears in the small bowel. Others believe that the small bowel may be seen before the gallbladder in patients who have eaten recently or who have been fasting for several hours.

PEARLS AND PITFALLS

- Provided the patient is in the appropriate fasting state (fasting for more than 4 hours but less than 24 hours), tracer should be seen in the gallbladder within 60 minutes for the study to be called normal. Appearance of the gallbladder after 60 minutes is more consistent with chronic cholecystitis.
- Clearance of tracer from the cardiac blood pool found on top of the left lobe of the liver is a good indicator of hepatocellular function. Delayed blood pool clearance may indicate that hepatocellular dysfunction is responsible for the lack of gallbladder visualization.
- Pooling of tracer in the small bowel overlying the gallbladder fossa may be confused with normal accumulation of tracer in the gallbladder. Tracer in the small bowel can be cleared by instructing the patient to drink a small amount of water. The water usually empties quickly from the stomach and washes away any tracer in the small bowel without stimulating cholecystokinin release.
- Look for signs of bowel obstruction, biliary reflux into the stomach, defects in the liver (metastases), and other serendipitous findings.
- Focal uptake of tracer in the region of the gallbladder that increases and decreases over time is very unlikely to be in the gallbladder. The gallbladder should not contract unless stimulated by cholecystokinin.
- The caliber of the biliary ducts cannot be accurately determined with biliary scintigraphy. Intense concentration of tracer in a duct of normal caliber can demonstrate "blooming" (through narrow-angle scatter), which makes the duct look larger than it is.
- The time between the last meal and imaging can be as little as 2 hours, but the specificity of the test may be diminished if imaging is done less than 4 hours after a meal.

Suggested Reading

Chen PFM, Nimeri A, Pham QHT, Yuh JN, Gusz JR, Chung RS. The clinical diagnosis of chronic acalculous cholecystitis. Surgery 2001;130(4):578–581, discussion 581–583

Hulse PA, Nicholson DA. Investigation of biliary obstruction. Br J Hosp Med 1994;52(2-3):103–107

Kalliafas S, Ziegler DW, Flancbaum L, Choban PS. Acute acalculous cholecystitis: incidence, risk factors, diagnosis, and outcome. Am Surg 1998;64(5):471–475

Ko CW, Lee SP. Gastrointestinal disorders of the critically ill. Biliary sludge and cholecystitis. Best Pract Res Clin Gastroenterol 2003;17(3):383–396

Lin EC, Kuni CC. Radionuclide imaging of hepatic and biliary disease. Semin Liver Dis 2001;21(2): 179–194

Saini S. Imaging of the hepatobiliary tract. N Engl J Med 1997;336(26):1889–1894

Singer AJ, McCracken G, Henry MC, Thode HC Jr, Cabahug CJ. Correlation among clinical, laboratory, and hepatobiliary scanning findings in patients with suspected acute cholecystitis [see comments]. Ann Emerg Med 1996;28(3):267–272

Warrington JC, Charron M. Pediatric gastrointestinal nuclear medicine. Semin Nucl Med 2007;37(4): 269–285

Weissmann HS, Badia J, Sugarman LA, Kluger L, Rosenblatt R, Freeman LM. Spectrum of 99m-Tc-IDA cholescintigraphic patterns in acute cholecystitis. Radiology 1981;138(1):167–175

Weissmann HS, Sugarman LA, Frank MS, Freeman LM. Serendipity in technetium-99m dimethyl iminodiacetic acid cholescintigraphy: diagnosis of nonbiliary disorders in suspected acute cholecystitis. Radiology 1980;135(2):449–454

Zuckier LS, Freeman LM. Selective role of nuclear medicine in evaluating the acute abdomen. Radiol Clin North Am 2003;41(6):1275–1288

CASE 121

Clinical Presentation

A 71-year-old man presents with a history of abdominal and chest pain. Myocardial infarction is ruled out (**Fig. 121.1**).

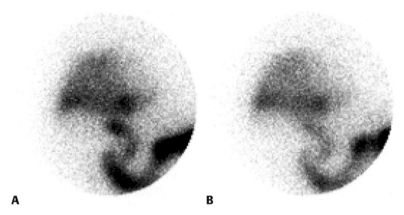

A   B

Fig. 121.1

Technique

- The patient should take nothing by mouth between less than 24 hours and more than 4 hours before the test.
- Immediately following the injection of 1.5 mCi of ^{99m}Tc-DISIDA, the patient is placed in a supine position beneath the gamma camera.
- Continuous images acquired in a 256 × 256 matrix are divided into 1-minute frames.
- Images are obtained in the left anterior oblique projection with a slant-hole collimator to better separate the small bowel from the liver. Straight anterior views may be obtained with a high-resolution, parallel-hole collimator if a slant-hole collimator is not available.
- Delayed static images may be acquired as necessary.

Image Interpretation

Serial 1-minute images (not shown) showed the prompt uptake of tracer by hepatocytes. Images at 60 minutes (**Fig. 121.1A**) and 75 minutes (**Fig. 121.1B**) show tracer in the liver and small bowel and a band of tracer ("rim sign") around the region of the gallbladder bed.

Differential Diagnosis

- Acute cholecystitis
- Gallbladder perforation
- Gangrenous cholecystitis
- Locally dilated biliary collecting system

Diagnosis and Clinical Follow-Up

The patient underwent surgery to remove a gangrenous gallbladder.

Discussion

The rim sign is a nonspecifc sign on biliary imaging that suggests gangrenous cholecystitis. Because the rim sign may be caused by inflammation, local biliary stasis, or local edema, the condition may warrant more immediate attention. The referring physician should be contacted and the significance of the finding communicated.

PEARLS AND PITFALLS⎯⎯⎯⎯⎯⎯⎯⎯⎯⎯⎯⎯⎯⎯⎯⎯⎯⎯⎯⎯⎯⎯⎯⎯⎯⎯⎯⎯⎯⎯⎯⎯⎯

- The rim sign may be related to hyperperfusion. Flow images obtained during tracer injection may provide additional information about local inflammatory changes.
- The rim sign is nonspecifc and may be caused by other structures, such as a prominent porta hepatis.

Suggested Reading

Aburano T, Yokoyama K, Taniguchi M, et al. Diagnostic values of gallbladder hyperperfusion and the rim sign in radionuclide angiography and hepatobiliary imaging. Gastrointest Radiol 1990;15(3):229–232

Bohdiewicz PJ. The diagnostic value of grading hyperperfusion and the rim sign in cholescintigraphy. Clin Nucl Med 1993;18(10):867–871

Dorio PJ. The rim sign. Radiology 1998;209(3):801–802

Joseph UA, Barron BJ, Lamki LM. Rim sign in Tc-99m sulfur colloid hepatic scintigraphy. Clin Nucl Med 2005;30(4):284–285

Meekin GK, Ziessman HA, Klappenbach RS. Prognostic value and pathophysiologic significance of the rim sign in cholescintigraphy. J Nucl Med 1987;28(11):1679–1682

Ziessman HA. Acute cholecystitis, biliary obstruction, and biliary leakage. Semin Nucl Med 2003;33(4):279–296

CASE 122

Clinical Presentation

A 23-year-old woman presents with a history of several weeks of intermittent abdominal and right upper quadrant pain (**Fig. 122.1**).

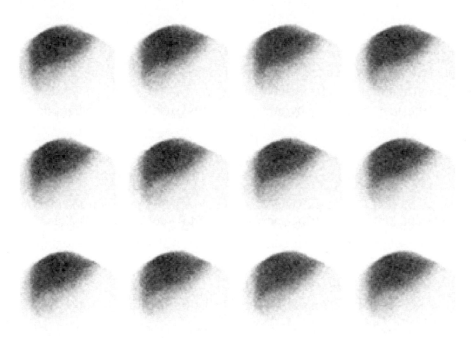

Fig. 122.1

Technique

- The patient should take nothing by mouth between less than 24 hours and more than 4 hours before the test.
- Immediately following the injection of 1.5 mCi of ^{99m}Tc-DISIDA, the patient is placed in a supine position beneath the gamma camera.
- Continuous images acquired in a 64 × 64 matrix are divided into 1-minute frames.
- Images are obtained in the left anterior oblique projection with a slant-hole collimator to better separate the small bowel from the liver. Straight anterior views may be obtained with a high-resolution, parallel-hole collimator if a slant-hole collimator is not available.
- Delayed static images may be acquired as necessary.

Image Interpretation

The images in **Fig. 122.1** are samples of the 1-minute frames obtained during imaging. The patient was imaged continuously for 90 minutes without a change in the distribution of tracer. These images show the rapid uptake and homogeneous distribution of tracer throughout the hepatic parenchyma. No movement of tracer into the biliary collecting system or bowel was noted during imaging.

Differential Diagnosis

- Choledocholithiasis
- Other causes of complete duct obstruction, such as carcinoma of the distal biliary tract, metastatic disease, and external compression of the common bile duct
- Drug cholestasis
- Hepatitis
- Biliary atresia

Diagnosis and Clinical Follow-Up

Common bile duct obstruction was diagnosed. Endoscopic retrograde cholangiopancreatography (ERCP) demonstrated an edematous, inflamed sphincter of Oddi. Laparotomy revealed two impacted gallstones at the sphincter of Oddi.

Discussion

This study demonstrates the typical appearance of complete common bile duct obstruction. Homogeneous uptake of tracer is seen in the liver because the hepatocytes are functioning normally, but the obstruction in the biliary collecting system causes intrahepatic cholestasis.

PEARLS AND PITFALLS

- The differential diagnosis includes any cause of intrahepatic cholestasis.
- Diffuse hepatocellular disease may prevent the excretion of tracer into the biliary collecting system. Prompt uptake of tracer within the first 15 minutes suggests normal hepatocellular function.
- Tracer activity in the kidneys or urinary collecting system can mimic excretion into the bowel.
- Rarely, hepatocellular disease may diminish the excretion of tracer into the collecting system, yet hepatocellular uptake of tracer is normal.
- In adults, delayed images of common bile duct obstruction, such as at 24 hours, have not been well studied. The appearance of tracer activity in the bowel or biliary collecting system on 24-hour delayed images should not be considered evidence of a nonobstructed biliary collecting system.

Suggested Reading

Donohoe KJ, Woolfenden JM, Stemmer JL. Biliary imaging suggesting common duct obstruction in acute viral hepatitis. Case report. Clin Nucl Med 1987;12(9):711–712

Iqbal M, Aggarwal S, Kumar R, et al. The role of 99mTc mebrofenin hepatobiliary scanning in predicting common bile duct stones in patients with gallstone disease. Nucl Med Commun 2004;25(3):285–289

Mathur SK, Soonawalla ZF, Shah SR, Goel M, Shikare S. Role of biliary scintiscan in predicting the need for cholangiography. Br J Surg 2000;87(2):181–185

Weltman DI, Zeman RK. Acute diseases of the gallbladder and biliary ducts. Radiol Clin North Am 1994;32(5):933–950

Yoon SN, Yoo BM, Hwang KH. Hepatobiliary scintigraphy showing acute complete common bile duct obstruction in a patient with acute hepatitis. Clin Nucl Med 2001;26(2):151–152

CASE 123

Clinical Presentation

A 63-year-old man presents with epigastric distress and a history of recent cholecystectomy (**Fig. 123.1**).

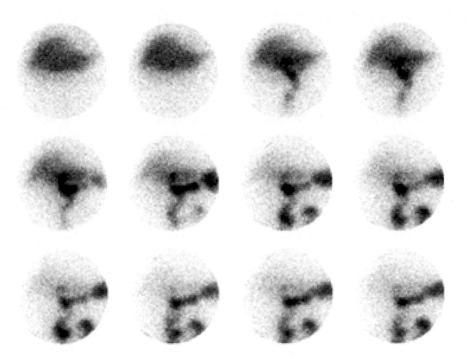

Fig. 123.1

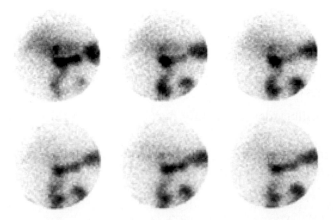

Fig. 123.2

Technique

- The patient should take nothing by mouth between less than 24 hours and more than 4 hours before the test.
- Immediately following the injection of 1.5 mCi of ^{99m}Tc-DISIDA, the patient is placed in a supine position beneath the gamma camera.
- Continuous images acquired in a 64 × 64 matrix are divided into 1-minute frames.
- Images are obtained in the left anterior oblique projection with a slant-hole collimator to better separate the small bowel from the liver. Straight anterior views may be obtained with a high-resolution, parallel-hole collimator if a slant-hole collimator is not available.
- Delayed static images may be acquired as necessary.

Image Interpretation

Selected 1-minute images (**Fig. 123.1**) obtained for 1 hour show uptake and excretion of tracer into the bowel. Reflux of tracer into the stomach is noted following the appearance of tracer activity in the bowel (**Fig. 123.2**).

Differential Diagnosis

- Normal variant
- Bile gastritis
- Superimposition of distal duodenum over stomach
- Biliary leak (from biliary tract or bowel perforation)

Diagnosis and Clinical Follow-Up

The images demonstrated reflux of bile into the stomach. No further workup of the reflux was obtained.

Discussion

The reflux of bile into the stomach can cause a gastritis that may be important in the diagnosis of epigastric discomfort. When bile reflux is noted on a biliary imaging study, it should be mentioned in the study report.

PEARLS AND PITFALLS_____

- Dynamic images displayed in cinematic format help to demonstrate the reflux of tracer into the stomach.
- Biliary leak following cholecystectomy may mimic gastric reflux. Filling of the stomach with bile and subsequent emptying of bile from the stomach will help rule out biliary leak.

Suggested Reading

Aydin M, Gumurdulu Y, Yapar AF, Reyhan M, Sukan A, Serin E. The significance of duodenogastric bile reflux seen during hepatobiliary scintigraphy. Eur J Nucl Med Mol Imaging 2006;33:S356–S357

Fountos A, Chrysos E, Tsiaoussis J, et al. Duodenogastric reflux after biliary surgery: scintigraphic quantification and improvement with erythromycin. ANZ J Surg 2003;73(6):400–403

Gerard PS, Gerczuk P, Finestone H. Bile reflux in the esophagus demonstrated by HIDA scintigraphy. Clin Nucl Med 2007;32(3):224–225

Hermans D, Sokal EM, Collard JM, Romagnoli R, Buts JP. Primary duodenogastric reflux in children and adolescents. Eur J Pediatr 2003;162(9):598–602

Jurgens MJ, Drane WE, Vogel SB. Dual-radionuclide simultaneous biliary and gastric scintigraphy to depict surgical treatment of bile reflux. Radiology 2003;229(1):283–287

Koek GH, Vos R, Flamen P, et al. Oesophageal clearance of acid and bile: a combined radionuclide, pH, and Bilitec study. Gut 2004;53(1):21–26

Obradovic VB, Artiko V, Chebib HY, Petrovic MN, Vlajkovic M, Petrovic NM. Estimation of the enterogastric reflux by modified scintigraphic method. Hepatogastroenterology 2000;47(33):738–741

Sundbom M, Hedenström H, Gustavsson S. Duodenogastric bile reflux after gastric bypass: a cholescintigraphic study. Dig Dis Sci 2002;47(8):1891–1896

Weissmann HS, Sugarman LA, Frank MS, Freeman LM. Serendipity in technetium-99m dimethyl iminodiacetic acid cholescintigraphy: diagnosis of nonbiliary disorders in suspected acute cholecystitis. Radiology 1980;135(2):449–454

CASE 124

Clinical Presentation

A 55-year-old man with a history of intravenous drug abuse presents with malaise and jaundice (**Fig. 124.1**).

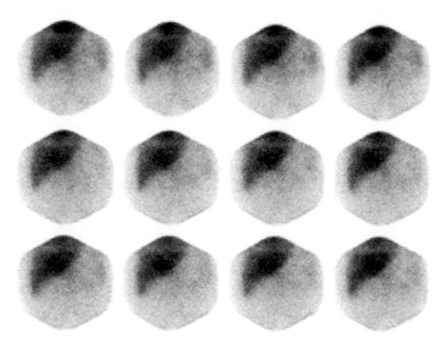

Fig. 124.1

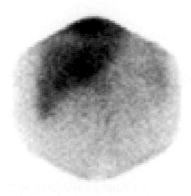

Fig. 124.2

Technique

- The patient should take nothing by mouth between less than 24 hours and more than 4 hours before the test.
- Immediately following the injection of 1.5 mCi of ^{99m}Tc-DISIDA, the patient is placed in a supine position beneath the gamma camera.
- Continuous images acquired in a 64 × 64 matrix are divided into 1-minute frames.
- Images are obtained in the left anterior oblique projection with a slant-hole collimator to better separate the small bowel from the liver. Straight anterior views may be obtained with a high-resolution, parallel-hole collimator if a slant-hole collimator is not available.
- Delayed static images may be acquired as necessary.

Image Interpretation

Figure 124.1 shows the uptake of tracer in the liver but also demonstrates tracer in the kidneys and persistent tracer activity in the blood pool. The delayed image obtained at 90 minutes also shows activity in the bowel (**Fig. 124.2**). The bowel activity was confirmed on cinematic display, which showed the tracer moving in a pattern consistent with small bowel.

Differential Diagnosis

- Choledocholithiasis
- Other causes of complete duct obstruction, such as carcinoma of the distal biliary tract, metastatic disease, and external compression of the common bile duct
- Drug cholestasis
- Hepatitis
- Biliary atresia

Diagnosis and Clinical Follow-Up

Viral hepatitis was diagnosed. No evidence of biliary obstruction was noted on further workup.

Discussion

Because the cardiac blood pool is usually just above the left lobe of the liver, the clearance of tracer from the blood pool can easily be monitored. Delayed clearance causes poor resolution of the liver contour and persistent diffuse background tracer activity. Although the kidneys are a secondary route of tracer excretion, they are posterior structures and therefore not seen very well on anterior views.

PEARLS AND PITFALLS

- Delayed hepatocellular uptake may also be seen if the radiopharmaceutical is not properly prepared.
- Make sure that the technologist begins imaging at the time of tracer injection or notifies you of any delay between the time of tracer injection and imaging. If technical difficulties with beginning imaging occurred immediately following the injection of tracer, the first image might suggest that tracer clearance was better than it actually was.
- If the hepatic concentration of tracer is poor, secondary excretion in the urinary collecting system may mimic activity in the bowel.

Suggested Reading

Aburano T, Yokoyama K, Shuke N, et al. 99mTc colloid and 99mTc IDA imagings in diffuse hepatic disease. J Clin Gastroenterol 1993;17(4):321–326

Caglar M, Sari O, Akcan Y. Prediction of therapy response to interferon-alpha in chronic viral hepatitis-B by liver and hepatobiliary scintigraphy. Ann Nucl Med 2002;16(7):511–514

Donohoe KJ, Woolfenden JM, Stemmer JL. Biliary imaging suggesting common duct obstruction in acute viral hepatitis. Case report. Clin Nucl Med 1987;12(9):711–712

el-Youssef M, Whitington PF. Diagnostic approach to the child with hepatobiliary disease. Semin Liver Dis 1998;18(3):195–202

Johnson K, Alton HM, Chapman S. Evaluation of mebrofenin hepatoscintigraphy in neonatal-onset jaundice. Pediatr Radiol 1998;28(12):937–941

Roca I, Ciofetta G. Hepatobiliary scintigraphy in current pediatric practice. Q J Nucl Med 1998;42(2): 113–118

Yoon SN, Yoo BM, Hwang KH. Hepatobiliary scintigraphy showing acute complete common bile duct obstruction in a patient with acute hepatitis. Clin Nucl Med 2001;26(2):151–152

CASE 125

Clinical Presentation

A 53-year-old woman experiences continued abdominal distension on postoperative day 3 after undergoing laparoscopic cholecystectomy (**Figs. 125.1** and **125.2**).

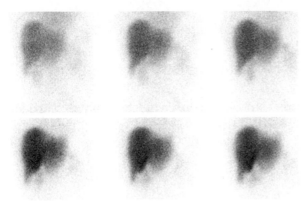

Fig. 125.1

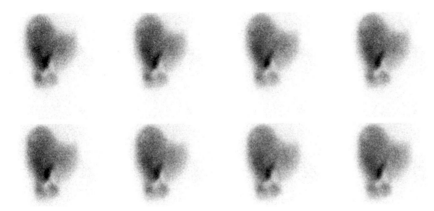

Fig. 125.2

Technique

- The patient should take nothing by mouth between less than 24 hours and more than 4 hours before the test.
- Immediately following the injection of 1.5 mCi of ^{99m}Tc-DISIDA, the patient is placed in a supine position beneath the gamma camera.
- Continuous images acquired in a 256 × 256 matrix are divided into 1-minute frames.
- Straight anterior views are obtained with a high-resolution, parallel-hole collimator.
- Delayed static images may be acquired as necessary.

Image Interpretation

Selected 1-minute dynamic images (**Fig. 125.1**) show the prompt uptake of tracer by the liver and subsequent appearance in the region of the gallbladder. Images later in the sequence (**Fig. 125.2**) show a vague focus of tracer concentration over the right lobe of the liver, lateral to the gallbladder. Also noted on these images is a change in the contour of the dome of the right lobe.

Differential Diagnosis

- Biliary tract leak
- Duodenal perforation
- Hepatoma (these findings are very rarely seen in hepatoma)

Diagnosis and Clinical Follow-Up

The accumulation of fluid lateral to the gallbladder is consistent with a bile leak (**Fig. 125.3**). CT shows a perihepatic accumulation of fluid surrounding the right lobe of the liver below the diaphragm (**Fig. 125.4**). Percutaneous drainage revealed the fluid to be bile.

Discussion

The biliary imaging study is an excellent test for demonstrating bile leak. In postoperative patients with a perihepatic accumulation of fluid, there may be a question regarding not only the source of the fluid but also, more importantly, whether the fluid is still accumulating. The biliary imaging study is the gold standard for demonstrating active bile leak. Although the static images shown in this case demonstrated the findings, cine display of the serial images made the abnormal sites of tracer accumulation much more readily apparent.

PEARLS AND PITFALLS

- If the leak is slow, delayed images may be necessary.
- If imaging is halted too early, a focal leak in the region of the gallbladder or bowel may be mistaken for expected excretion into normal structures. Continued imaging may be needed to show that local accumulation does not demonstrate the contour of normal structures.
- Cine display facilitates the diagnosis of abnormal sites of tracer accumulation.

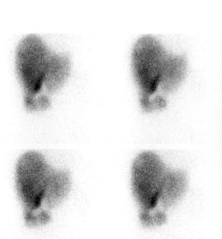

Fig. 125.3

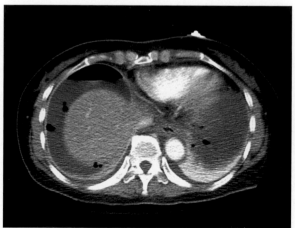

Fig. 125.4

Suggested Reading

Balakrishnan VB, Kumar R, Dhanpathi H, et al. Hepatobiliary scintigraphy in detecting lesser sac bile leak in postcholecystectomy patients: the need to recognize as a separate entity. Clin Nucl Med 2008;33(3):161–167

Bohnen NI, Gross MD, Shapiro B. Gallbladder bed photopenic halo on hepatobiliary scintigraphy: a sign of biliary leakage. Clin Nucl Med 1999;24(1):70–71

Goletti O, Boni G, Lippolis PV, et al. Scintigraphic evaluation of biliary leakage following laparoscopic cholecystectomy. Surg Laparosc Endosc 1993;3(4):286–289

Iqbal S, Khalid A, Weng LJ, Mansour M. Assessing the response to drainage for biliary leak: falsely positive HIDA scan. Am J Gastroenterol 2006;101(9):730

Johnston TD, Gates R, Reddy KS, Nickl NJ, Ranjan D. Nonoperative management of bile leaks following liver transplantation. Clin Transplant 2000;14(4 Pt 2):365–369

Mittal BR, Sunil HV, Bhattacharya A, Singh B. Hepatobiliary scintigraphy in management of bile leaks in patients with blunt abdominal trauma. ANZ J Surg 2008;78(7):597–600

Mortazavi N, Chaumet-Riffaud P, Chauffet-Riffaud P, Archambaud F, Prigent A. Biliary leak in a child after liver transplant and value of delayed images. Clin Nucl Med 2008;33(1):44–45

Peters JH, Ollila D, Nichols KE, et al. Diagnosis and management of bile leaks following laparoscopic cholecystectomy. Surg Laparosc Endosc 1994;4(3):163–170

Ramachandran A, Gupta SM, Johns WD. Various presentations of postcholecystectomy bile leak diagnosed by scintigraphy. Clin Nucl Med 2001;26(6):495–498

Young SA, Sfakianakis GN, Pyrsopoulos N, Nishida S. Hepatobiliary scintigraphy in liver transplant patients: the "blind end sign" and its differentiation from bile leak. Clin Nucl Med 2003;28(8):638–642

CASE 126

Clinical Presentation

A 71-year-old man who has pancreatic cancer presents with right upper quadrant pain. The patient is given narcotic analgesia before biliary scintigraphy is started (**Fig. 126.1**).

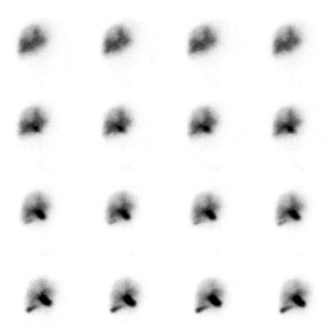

Fig. 126.1

Technique

- The patient should take nothing by mouth between less than 24 hours and more than 4 hours before the test.
- Immediately following the injection of 1.5 mCi of ^{99m}Tc-DISIDA, the patient is placed in a supine position beneath the gamma camera.
- Continuous images acquired in a 64 × 64 matrix are divided into 1-minute frames.
- Images are obtained in the left anterior oblique projection with a slant-hole collimator to better separate the small bowel from the liver. Straight anterior views may be obtained with a high-resolution, parallel-hole collimator if a slant-hole collimator is not available.
- Delayed static images may be acquired as necessary.

Image Interpretation

Selected 1-minute images (**Fig. 126.1**) immediately after the injection of tracer demonstrate irregular uptake of tracer in the liver. The defects in the liver correspond to lesions noted on CT scan. The gallbladder is visualized, but no activity is seen in the bowel at 1 hour. The lack of small-bowel visualization may be secondary to contraction of the sphincter of Oddi caused by narcotics. A prominent hepatic duct is noted. This may be secondary to the pooling of tracer in a normal-caliber duct, however, and is not necessarily a sign of a dilated or obstructed duct.

429

Differential Diagnosis

- Hemangioma
- Hepatic cyst
- Metastasis
- Abscess
- Hepatoma

Diagnosis and Clinical Follow-Up

Biopsy demonstrated that the liver defects seen on the biliary study were secondary to metastases of pancreatic cancer.

Discussion

Biliary imaging studies may provide information about causes of right upper quadrant abdominal pain other than cholecystitis. Early images of tracer uptake in the liver can demonstrate not only diffuse hepatocellular dysfunction but also focal abnormalities in the liver. Intrahepatic lesions may also cause the regional obstruction of bile flow. This may be demonstrated by delayed or absent emptying of tracer from one or more hepatic segments. If complete cholestasis is present in the obstructed segment, the visualization of tracer in a dilated biliary tree is unlikely.

PEARLS AND PITFALLS

- Focal defects in the liver are nonspecific and should be followed with more anatomic imaging, such as CT.
- Photomultiplier tube malfunction can mimic focal hepatic lesions. The daily review of flood images before patient studies are acquired will help eliminate this problem.
- Concentrated tracer in a normal-caliber duct may cause a "blooming" artifact, which makes the duct look dilated. Therefore, the caliber of ducts should not be inferred from a scintigraphic study.

Suggested Reading

Kinnard MF, Alavi A, Rubin RA, Lichtenstein GR. Nuclear imaging of solid hepatic masses. Semin Roentgenol 1995;30(4):375–395

Liu CH, Yen RF, Liu KL, Jeng YM, Pan MH, Yang PM. Biliary hamartomas with delayed 99mTc-diisopropyl iminodiacetic acid clearance. J Gastroenterol 2005;40(5):540–544

Salvatori M. Imaging of hepatic focal lesions by nuclear medicine. J Surg Oncol Suppl 1993;3:189–191

CASE 127

Clinical Presentation

A 53-year-old woman who has hepatitis C presents with right upper quadrant pain associated with meals (**Figs. 127.1** and **127.2**).

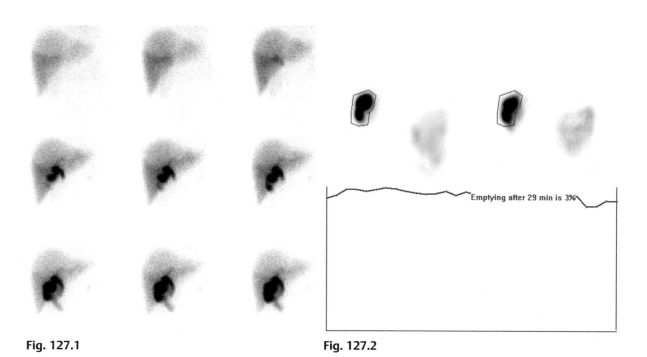

Fig. 127.1   **Fig. 127.2**

Technique

- The patient should take nothing by mouth between less than 24 hours and more than 4 hours before the test.
- Immediately following the injection of 5 mCi of ^{99m}Tc-DISIDA, the patient is placed in a supine position beneath the gamma camera.
- Continuous images acquired in a 256 × 256 matrix for 1 hour are divided into 1-minute frames.
- Images are obtained with a high-resolution, parallel-hole collimator.
- Following the collection of images for 1 hour, sincalide (0.02 µg/kg) is administered intravenously over 60 minutes while a second series of 1-minute images is obtained.

Image Interpretation

Selected 1-minute images (**Fig. 127.1**) immediately after the injection of tracer demonstrate normal uptake of tracer in the liver and subsequent excretion into the gallbladder. The gallbladder contour is slightly irregular, which may be secondary to a fold, or "Phrygian cap."

Following the intravenous administration of sincalide, there is minimal change in tracer activity in the gallbladder, indicated by the lack of change in activity within the region-of-interest in **Fig. 127.2**.

Differential Diagnosis

- Biliary dyskinesia
- Excessively rapid injection of sincalide (< 30 minutes)
- Choledochal cyst
- Duodenal diverticulum
- Biloma in the gallbladder fossa

Diagnosis and Clinical Follow-Up

Cholecystectomy revealed chronic cholecystitis. No gallstones or acute obstruction was noted. The symptoms of meal intolerance resolved following cholecystectomy.

Discussion

The cause of right upper quadrant abdominal pain can be difficult to diagnose. When the gallbladder is the suspected cause, ultrasonography and CT are often used to look for anatomic abnormalities, such as thickening of the gallbladder wall, gallstones, and edema around the gallbladder. Anatomic imaging findings may be normal in patients with biliary dyskinesia.

Contraction of the gallbladder is initiated by cholecystokinin (CCK), which is secreted by the proximal small bowel following stimulation by a meal containing lipid. If the sensitivity or distribution of CCK receptors in the gallbladder and cystic duct is abnormal, there may not be coordinated contraction of the gallbladder, which may result in postprandial pain.

Recently, concerns have arisen about the supraphysiologic concentrations of sincalide in the blood associated with rapid injection (< 30 minutes), which may lead to dyskinesia. A multi-institutional study recently concluded suggests that the optimal method for administering sincalide is over 60 minutes with a normal gallbladder ejection fraction being greater than 38% at one hour following the beginning of sincalide administration.

PEARLS AND PITFALLS

- Normal filling of the gallbladder does not rule out chronic cholecystitis or biliary dyskinesia.
- CCK (or an analog) must be injected slowly to avoid supraphysiologic levels, which may cause abnormal gallbladder contraction and a false-positive test result.
- Overlying bowel or patient motion may affect counts in the gallbladder region-of-interest during calculation of the ejection fraction. Review of the cine images is essential to ensure that the calculated ejection fraction accurately reflects change in tracer activity within the gallbladder.

Suggested Reading

Gurusamy KS, Junnarkar S, Farouk M, Davidson BR. Cholecystectomy for suspected gallbladder dyskinesia. Cochrane Database Syst Rev 2009(1)CD.

Vassiliou MC, Laycock WS. Biliary dyskinesia. Surg Clin North Am 2008;88(6):1253–1272, viii–ix

Ziessman HA. Cholecystokinin cholescintigraphy: clinical indications and proper methodology. Radiol Clin North Am 2001;39(5):997–1006, ix

Ziessman HA, Muenz LR, Agarwal A. The importance of establishing normal gallbladder ejection fraction (GBEF) values for sincalide (CCK) cholescintigraphy. J Nucl Med 2001;42(5):316

Ziessman HA, Muenz LR, Agarwal AK, ZaZa AAM. Normal values for sincalide cholescintigraphy: comparison of two methods. Radiology 2001;221(2):404–410

Ziesman HA, Tulchinsky M, Lavely WC, Gaughan JP, Allen TW, Maru A, Parkman HP, Maurer AH. Sincalide-stimulated cholescintigraphy: a multicenter investigation to determine optimal infusion methodology and gallbladder ejection fraction normal values. J Nucl Med 2010:51(2):277–281

Section X

Lymphoscintigraphy

Annick D. Van den Abbeele and Kevin J. Donohoe

CASE 128

Clinical Presentation

A 50-year-old woman has a history of breast cancer treated with left breast lumpectomy, axillary lymph node dissection, and radiation. She presents with progressive swelling of the ipsilateral arm and forearm. Results of Doppler studies are normal. She is referred for lymphoscintigraphy to evaluate lymphatic drainage.

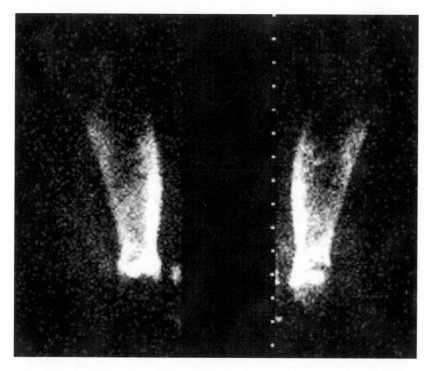

A **B**

Fig. 128.1

Technique

- The radiopharmaceutical is filtered (0.22 µm filter) sulfur colloid labeled with ^{99m}Tc-sulfur colloid. It is administered at a concentration of 10 mCi (370 MBq)/mL and at a dose of 0.5 mCi (18.5 MBq) per injection site.
- Administer two 0.05-mL intradermal injections of filtered ^{99m}Tc-sulfur colloid in the dorsum (as opposed to the web space) of the hand with sterile technique. The contralateral extremity is sometimes injected to provide a comparison. The patient is then asked to exercise the hand and arm to aid lymphatic drainage from the injection site.
- Static images of the forearm, arm, and shoulder are acquired for 15 minutes each, with the injection sites left just outside the field of view. Images are obtained over the first 90 minutes after injection or until the lymph vessels and nodal groups are visualized. Delayed views (2–3 hours after the injection) are also obtained to assess for dermal backflow, or "cutaneous flare."

Image Interpretation

Anterior (**Fig. 128.1A**) and posterior (**Fig. 128.1B**) delayed views of the left arm are shown. The hand is outside the lower end of the field of view. The images demonstrate nonvisualization of the deep lymphatic vessels and diffuse dermal backflow, or cutaneous flare, extending from the wrist up to the elbow region. Two faint brachial nodes are seen on the anterior view in the distal aspect of the arm.

Differential Diagnosis

* Lymphedema
* Cellulitis
* Edema secondary to a vascular cause

Diagnosis and Clinical Follow-Up

The findings were consistent with lymphedema and severe functional impairment of the lymphatic drainage of the left upper extremity.

Discussion

Radionuclide lymphoscintigraphy is a physiologic, noninvasive technique that can be easily performed and readily repeated. This diagnostic tool provides unique functional information about lymphatic channels and nodes. Because it does not require direct intralymphatic administration, it can be applied in diverse clinical situations and in anatomic sites that may not be accessible to contrast lymphangiography. It is based on the principle that radiolabeled colloid or macromolecules of appropriate size and properties introduced into appropriate tissue planes are transported into lymphatic channels and drain into lymphatic nodes. This allows anatomic and functional visualization of the lymphatic system under normal and abnormal conditions (Ege, 1996). It has also been useful in assessing lymphatic drainage before and after reconstructive and plastic surgery (Slavin et al., 1997 and 1999).

Typically, lymphoscintigraphy of a normal upper extremity will show rapid migration from the injection sites into the ulnar or radial vessels, or both, as well as a few main channels over the posterior wrist and forearm within a few minutes after the injection. The radiocolloid will then transit medially through the antecubital fossa into a brachial vessel in the medial upper arm and then into the axillary lymph node basin. Besides axillary nodes, epitrochlear and brachial nodes can be visualized.

PEARLS AND PITFALLS

* Two tuberculin syringes (one per injection site) are prepared equipped with a 26-gauge needle, each containing 50 µL of the filtered sulfur colloid preparation, topped with 50 µL of air. The small volume minimizes the pain or burning sensation that may be felt during the intradermal injection, and the air pushes the entire volume in, preventing loss of tracer in the tip of the syringe or within the needle.
* Delayed views are essential in the evaluation of lymphedema because it takes longer for the superficial lymphatic vessels to fill in.
* There are several stages of lymphedema. Early changes include tortuosity and collateralization of the lymphatic vessels, followed by focal flare, usually in the elbow region. As lymphedema increases, the cutaneous flare extends over the extremity, and there is decreased or nonvisualization of the deep lymphatic vessels and lymph node groups.

- It is important to use sterile technique during the injection because lymphedematous areas are extremely susceptible to infection. The development of cellulitis may quickly lead to systemic infection, and aggressive intravenous antibiotic therapy with a hospital stay is usually needed.
- The assessment of lymphedema with lymphoscintigraphy may not be current practice in many nuclear medicine practices. However, conservative surgeries, newly developed reconstructive and plastic surgical techniques, as well as new drugs may help alleviate lymphedema. Lymphoscintigraphy makes it possible to evaluate lymph vessel patency and the severity of lymphedema. This may help identify which patients will benefit from such treatment.

Suggested Reading

Browse NL. The diagnosis and management of primary lymphedema. J Vasc Surg 1986;3(1):181–184

Ege GN. Lymphoscintigraphy in oncology. In: Henkin RE, Boles MA, Dillehay GL, et al., eds. Nuclear Medicine. St. Louis, MO: Mosby Year Book; 1996:1504–1523

Gloviczki P, Calcagno D, Schirger A, Pairolero PC, Cherry KJ, Hallett JW, Wahner HW. Noninvasive evaluation of the swollen extremity: experiences with 190 lymphoscintigraphic examinations. J Vasc Surg 1989;9(5):683–689, discussion 690

Golueke PJ, Montgomery RA, Petronis JD, Minken SL, Perler BA, Williams GM. Lymphoscintigraphy to confirm the clinical diagnosis of lymphedema. J Vasc Surg 1989;10(3):306–312

Hung JC, Wiseman GA, Wahner HW, Mullan BP, Taggart TR, Dunn WL. Filtered technetium-99m-sulfur colloid evaluated for lymphoscintigraphy. J Nucl Med 1995;36(10):1895–1901

Slavin SA, Upton J, Kaplan WD, Van den Abbeele AD. An investigation of lymphatic function following free-tissue transfer. Plast Reconstr Surg 1997;99(3):730–741, discussion 742–743

Slavin SA, Van den Abbeele AD, Losken A, Swartz MA, Jain RK. Return of lymphatic function after flap transfer for acute lymphedema. Ann Surg 1999;229(3):421–427

Ter SE, Alavi A, Kim CK, Merli G. Lymphoscintigraphy: a reliable test for the diagnosis of lymphedema. Clin Nucl Med 1993;18(8):646–654

Vendrell-Torné E, Setoain-Quinquer J, Doménech-Torné FM. Study of normal mammary lymphatic drainage using radioactive isotopes. J Nucl Med 1972;13(11):801–805

CASE 129

Clinical Presentation

A 42-year-old woman underwent pelvic surgery 2.5 years ago. There has been a gradual onset of left lower extremity edema without a venous explanation. Lymphatic drainage is to be evaluated.

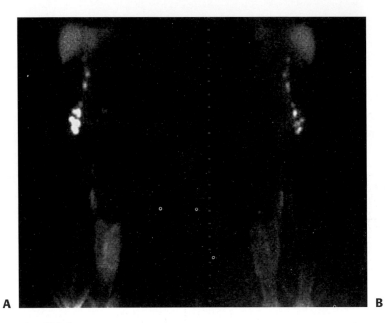

Fig. 129.1

Technique

- Filtered (0.22 μm filter) sulfur colloid labeled with 99mTc-sulfur colloid is administered at a concentration of 10 mCi (370 MBq)/mL and at a dose of 0.5 mCi (18.5 MBq) per injection site.
- Administer two 0.05-mL intradermal injections of 99mTc-sulfur colloid into the dorsum (as opposed to the web space) of each foot with sterile technique. The contralateral extremity is injected to provide a comparison. The patient is then asked to go up and down a flight of stairs to aid lymphatic drainage from the injection site.
- Successive anterior and posterior whole-body images are acquired at 8 cm/min up to the level of the chest, with the injection sites left out of the field of view. Images are obtained over the first 90 minutes after the injection until the lymph vessels and nodal groups are visualized up to the cisterna chyli and until the liver is visualized. Delayed views (2–3 hours after the injection) are also obtained to assess for dermal backflow, or "cutaneous flare." This is important in the diagnosis of lymphedema and may not be evident on the earlier set of images.
- The end point of an examination occurs when the clinical question has been answered.

Image Interpretation

Delayed anterior (**Fig. 129.1A**) and posterior (**Fig. 129.1B**) whole-body views show a normal right lower extremity lymphoscintigraphy. Visualization of the deep lymphatic vessels along the right lower extremity is followed by filling of the right inguinal and iliac nodes and progression of the tracer into the right para-aortic nodal chain up to the level of the cisterna chyli. The liver is also visualized.

There is only faint visualization of the deep lymphatic vessels in the left lower extremity, and diffuse cutaneous flare is seen from the knee to the ankle. Two areas of more focal flare are also seen in the medial aspect of the left thigh. There is only faint visualization of an inguinal lymph node and no further progression of activity beyond the inguinal region. The posterior view shows a left popliteal lymph node.

Differential Diagnosis

- Low plasma osmotic pressure
- Obstruction of venous return
- Obstruction of lymphatic return

Diagnosis and Clinical Follow-Up

The findings were consistent with severe functional impairment of the lymphatic drainage in the left lower extremity and lymphedema in the lower portion of the extremity with progression into the thigh.

Discussion

A normal study, as demonstrated in the right lower extremity in this case, should demonstrate the major lymph vessels along the entire extremity and lymph node groups in the inguinal, iliac, and para-aortic regions up to the cisterna chyli. Occasionally, popliteal lymph nodes are seen. From the cisterna chyli, lymph drains into the thoracic duct and left subclavian vein. Visualization of the liver, therefore, confirms patent communication between the lymphatic and venous systems.

Generally, edema in an extremity has three main causes: low plasma osmotic pressure (usually seen in kidney or liver failure but also in inflammation and associated increased vascular permeability), obstruction of venous return (with causes ranging from heart failure to venous thrombus), and obstruction of lymphatic return. Some of the more commonly encountered causes of impaired lymphatic return include congenital deficiency of lymphatic vessels, luminal obstruction by lymphadenopathy (because of tumor or infection), compression of a lymphatic vessel lumen by fibrosis (secondary to radiation therapy) or edema (often with a venous etiology) in the surrounding tissues, and node dissection associated with radiation therapy (frequently observed in patients with breast or pelvic cancers).

A study of 17 patients (20 extremities) referred for evaluation of lymphedema resulted in 8 true-positive, 9 true-negative, 0 false-positive, and 3 false-negative images of an extremity; the 3 false-negative images were not obtained within the first hour, decreasing the sensitivity for detecting subtle pedal lymphedema and crossover filling of major lymph nodes (Ter et al., 1993). Another study of 115 patients (190 extremities) referred for the evaluation of extremity edema showed lymphoscintigraphy to be 92% sensitive and 100% specific for the diagnosis of lymphedema (Gloviczki et al., 1989).

PEARLS AND PITFALLS

- Exercising the limb immediately after the injection, such as by walking or preferably by going up and down a flight of stairs, usually results in rapid drainage from the injection site, which significantly shortens the early imaging sessions. Delayed images should still be obtained, however, to assess for lymphedema.

- There is no need to inject the web space. Injection in the lateral aspect of the dorsum of each foot close to the toes is just as efficient and much better tolerated by patients.
- Visualization of the liver confirms patent communication between the lymphatic and venous systems.
- Lymphoscintigraphy is also useful in assessing lymphoceles, chylous leaks, and lymphatic drainage before and after reconstructive and plastic surgery (Slavin et al., 1997).
- If it appears that tracer has failed to migrate from the injection site, the dermal layer (which contains most of the lymphatic tissue) may not have been injected. If an epidermal or subdermal injection is suspected, the injections should be repeated.
- Lymphoscintigraphy is the diagnostic study of choice to evaluate lymphedema. Although conventional lymphangiography better demonstrates lymph vessel morphology, lymphoscintigraphy can readily demonstrate the presence of lymphedema, the location of major nodal groups, and the lymphatic drainage patterns at a lower price and with less radiation exposure for the patient. Also, lymphangiography is technically more difficult to perform, provides little functional information, and may have significant side effects (including local tissue necrosis, contrast reaction, and exacerbation of lymphedema).

Suggested Reading

Browse NL. The diagnosis and management of primary lymphedema. J Vasc Surg 1986;3(1):181–184

Ege GN. Lymphoscintigraphy in oncology. In: Henkin RE, Boles MA, Dillehay GL, et al., eds. Nuclear Medicine. St. Louis, MO: Mosby Year Book; 1996:1504–1523

Gloviczki P, Calcagno D, Schirger A, Pairolero PC, Cherry KJ, Hallett JW, Wahner HW. Noninvasive evaluation of the swollen extremity: experiences with 190 lymphoscintigraphic examinations. J Vasc Surg 1989;9(5):683–689, discussion 690

Golueke PJ, Montgomery RA, Petronis JD, Minken SL, Perler BA, Williams GM. Lymphoscintigraphy to confirm the clinical diagnosis of lymphedema. J Vasc Surg 1989;10(3):306–312

Hung JC, Wiseman GA, Wahner HW, Mullan BP, Taggart TR, Dunn WL. Filtered technetium-99m-sulfur colloid evaluated for lymphoscintigraphy. J Nucl Med 1995;36(10):1895–1901

Slavin SA, Upton J, Kaplan WD, Van den Abbeele AD. An investigation of lymphatic function following free-tissue transfer. Plast Reconstr Surg 1997;99(3):730–741, discussion 742–743

Ter SE, Alavi A, Kim CK, Merli G. Lymphoscintigraphy: a reliable test for the diagnosis of lymphedema. Clin Nucl Med 1993;18(8):646–654

Vendrell-Torné E, Setoain-Quinquer J, Doménech-Torné FM. Study of normal mammary lymphatic drainage using radioactive isotopes. J Nucl Med 1972;13(11):801–805

CASE 130

Clinical Presentation

A 38-year-old woman presents 2 weeks after undergoing excisional biopsy of a level 3 melanoma on her right flank. She has no palpable nodal disease and is scheduled for wide local excision on the day of this study.

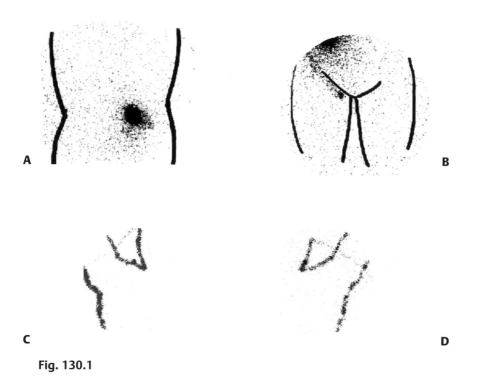

Fig. 130.1

Technique

- Two to four 100- to 200-µCi doses of filtered sulfur colloid (0.22-µm filter) labeled with ^{99m}Tc are diluted in a volume of 0.1 to 0.2 mL. The use of 1-mL syringes with 25-gauge needles is recommended. Drawing approximately 0.1 mL of air behind the tracer solution will ensure that the dose is emptied from the syringe during injection.
- For injection, it is helpful to bend the needle to a 45-degree angle, using the loosened cap as a sterile tool. The application of standard sterile povidone-iodine (Betadine) followed by an alcohol preparation is recommended.
- Draping the field will reduce the chance of skin contamination.
- Use a high-resolution collimator.
- Energy window 20% centered on 140 keV.
- Imaging time is 60 seconds per view.
- After sterile preparation of the injection site, inject the tracer intradermally at four sites surrounding the lesion and within 1.5 cm of the lesion. Intradermal injections usually raise a "wheal" or bump of tense skin at the injection site. Before withdrawing the needle from the skin, place a 2 × 2

443

or 4 × 4 gauze pad over the injection site to prevent the injectate from spraying back out of the puncture wound when the needle is withdrawn. Consider SPECT or SPECT/CT for improved localization of the site(s) of tracer uptake.

Image Interpretation

Figure 130.1A is a posterior abdominal view obtained immediately after injection showing confluence of the injection sites. The patient received a total of four injections because the first two injections were not clearly intradermal. **Figure 130.1B** is an image obtained 10 minutes after injection and shows intensely increased uptake in a single groin node medially. Right and left anterior axillary views (**Figs. 130.1C** and **130.1D**) acquired at 18 and 20 minutes after injection are negative (rough outlines of the arm and neck were drawn with a radioactive marker).

Differential Diagnosis

- Sentinel lymph node
- Skin contamination
- Tortuous lymphatic channel with transient "hang-up" of tracer
- Secondary lymph node

Diagnosis and Clinical Follow-Up

A pathologic examination of this inguinal node was negative for melanoma.

Discussion

Malignant melanoma is a cancerous transformation of melatonin cells. The extent of disease is categorized according to the thickness of the primary lesion and the presence of lymph node or distant metastases. Melanoma cells spread via lymphatic (more common) and hematogenous routes. The surgical management of the primary lesion is wide local dermal excision. A radical lymph node dissection is indicated for palpable nodes. Elective lymph node dissection is indicated only in cases in which the thickness of the primary lesions is 1 to 4 mm and there is no clinical evidence of metastases. The overall benefit of elective lymph node dissection is controversial and under investigation.

Lymphoscintigraphy is important because lymph drainage patterns are quite variable, particularly in lesions of the head, neck, and trunk. For all nodal groups, identification and biopsy of the primary draining node (sentinel node) can preempt further exploration if the sentinel node is negative for tumor. The use of a gamma probe is helpful for the localization of radioactive nodes during surgery.

PEARLS AND PITFALLS

- Additional views (lateral and oblique) of a sentinel node to determine its depth will aid in intraoperative localization. These extra views are strongly recommended for axillary nodes. SPECT (particularly the cinematic projections) can also aid in obtaining a more definitive localization.
- Poor progression of tracer beyond the injection site can be due to an inadvertently subcutaneous injection; a repeated injection is recommended if a small, tense wheal is not evident. The covering epidermis on the palms and soles is relatively thick and requires a deeper injection.
- Delayed imaging (at 2–4 hours) has been recommended to increase the intraoperative target-to-background count ratios.

- Contamination of the skin or clothing can cause false-positive results. Great care should be taken to avoid contamination; draping the field with an opening only for the injection site should be considered.
- Sentinel node lymphoscintigraphy is well established for the staging of malignant melanoma and breast cancer. The injection technique for breast cancer remains controversial. Some investigators prefer injecting around the tumor while others believe peri-areolar injections are simpler and just as accurate for identifying the sentinel node.

Suggested Reading

Albertini JJ, Cruse CW, Rapaport D, Wells K, Ross M, DeConti R, Berman CG, Jared K, Messina J, Lyman G, Glass F, Fenske M, Reintgen DS. Intraoperative radio-lympho-scintigraphy improves sentinel lymph node identification for patients with melanoma. Ann Surg 1996;223(2):217–224

Krag DN. Meijer SJ, Weaver DL, Loggie BW, Harlow SP, Tanabe KK, Laughlin EH, Alex JC. Minimal-access surgery for staging of malignant melanoma. Arch Surg 1995;130(6):654–658, discussion 659–660

Krag D, Weaver D, Ashikaga T, Moffat F, Klimberg VS, Shriver C, Feldman S, Kusminsky R, Gadd M, Kuhn J, Harlow S, Beitsch P. The sentinel node in breast cancer—a multicenter validation study. N Engl J Med 1998;339(14):941–946

Morton DL, Wen DR, Wong JH, Economov JS, Cagle LA, Storm FK, Foshag LJ, Cochran AJ, McCarthy WH. Technical details of intraoperative lymphatic mapping for early stage melanoma. Arch Surg 1992;127(4):392–399

O'Brien CJ, Uren RF, Thompson JF, Howman-Giles RB, Petersen-Schaefer K, Shaw HM, Quinn MJ. Prediction of potential metastatic sites in cutaneous head and neck melanoma using lymphoscintigraphy. Am J Surg 1995;170(5):461–466

CASE 131

Clinical Presentation

A 36-year-old man presents 18 months after noticing a change in the appearance of a mole on his back. An excisional biopsy performed 3 weeks before this presentation showed a 1.04-mm level 3 malignant melanoma.

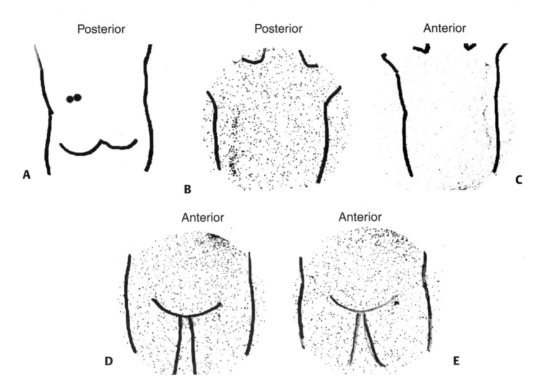

Fig. 131.1

Technique

- Two to four 100- to 200-µCi doses of filtered sulfur colloid (0.22–µm filter) labeled with ^{99m}Tc are diluted in a volume of 0.1 to 0.2 mL. The use of 1-mL syringes with 25-gauge needles is recommended. Drawing approximately 0.1 mL of air behind the tracer solution will ensure that the dose is emptied from the syringe during injection.
- For injection, it is helpful to bend the needle to a 45-degree angle using the loosened cap as a sterile tool. The application of standard sterile povidone-iodine (Betadine) followed by an alcohol preparation is recommended.
- Draping the field will reduce the chance of skin contamination.
- Use a high-resolution collimator.
- Energy window 20% centered on 140 keV.
- Imaging time is 60 seconds per view.

- After sterile preparation of the injection site, inject the tracer intradermally at four sites surrounding the lesion and within 1.5 cm of the lesion. Intradermal injections usually raise a "wheal" or bump of tense skin at the injection site. Before withdrawing the needle from the skin, place a 2 × 2 or 4 × 4 gauze pad over the injection site to prevent the injectate from spraying back out of the puncture wound when the needle is withdrawn. Consider SPECT or SPECT/CT for improved localization of the site(s) of tracer uptake.

Image Interpretation

Figure 131.1A is a posterior abdominal view obtained immediately after injection showing the two sites of intradermal injection over the left flank. Eight minutes after injection, a posterior view of the trunk **(Fig. 131.1B)** demonstrates a prominent lymph channel on the left side ascending to the left axilla. Fourteen minutes after injection, an axillary node is seen on the anterior chest view **(Fig. 131.1C)**. Eighteen minutes after injection, faint uptake is seen in a node in the left groin **(Fig. 131.1D)**. Fifteen minutes later, this node is more prominent **(Fig. 131.1E)**.

Differential Diagnosis

- Sentinel lymph node
- Skin contamination
- Tortuous lymphatic channel with transient "hang-up" of nuclide
- Secondary lymph node

Diagnosis and Clinical Follow-Up

Pathologic examination of the axillary and inguinal nodes showed no evidence of lymphatic spread of disease.

Discussion

This case is an example of the unpredictability of lymph drainage patterns, particularly in the trunk at approximately the level of the umbilicus and in any midline location in the back or the anterior chest and abdomen. Lymph drainage patterns are also quite variable in the head and neck. There are two sentinel nodes in this case: one in the ipsilateral axilla and one in the groin. Drainage to two or more lymph node beds is observed in approximately 60% of cases; drainage to three or more nodal groups occurs in 10% of cases. Lymphoscintigraphy can identify sentinel nodes in several distant nodal beds.

PEARLS AND PITFALLS

- Rapid imaging under direct supervision is important for the successful use of this technique. Nodes can appear at several locations within minutes of one another. Careful skin marking and conscientious communication of the findings to the surgeon are very important.
- Cleaning any contaminated area will help decrease confusion for the surgeon using the radiation probe during surgery.
- Covering the injection site with a 4 × 4-cm gauze pad while removing the needle will decrease the chances of tracer spraying or leaking out of the injection site to contaminate the surrounding area.
- The importance of tracer uptake in nodes distal to the first visualized node has been debated. Some surgeons pursue any nodes with radiotracer; some are primarily interested in the first node visualized in any single nodal group.

Suggested Reading

McCarthy WH, Shaw HM, Cascinelli N, Santinami M, Belli F. Elective lymph node dissection for melanoma: two perspectives. World J Surg 1992;16(2):203–213

Slingluff CL Jr, Stidham KR, Ricci WM, Stanley WE, Seigler HF. Surgical management of regional lymph nodes in patients with melanoma: experience with 4682 patients. Ann Surg 1994;219(2):120–130

Uren RF, Howman-Giles RB, Shaw HM, Thompson JF, McCarthy WH. Lymphoscintigraphy in high-risk melanoma of the trunk: predicting draining node groups, defining lymphatic channels and locating the sentinel node. J Nucl Med 1993;34(9):1435–1440

Uren RF, Howman-Giles RB, Thompson JF, Malouf D, Ramsey-Stewart G, Niesche FW, Renwick RB. Mammary lymphoscintigraphy in breast cancer. J Nucl Med 1995;36(10):1775–1780

Wells KE, Cruse CW, Daniels S, Berman C, Norman J, Reintgen DS. The use of lymphoscintigraphy in melanoma of the head and neck. Plast Reconstr Surg 1994;93(4):757–761

Section XI

CNS Scintigraphy

Rachel A. Powsner

CASE 132

Clinical Presentation

A 62-year-old woman presents with short-term memory loss that has increased over the past 3 years. A radionuclide brain perfusion SPECT study is ordered to evaluate the perfusion pattern.

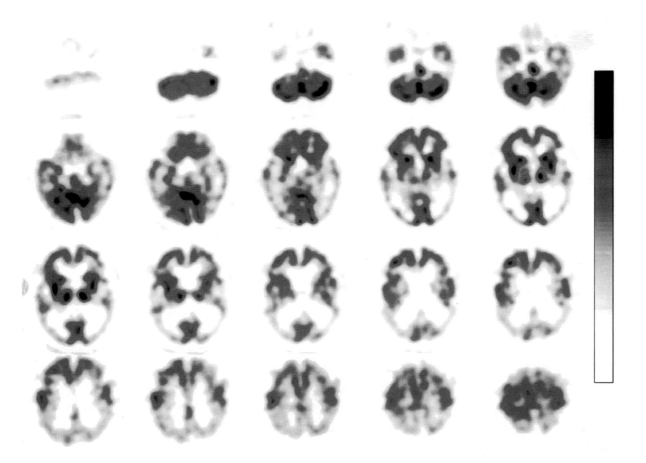

Fig. 132.1

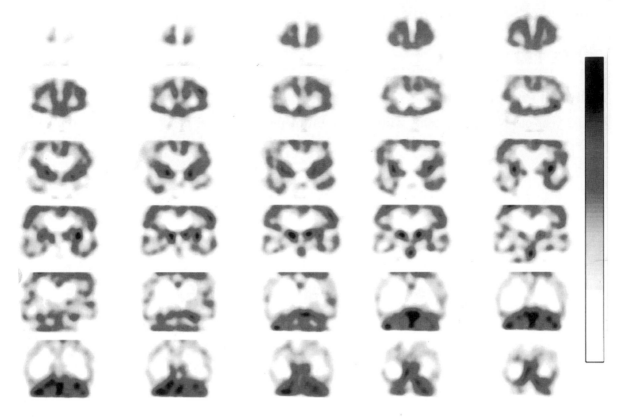

Fig. 132.2

Technique

- Approximately 20 mCi of ^{99m}Tc-HMPAO or ^{99m}Tc-ECD is injected intravenously.
- Imaging time is 20 to 30 minutes after injection (1 hour if ^{99m}Tc-ECD is used).
- Acquisition protocol is 30 minutes with a 360-degree SPECT rotation.
- The patient should be supine, with the head slightly elevated and eyes closed. The head should be as close to the camera as possible and strapped tightly with a nonattenuating material such as Velcro, rubber, or elastic to avoid head motion.
- During injection and image acquisition, the room should be quiet, with the lights dimmed.
- The head should be in the center of the axis of rotation.

Image interpretation

The axial (**Fig. 132.1**) and coronal (**Fig. 132.2**) views display a global reduction in radiotracer uptake with increased background activity. Lateral frontal perfusion defects are seen on the left side. Marked reduction in the perfusion to the temporal lobes (medial, lateral, and inferior aspects) is seen bilaterally in the axial and coronal slices. The left side is more affected than the right side. Marked reduction in the perfusion to the entire parietal cortex is noted bilaterally. Symmetric radiotracer uptake is visible in the basal ganglia and thalami.

Differential Diagnosis

- Alzheimer disease
- Dementia with Lewy bodies

- Parkinson disease with Alzheimer dementia
- Multiple-infarct dementia
- Progressive subcortical gliosis

Diagnosis and Clinical Follow-Up

The bilateral temporoparietal perfusion defects, seen on the left more than right, were in a pattern consistent with Alzheimer disease.

Discussion

The pattern of uptake in the SPECT and PET imaging of Alzheimer disease is classically described as hypoperfusion of the superior parietal cortices in the initial stages, with involvement of both temporoparietal regions and eventually the frontal cortices as the disease progresses. Early in the disease, the defects can be asymmetric and of variable intensity. As the disease progresses, the defects become more prominent, with relative sparing of the motor cortex, basal ganglia, and cerebellum. Like those detected with PET imaging, perfusion abnormalities detected with SPECT imaging in patients with Alzheimer disease correlate with the severity of the disease.

Advances in the quantitative software evaluation of both SPECT and PET images of the brain have aided the diagnosis of Alzheimer disease, which has been associated with decreased uptake in the posterior cingulate gyrus, a finding difficult to discern by visual inspection alone.

PEARLS AND PITFALLS

- Sulci, gyri, and ventricles tend to appear larger in older patients because of atrophy. This is a common finding.
- The uptake of ^{99m}Tc-HMPAO and ^{99m}Tc-ECD during SPECT and of ^{18}F-FDG during PET is greater in gray matter (neuronal cell bodies) than in white matter (neuronal axons). This is because gray matter is more vascular and has a higher metabolic rate than white matter. As a result, it can be difficult to distinguish the ventricles from the white matter when images are interpreted.
- All functional brain imaging should be coregistered or visually compared with anatomic imaging studies, such as CT and/or MRI. This is because anatomic findings such as cerebral infarcts or atrophy cannot be distinguished from Alzheimer disease or other functional perfusion defects on SPECT or ^{18}F-FDG-PET imaging alone.
- Temporal lobe perfusion defects can be missed on axial images. Coronal slices are useful for evaluation of the temporal lobes.
- Brain perfusion scans are normalized to the cerebellum. Any visible defect below 60% of the cerebellar activity noted over a span of two adjacent slices should be considered abnormal.
- It is normal to observe a few small perfusion defects in healthy subjects caused by sulci and wide gyri.
- Consider one of the frontotemporal dementias, such as Pick disease, if there is involvement of frontal and occasionally the temporal lobes.
- Always check for image orientation (left and right sides of the patient) before correlating with MRI, CT, or other SPECT studies because the protocols used for image processing may differ.
- Patient motion as well as a tilted axis can be the source of perceived perfusion defects in different views. Always correlate the asymmetry with the slice above and the slice below and also with corresponding views in other planes.
- The reported accuracy of SPECT in early Alzheimer disease has varied widely. Recent data, however, suggest a high accuracy rate, even in very mild disease.

Suggested Reading

Bonte FJ, Harris TS, Roney CA, Hynan LS. Differential diagnosis between Alzheimer's and frontotemporal disease by the posterior cingulate sign. J Nucl Med 2004;45(5):771–774

Hoffman JM, Welsh-Bohmer KA, Hanson M, et al. FDG PET imaging in patients with pathologically verified dementia. J Nucl Med 2000;41(11):1920–1928

Silverman DH, Small GW, Chang CY, et al. Positron emission tomography in evaluation of dementia: regional brain metabolism and long-term outcome. JAMA 2001;286(17):2120–2127

van Dyck CH, Lin CH, Smith EO, et al. Comparison of technetium-99m-HMPAO and technetium-99m-ECD cerebral SPECT images in Alzheimer's disease. J Nucl Med 1996;37(11):1749–1755

CASE 133

Clinical Presentation

A 34-year-old woman who has had intractable complex partial seizures since the age of 22 years and has undergone a prior left temporal lobectomy is admitted for evaluation of the seizure focus. Depth electrode placement shows spike activity in the frontal and temporal lobes.

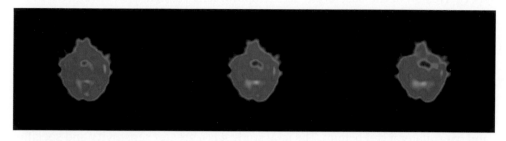

Fig. 133.1 Ictal Imaging.

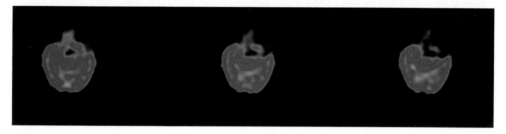

Fig. 133.2 Interictal imaging.

Technique

- Approximately 20 mCi of ^{99m}Tc-HMPAO or ^{99m}Tc-ECD is injected intravenously.
- Imaging time is 20 to 30 minutes after injection (1 hour if ^{99m}Tc-ECD is used).
- Acquisition protocol is 30 minutes with a 360-degree SPECT rotation.
- The patient should be supine, with the head slightly elevated and eyes closed. The head should be as close to the camera as possible and strapped tightly with a nonattenuating material such as Velcro, rubber, or elastic to avoid head motion.
- During injection and image acquisition, the room should be quiet, with the lights dimmed (avoid disturbances and noise).
- The head should be in the center of the axis of rotation.
- For ictal imaging, the patient is preferably injected during a seizure (an intravenous line should be ready). Seizure in this case was induced by voice activation.

Image Interpretation

The ictal perfusion study (**Fig. 133.1**) demonstrates marked hyperperfusion in the base of the residual left temporal lobe. The interictal (baseline) study (**Fig. 133.2**) shows areas of relatively symmetric perfusion in the bases of the temporal lobes bilaterally.

Differential Diagnosis

- Epileptic focus
- Encephalitis
- Tumor
- Luxury perfusion
- Hallucinations secondary to dementia or schizophrenia

Diagnosis and Clinical Follow-Up

The diagnosis was hyperperfusion in the base of the left temporal lobe remnant, consistent with seizure focus.

Discussion

Combined positive ictal and interictal imaging studies are highly specific for the localization of a temporal lobe seizure focus. The ictal study in temporal lobe epilepsy will reveal hyperperfusion of the temporal lobe, often with extension into the ipsilateral basal ganglia and thalamus and sometimes ipsilateral motor cortex and contralateral cerebellum. The ictal study has a greater sensitivity and specificity for the detection of temporal lobe epilepsy than does the interictal study; however, it is frequently very difficult to coordinate an injection of tracer with the start of a seizure. The interictal study, when positive, will demonstrate a focus of hypoperfusion at the seizure site.

PEARLS AND PITFALLS

- There are some important differences between HMPAO and ECD. Both agents are blood flow tracers and useful for the localization of epileptogenic foci; however, ECD may be a less effective flow tracer at high flow rates and may reflect metabolism in addition to flow.
- While evaluating disease progress by comparing with previous studies, be aware of the differences between the perfusion patterns of HMPAO studies and those of ECD studies.
- Fusion of SPECT images and CT or MRI is useful for determining the exact anatomic location of a seizure focus.
- Head motion can introduce artifactual defects.

Suggested Reading

Asenbaum S, Brücke T, Pirker W, Pietrzyk U, Podreka I. Imaging of cerebral blood flow with technetium-99m-HMPAO and technetium-99m-ECD: a comparison. J Nucl Med 1998;39(4):613–618

Camargo EE. Brain SPECT in neurology and psychiatry. J Nucl Med 2001;42(4):611–623

Devous MD Sr, Thisted RA, Morgan GF, Leroy RF, Rowe CC. SPECT brain imaging in epilepsy: a meta-analysis. J Nucl Med 1998;39(2):285–293

Oku N, Matsumoto M, Hashikawa K, et al. Intra-individual differences between technetium-99m-HMPAO and technetium-99m-ECD in the normal medial temporal lobe. J Nucl Med 1997;38(7):1109–1111

Oommen KJ, Saba S, Oommen JA, Francel PC, Arnold CD, Wilson DA. The relative localizing value of interictal and immediate postictal SPECT in seizures of temporal lobe origin. J Nucl Med 2004;45(12):2021–2025

CASE 134

Clinical Presentation

A 25-year-old woman in otherwise good health presents with several episodes of severe headache. MRI demonstrates a small area of enhancement in the right thalamus, and stereotactic biopsy confirms the diagnosis of grade 3 astrocytoma. A ¹⁸F-FDG-PET study is performed to define the metabolic extent of the lesion, determine if additional lesions are present, and serve as a baseline for monitoring the effect of radiation therapy. The four images below are axial slices obtained at the same location in the brain at different time points: 134.1A was obtained prior to therapy; 134.1B is mid-way through radiation therapy; 134.1C is done at the completion of therapy; 134.1D is 6 months following the completion of therapy.

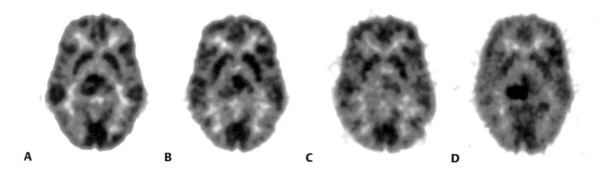

A   B   C   D

Fig. 134.1

Technique

- The patient should take nothing by mouth for 12 hours before the radiopharmaceutical is administered. Switch all glucose-containing intravenous solutions to normal saline on the day before imaging.
- During injection and acquisition, the room should be quiet, with the lights dimmed (avoid disturbances and noise).
- ¹⁸F-FDG (dose determined by type of imaging system and patient weight) is administered intravenously 45 minutes before image acquisition.
- The imaging device is a dedicated PET camera or PET/CT scanner.
- Carefully position the patient in a head holder.

Image Interpretation

Before therapy, the transaxial ¹⁸F-FDG-PET image of the brain demonstrates an intense focus of increased accumulation in the anterior aspect of the right thalamus (**Fig. 134.1A**). The location of this lesion corresponds well with the area of enhancement on MRI. Midway into a course of radiation therapy, the degree and extent of the hypermetabolic focus decrease (**Fig. 134.1B**). In a study performed after the completion of therapy (**Fig. 134.1C**), further regression of the tumor is evident. However, 6 months after completion of therapy, the PET study reveals intense focal hypermetabolism in the posterior aspect of the right thalamus (**Fig. 134.1D**).

Diagnosis and Clinical Follow-Up

After radiation therapy, the patient's symptoms decreased. However, 6 months later, at the time of the fourth study, the symptoms recurred, and she died several weeks later.

Discussion

Radiolabeled amino acids such as ^{11}C-methionine and ^{11}C-tyrosine are used as tracers for brain tumor imaging and have the added advantage of low background activity in normal brain tissue. However, they are not commercially available at this time. ^{18}F-FDG is the "workhorse" of clinical PET, even though its high background activity in normal brain tissue can interfere with detection of less metabolically active, lower-grade tumors. Normal ^{18}F-FDG uptake in the brain in this study illustrates the importance of correlation with anatomic imaging studies. The uptake of ^{18}F-FDG is usually more intense in high-grade gliomas than in low-grade gliomas. Its sensitivity for the detection of high-grade tumors has been reported to be as high as 94%. Its lower specificity of 77% is due largely to intensely increased uptake in some lower-grade tumors, such as low-grade oligodendrogliomas and pilocytic astrocytomas.

In addition to assessing the degree of malignancy and providing initial prognostic information, ^{18}F-FDG PET can be useful in differentiating radiation necrosis from recurrent high-grade gliomas. Radiation therapy to the brain may cause dramatic tissue necrosis that is indistinguishable from tumor recurrence by anatomic imaging with CT or MRI. Recurrent high-grade tumors demonstrate increased ^{18}F-FDG uptake, whereas necrotic tissue demonstrates reduced ^{18}F-FDG uptake, with a sensitivity of 75% and a specificity of 81%.

PEARLS AND PITFALLS

- Patients must fast, and all intravenous solutions containing glucose must be stopped for at least 4 hours before an injection of ^{18}F-FDG. It is important to determine that all intravenous drugs (antibiotics, chemotherapy agents) administered before and during the study do not contain glucose.
- The uptake of ^{18}F-FDG is generally more intense in higher-grade gliomas and less intense in lower-grade gliomas.
- Longer delays between time of injection and imaging can improve the tumor-to-background uptake ratio in gliomas.
- The imaging of many low-grade gliomas with ^{18}F-FDG is hampered by the high background uptake of ^{18}F-FDG in normal brain tissue.
- The ratio of tumor to white matter or of tumor to gray matter is considered more reliable than the standard uptake value (SUV) for quantifying ^{18}F-FDG activity in a tumor.

Suggested Reading

Bénard F, Romsa J, Hustinx R. Imaging gliomas with positron emission tomography and single-photon emission computed tomography. Semin Nucl Med 2003;33(2):148–162

De Witte O, Lefranc F, Levivier M, Salmon I, Brotchi J, Goldman S. FDG-PET as a prognostic factor in high-grade astrocytoma. J Neurooncol 2000;49(2):157–163

Jacobs AH, Kracht LW, Gossmann A, et al. Imaging in neurooncology. NeuroRx 2005;2(2):333–347

Minn H. PET and SPECT in low-grade glioma. Eur J Radiol 2005;56(2):171–178

Spence A, Muzi M, Mankoff D, et al. ^{18}F-FDG PET of gliomas at delayed intervals: improved distinction between tumor and normal gray matter. J Nucl Med 2004;45:1653–1659

CASE 135

Clinical Presentation

A 34-year-old woman presents 2 weeks after a subarachnoid hemorrhage. Two hours before the first brain scintigraphic study, she has a sudden deterioration in mental status and no clinical evidence of cerebral or brain stem function. A second scintigraphic study of the brain is repeated 17 hours after the first study. **Figures 135.1A, B, C, D, E** show flow and static images for the first study. **Figures 135.1F, G, H, I, J** show flow and static images from the second study.

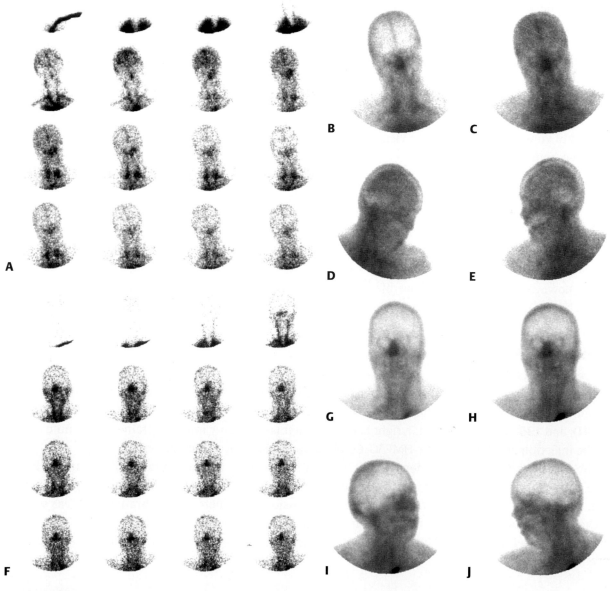

Fig. 135.1

Technique

- Flow (only) imaging agent may be used. The most common is the following (adults):
  - 15 to 20 mCi (555–740 MBq) of ^{99m}Tc-DTPA
- Brain-specific agents may also be used in combination with a flow agent or separately. The two currently available brain-specific agents are the following:
  - 10 to 30 mCi (370–1110 MBq) of ^{99m}Tc-HMPAO
  - 10 to 30 mCi (370–1110 MBq) of ^{99m}Tc-ECD. Plan on divided doses with the brain-specific agents if DTPA is not used for flow imaging (see below).
- **Quantity of injectate:** A volume of 1 mL or less of injectate is preferable to ensure a good-quality bolus for the flow portion of the examination. A 20 mCi dose of ^{99m}Tc-DTPA can easily be prepared in this small quantity. The brain-specific agents (^{99m}Tc-HMPAO and ^{99m}Tc-ECD) usually cannot be reconstituted in as concentrated a solution. If one of these latter agents is to be used for both the flow phase and subsequent static phase (see below) of imaging, it is recommended that a 1-mL portion of the dose (containing no less than 10 mCi) be used for the flow portion of the examination. The remainder of the dose (up to a total dose of 30 mCi) is injected after the flow imaging and before the static imaging.
- **Procedure:** A rapid bolus of radiopharmaceutical is followed by a minimum of 10 mL of normal saline flush; a three-way stopcock can facilitate this maneuver. Injection into a central line is preferred; peripheral access results in a poorer-quality bolus.
- Use a high-resolution collimator.
- The patient should be placed in a supine position with the top of the head just below the top of the field of view to allow maximum visualization of the internal carotid artery flow.
- Views and framing rates
  - **Flow imaging:** 60- to 90-second dynamic at 1 second per frame in the anterior projection. Begin acquisition just before injection of dose.
  - **Static imaging:** Wait about 5 minutes if ^{99m}Tc-DTPA is used and obtain an anterior view of the head for 3 to 5 minutes. Wait for 20 minutes after injection if ^{99m}Tc-ECD or ^{99m}Tc-HMPAO is used before commencing static imaging at 3 to 5 minutes per frame. Acquire images in the anterior, right and left lateral, and posterior projections. SPECT imaging is recommended if possible; however, the use of extensive life support equipment, which impedes rotation of the camera head(s), combined with the fragile state of these patients often precludes SPECT imaging.

Image Interpretation

Figure 135.1A is the flow study compressed into 3-second frames. Carotid flow is normal bilaterally; middle and anterior cerebral artery flow is reduced, but a "blush" of tracer activity in the brain is seen. An immediate ^{99m}Tc-DTPA static image (**Fig. 135.1B**) demonstrates sagittal sinus uptake. **Figures 135.1C, 135.1D,** and **135.1E** are the anterior, right lateral, and left lateral static images obtained 10 minutes after the injection of 10 mCi of ^{99m}Tc-HMPAO. Cerebral uptake is reduced but present.

The patient returned to the department 17 hours later for a repeated brain flow scan. At that time, both carotid arteries were visualized, but there was no anterior or middle cerebral artery flow (**Fig. 135.1F**). The "hot nose" sign was noted (see discussion), and there was no brain "blush," as seen in the earlier study. There was no uptake in the sagittal sinus on the immediate ^{99m}Tc-DTPA static anterior image (**Fig. 135.1G**). The ^{99m}Tc-HMPAO images (**Figs. 135.1H, 135.1I,** and **135.1J**) showed no cerebral uptake.

Differential Diagnosis

- Brain death
- Poor tracer preparation resulting in lack of accumulation in the central nervous system (may cause false-positive static images but will not alter accuracy of flow images)
- Attenuation artifact, such as metallic skull implant or metal between head and camera

Diagnosis and Clinical Follow-Up

The patient had no spontaneous respiration on the apnea test. She was declared brain-dead immediately after the second study.

Discussion

Brain death is inevitably followed by cardiopulmonary death. The criteria for a determination of brain death include absence of brain stem reflexes (gag, corneal, oculovestibular, and others) and lack of spontaneous respiration with the apnea test. Confirmation of the diagnosis can also include an electroencephalogram, contrast arteriography, Doppler echocardiography, and/or brain flow imaging.

Reservations about the use of ^{99m}Tc-HMPAO, in particular, as an imaging agent for brain death originated from concern about the labeling stability of this agent in its original form, which did not include a stabilizing agent. A false-positive test because of poor labeling, however, is very unlikely with use of the stabilizing agent methylene blue as long as the radiopharmaceutical is administered within 4 hours of preparation. As an additional precaution, ^{99m}Tc-HMPAO must be prepared with the ^{99m}Tc-pertechnetate eluted from the molybdenum-technetium generator no more than 24 hours before use. A good-quality flow study before static imaging (the carotid arteries should be distinctly visualized) is another means of ensuring accurate interpretation.

The "hot nose" sign is not pathognomonic for cessation of brain flow. It is, however, frequently seen in cases of brain death. This finding has been attributed to external carotid collateral flow through the facial and ophthalmic arteries once internal carotid flow is interrupted by an elevated intracranial pressure. Similarly, what appears to be visualization of the sagittal sinus in the absence of arterial flow may represent increased blood supply to the falx from the external carotid system (eg, anterior facial arteries).

This case illustrates the importance of waiting for several hours to image after clinical evidence of brain death appears. Cerebral blood flow can be visualized in the time period in which the intracranial pressure has risen enough to affect brain stem function but is not yet elevated enough to interrupt internal carotid artery flow.

PEARLS AND PITFALLS

- A tourniquet wrapped tightly around the head above the eyes and ears can reduce overlying scalp activity and improve diagnostic confidence. Use of a tourniquet, however, is not recommended for patients with skull wounds or fractures (surgical or traumatic) because the intracranial pressure may rise with application of the tourniquet.
- A systolic blood pressure of less than 60 mm Hg may invalidate the test.
- Imaging too early (~6 hours within cessation of brain function) can result in a false-negative test.
- Careful examination of the patient and review of the correlative brain imaging are important because scalp and cerebral bleeding can lead to false-negative readings.

- Small isolated areas of residual cerebral, cerebellar, midbrain, or brain stem uptake seen on ^{99m}Tc-HMPAO or ^{99m}Tc-ECD static images have, to date, always been a precursor to complete absence of brain uptake on follow-up studies. However, some facilities are reluctant to make the diagnosis of brain death with any evidence of residual brain or brain stem perfusion.

Suggested Reading

Conrad GR, Sinha P. Scintigraphy as a confirmatory test of brain death. Semin Nucl Med 2003;33(4):312–323

Donohoe KJ, Frey KA, Gerbaudo VH, Mariani G, Nagel JS, Shulkin B. Procedure guideline for brain death scintigraphy. J Nucl Med 2003;44(5):846–851

Lee VW, Hauck RM, Morrison MC, Peng TT, Fischer E, Carter A. Scintigraphic evaluation of brain death: significance of sagittal sinus visualization. J Nucl Med 1987;28(8):1279–1283

Wijdicks EFM. The diagnosis of brain death. N Engl J Med 2001;344(16):1215–1221

CASE 136

Clinical Presentation

A 70-year-old man with a history of anterior cerebral artery aneurysm has a new onset of seizures. The patient is unresponsive.

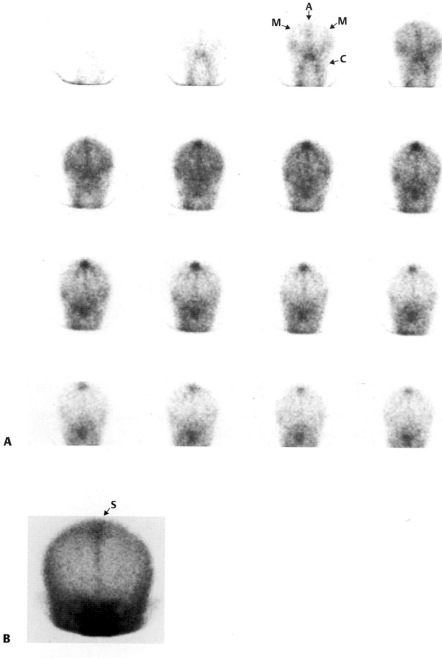

Fig. 136.1

Technique

- A 20 mCi dose of ^{99m}Tc-DTPA is administered as a rapid intravenous bolus.
- Use a high-resolution collimator.
- Patient position: anterior with top of skull just below the top of the field of view.
- Imaging time: for flow, 60-second dynamic at 1 second per frame; for static images, 3 minutes per frame.

Image Interpretation

Figure 136.1A shows the ^{99m}Tc-DTPA flow study in sequential 3-second frames. The carotid (*C*), middle cerebral (*M*), and anterior cerebral (*A*) arteries are marked. Note that the anterior cerebral vessels are seen as a single structure. Sagittal sinus filling (*S*) can be seen on the immediate static image (**Fig. 136.1B**).

Differential Diagnosis

- Normal brain blood flow
- False-negative result because study was obtained too soon after loss of cerebral function

Diagnosis and Clinical Follow-Up

The diagnosis was normal brain blood flow. There was no further follow-up.

Discussion

Compared with Case 135, the carotid, anterior, and middle cerebral arteries are clearly visualized.

Suggested Reading

Conrad GR, Sinha P. Scintigraphy as a confirmatory test of brain death. Semin Nucl Med 2003;33(4): 312–323

Donohoe KJ, Frey KA, Gerbaudo VH, Mariani G, Nagel JS, Shulkin B. Procedure guideline for brain death scintigraphy. J Nucl Med 2003;44(5):846–851

Lee VW, Hauck RM, Morrison MC, Peng TT, Fischer E, Carter A. Scintigraphic evaluation of brain death: significance of sagittal sinus visualization. J Nucl Med 1987;28(8):1279–1283

Wijdicks EFM. The diagnosis of brain death. N Engl J Med 2001;344(16):1215–1221

CASE 137

Clinical Presentation

A 48-year-old woman with subarachnoid hemorrhage presents with decerebrate posturing to sternal rub, lower extremity withdrawal to pain, and absent brain stem reflexes (corneal, gag, oculocephalic). Her electroencephalogram (EEG) demonstrates no evidence of cerebral cortical activity.

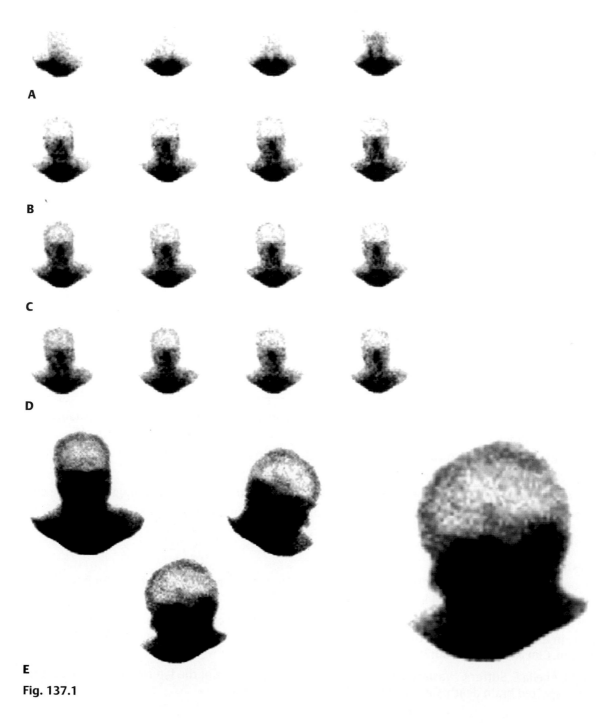

A

B

C

D

E

Fig. 137.1

Technique

- Use a high-resolution collimator.
- Patient position: anterior with top of skull just below the top of the field of view
- Imaging time: 60-second dynamic at 1 second per frame; for static images, 3 minutes per frame

Image Interpretation

The cerebral flow study in **Fig. 137.1A** demonstrates adequate carotid artery flow and no evidence of middle or anterior cerebral artery flow. The 15-minute delayed static images (**Figs. 137.1B, 137.1C, and 137.1D**) demonstrate uptake in the deep gray matter, seen best on the lateral views just above the intense activity at the base of the skull (**Fig. 137.1E**).

Differential Diagnosis

- Evolving brain death
- Bilateral subdural hematomas
- Faulty radiopharmaceutical preparation (although even faulty radiopharmaceutical preparation would show a normal flow phase)

Diagnosis and Clinical Follow-Up

The subsequent apnea test demonstrated spontaneous breathing on withdrawal from assisted ventilation. The patient expired 5 hours later.

Discussion

This is an example of residual cerebral uptake of radionuclide in the absence of middle and anterior cerebral blood flow on the anterior flow images. The patient's clinical status was consistent with minimal residual cerebral function. The clinical significance of this finding is unclear because the patient progressed to complete brain death within several hours.

PEARLS AND PITFALLS

- A careful examination of computer images with varied windowing is important for the visualization of subtle findings.
- Medications such as barbiturates, which cause false-positive EEG findings, do not affect radionuclide cerebral angiography studies.
- Intracranial or extracranial bleeding can mimic cerebral uptake of tracer; all findings should be correlated with the physical examination findings and available anatomic imaging.

Suggested Reading

Donohoe KJ, Frey KA, Gerbaudo VH, Mariani G, Nagel JS, Shulkin B. Procedure guideline for brain death scintigraphy. J Nucl Med 2003;44(5):846–851

Kurtek RW, Lai KK, Tauxe WN, Eidelman BH, Fung JJ. Tc-99m hexamethylpropylene amine oxime scintigraphy in the diagnosis of brain death and its implications for the harvesting of organs used for transplantation. Clin Nucl Med 2000;25(1):7–10

Spieth M, Abella E, Sutter C, Vasinrapee P, Wall L, Ortiz M. Importance of the lateral view in the evaluation of suspected brain death. Clin Nucl Med 1995;20(11):965–968

CASE 138

Clinical Presentation

A 26-year-old man in whom a right frontal anaplastic oligodendroglioma was diagnosed 5 years earlier underwent surgical resection initially, followed by radiation therapy. He now presents for repeated imaging with ^{201}TI (**Fig. 138.1**) because of evidence of recurrence on MRI.

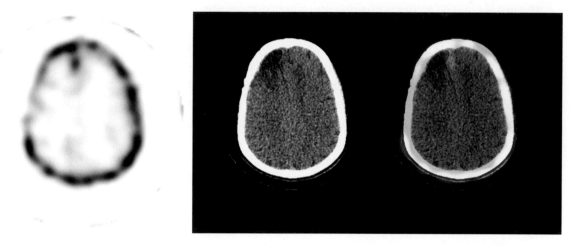

Fig. 138.1

Technique

- A 3 mCi dose of ^{201}TI is injected intravenously.
- Imaging begins 20 to 30 minutes after injection.
- Acquisition protocol: 30 minutes with SPECT/CT

Image Interpretation

Images show an abnormal area of increased thallium uptake involving the right frontal region just adjacent to midline (**Fig. 138.1**). No other areas of abnormally increased thallium accumulation are noted.

Differential Diagnosis

- Recurrent brain tumor
- Cerebral sarcoid (rare)
- Meningioma (rare)

Diagnosis and Clinical Follow-Up

The increased thallium uptake indicated a high probability of solid tumor recurrence. Radiation therapy felt that the thallium uptake was outside the previous therapy port. MRI suggested recurrence at the same site. The patient was lost to follow-up.

Discussion

Neurosurgeons and neuro-oncologists use ^{201}Tl to assess for residual disease following surgical resection, to evaluate response to therapy, and to differentiate radiation necrosis from recurrent disease. In a patient with a large abnormality on CT or MRI, ^{201}Tl also helps to guide biopsy and minimize sampling error by directing the surgeon to the site of focal thallium uptake that most likely represents the site of recurrence. SPECT/CT is very helpful for localizing the site of tracer uptake and for allowing correlation with the results of other anatomic imaging tests, such as MRI.

PEARLS AND PITFALLS

- The uptake of ^{201}Tl on brain imaging is useful in distinguishing post-radiation necrosis from residual or recurrent tumor.
- The uptake of ^{201}Tl is generally greater in high-grade tumors than in low-grade gliomas.
- There is very little uptake of ^{201}Tl in normal brain tissue.
- Tumor uptake indices (ratio of lesion uptake to uptake in contralateral normal brain, or ratio of lesion uptake to uptake in contralateral scalp) can be useful for assessing thallium uptake.
- The finding of increased thallium uptake and decreased perfusion (with ^{99m}Tc-HMPAO or ^{99m}Tc-ECD) is very specific for tumor recurrence.
- Previous MRI and SPECT studies, if available, should be routinely evaluated. Such comparative evaluation offers significant information regarding progress of the lesion and aids in defining new regions of thallium uptake.

Suggested Reading

Schwartz RB, Carvalho PA, Alexander E III, et al. Radiation necrosis vs high grade re-current glioma: differentiation using dual isotope SPECT with TI and TcHMPAO. AJNR Am J Neuroradiol 1991;12(6): 1187–1192

Sun D, Liu Q, Liu W, Hu W. Clinical application of 201Tl SPECT imaging of brain tumors. J Nucl Med 2000;41(1):5–10

Vos MJ, Hoekstra OS, Barkhof F, et al. Thallium-201 single-photon emission computed tomography as an early predictor of outcome in recurrent glioma. J Clin Oncol 2003;21(19):3559–3565

Section XII

Gastrointestinal Scintigraphy

Harvey A. Ziessman and Kevin J. Donohoe

CASE 139

Clinical Presentation

A 54-year-old woman presents with dysphagia.

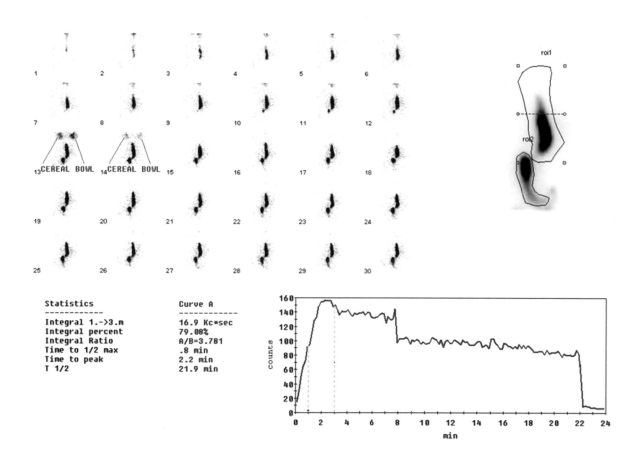

Statistics

Integral 1.->3.m	16.9 Kc*sec
Integral percent	79.08%
Integral Ratio	A/B=3.781
Time to 1/2 max	.8 min
Time to peak	2.2 min
T 1/2	21.9 min

Fig. 139.1

Technique

- A 0.3 mCi dose of ^{99m}Tc-DTPA is mixed with cornflakes and milk.
- Posterior view imaging begins just after ingestion of the meal.
- Images are acquired at 10 seconds per frame for 30 minutes.
- A region-of-interest is drawn on the computer for the esophagus.
- A time–activity curve is generated.
- Esophageal retention is quantified.

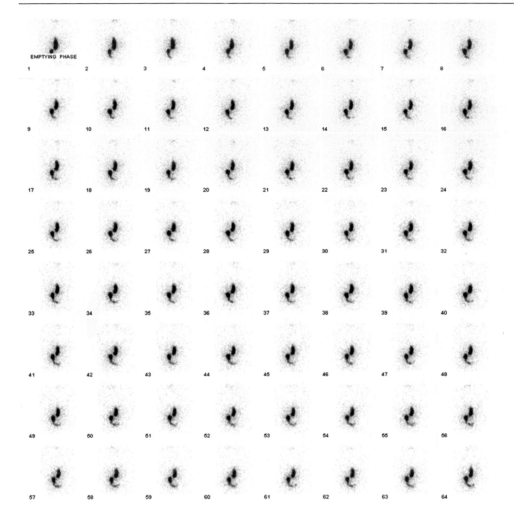

Fig. 139.2

Image Interpretation

Sequential posterior images (**Fig. 139.1**) demonstrate delayed clearance from the esophagus, with a minimal amount of radiolabeled meal reaching the stomach.

A region-of-interest is drawn around the esophagus (**Fig. 139.2**). Frames 13 and 14 have scatter from the cereal bowel in the field of view. The time-activity curve confirms delayed clearance. Emptying occurs at the end of the study after the ingestion of soda. Although a value for $t_{1/2}$ is calculated, we routinely report the percentage of retention (63% at 20 minutes; normal retention, < 5%).

Differential Diagnosis

- Anatomic obstruction
- Achalasia
- Hiatal hernia
- Scleroderma
- Diabetic enteropathy
- Presby-esophagus

Diagnosis and Clinical Follow-Up

Achalasia, with prominent esophageal retention of food. The patient was treated with esophageal dilation. This study will be used as a baseline for subsequent follow-up.

Discussion

Dysphagia is the most common symptom of abnormal esophageal motility. The diagnosis is most often made with barium swallow studies and esophageal manometry. Radiographic studies show retention of contrast in the distended esophagus, a narrowed sphincter, and very delayed clearance. Manometry is usually diagnostic, demonstrating an absence of peristalsis in the distal two-thirds of the esophagus, elevated pressure in the lower esophageal sphincter, and poor sphincter relaxation with swallowing. Esophageal motility scintigraphy is sometimes used as a screening test and can suggest certain diagnoses (eg, esophageal spasm, achalasia), but it is most commonly requested to determine the effectiveness of therapy.

Achalasia is a primary esophageal motor disorder manifested by partial or absent relaxation of the lower esophageal sphincter and loss of esophageal body peristalsis due to the degeneration of neurons in the esophageal wall. Food is retained in the esophagus, resulting in dilation and symptoms of weight loss, nocturnal regurgitation, cough, and aspiration. Scintigraphy can quantify the amount of retention and be valuable for judging the effectiveness of therapy.

PEARLS AND PITFALLS

- A clear liquid (eg, water) is the most common meal used for esophageal scintigraphy; however, data suggest that semisolid meals are more sensitive for detecting motility disorders.
- Rapid image acquisition (eg, 5–10 seconds per frame) is necessary to diagnose most motility disorders. Achalasia is an exception. The esophageal retention can usually be seen on images acquired for one minute per frame.
- All images should be reviewed. Cinematic display can be quite helpful. Quantification is usually performed.

Suggested Reading

Mariani G, Boni G, Barreca M, et al. Radionuclide gastroesophageal motor studies. J Nucl Med 2004;45(6):1004–1028

Parkman HP, Maurer AH, Caroline DF, Miller DL, Krevsky B, Fisher RS. Optimal evaluation of patients with nonobstructive esophageal dysphagia: manometry, scintigraphy, or videoesophagography? Dig Dis Sci 1996;41(7):1355–1368

Tatsch K, Voderholzer WA, Weiss MJ, Schröttle W, Hahn K. Reappraisal of quantitative esophageal scintigraphy by optimizing results with ROC analyses. J Nucl Med 1996;37(11):1799–1805

CASE 140

Clinical Presentation

A 1-month-old premature infant presents with pneumonia and failure to thrive.

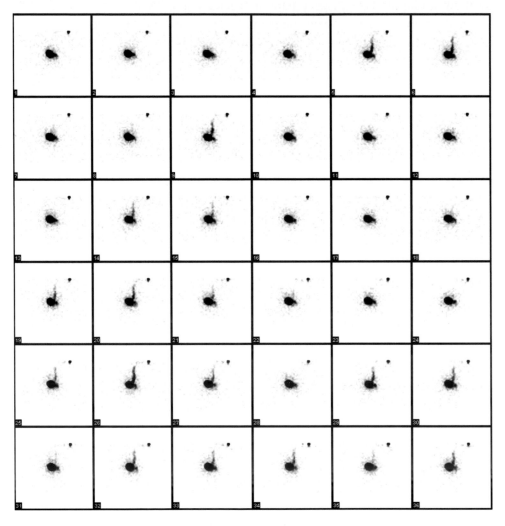

Figs. 140.1

Technique

- A 200- to 300-μCi dose of ^{99m}Tc-sulfur colloid is mixed with formula or milk.
- The patient is imaged supine with the gamma camera placed posteriorly.
- Images are acquired at 10 seconds per frame for 1 hour.
- Gastroesophageal reflux is quantified by counting the number of reflux events and categorizing them as occurring at a high (higher than the mid-esophagus) or low level and as short or long (> 10 seconds).
- Delayed images of the chest are obtained to look for aspiration.

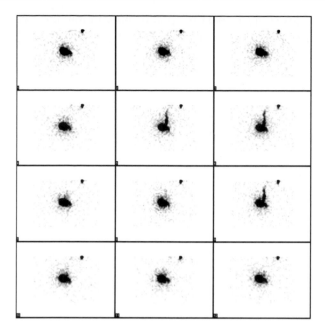

Figs. 140.2

Image Interpretation

Sequential 10-second frames (**Figs. 140.1** and **140.2**) show frequent reflux events. The "hot spot" in the right upper corner of each image is a radioactive marker at the level of the mouth. Most of the reflux events are high, and many are long (> 10 seconds).

Differential Diagnosis

- Gastroesophageal reflux
- Physiologic neonatal reflux

Diagnosis and Clinical Follow-Up

Although all babies have some reflux and normal values are not available, the frequency of reflux events in this patient was definitely abnormal. The neonate was treated symptomatically with the hope that the problem will resolve as the child gets older.

Discussion

Although reflux occurs in normal infants, it usually resolves by 7 to 8 months. Even when reflux is persistent, the course is benign in most children. However, one-third of patients may have persistent symptoms, and serious sequelae (strictures and inanition) develop in 5 to 10%.

Although the radionuclide gastroesophageal reflux study is very sensitive for reflux events, it is not very sensitive for the detection of aspiration. The radionuclide "salivagram" has a better sensitivity for the detection of aspiration. It is performed similarly to an esophageal motility study. A small volume of water with ^{99m}Tc-sulfur colloid is placed in the posterior pharynx, and images are acquired during and after the swallow.

All images should be reviewed. Cinematic display can be helpful for detecting reflux events. The more reflux events there are, and the longer and higher they are, the more clinically significant they are. Gastric emptying is often calculated during the reflex study at two time points: 60 minutes and two hours. For neonates, normal emptying for the pediatric population is considered to be greater than 50% at 1 hour and 75% at 2 hours.

PEARLS AND PITFALLS

- The symptoms of gastroesophageal reflux in children are often different from those in adults (eg, respiratory symptoms, iron deficiency anemia, and failure to thrive).
- The radionuclide gastroesophageal reflux study is most commonly requested in neonates to confirm the clinical diagnosis, although it can be used in adults.
- The detection of short reflux events requires a rapid framing rate (eg, 5–10 seconds per frame).
- Although the test is very sensitive for reflux events, it is much less sensitive for aspiration. A "salivagram" can be useful to detect aspiration if it is not seen on the reflux study and is strongly suspected clinically.

Suggested Reading

Gelfand MJ, Wagner GG. Gastric emptying in infants and children: limited utility of 1-hour measurement. Radiology 1991;178(2):379–381

Heyman S, Respondek M. Detection of pulmonary aspiration in children by radionuclide "salivagram." J Nucl Med 1989;30(5):697–699

Shay SS, Eggli D, Johnson LF. Simultaneous esophageal pH monitoring and scintigraphy during the postprandial period in patients with severe reflux esophagitis. Dig Dis Sci 1991;36(5):558–564

CASE 141

Clinical Presentation

A 30-year-old man volunteered for a gastric emptying study to establish normal values. There was no history of gastric complaints.

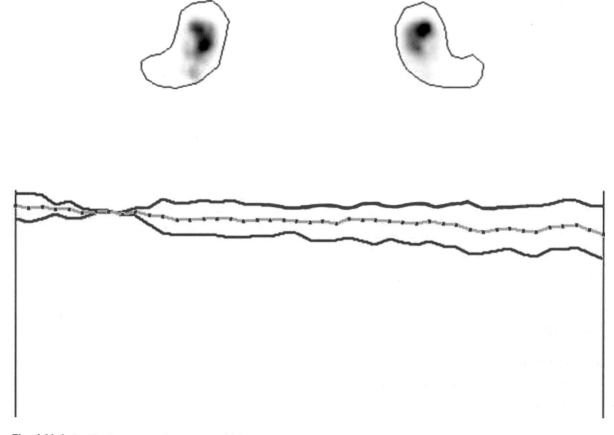

Fig. 141.1 0–45 minutes continuous acquisition.

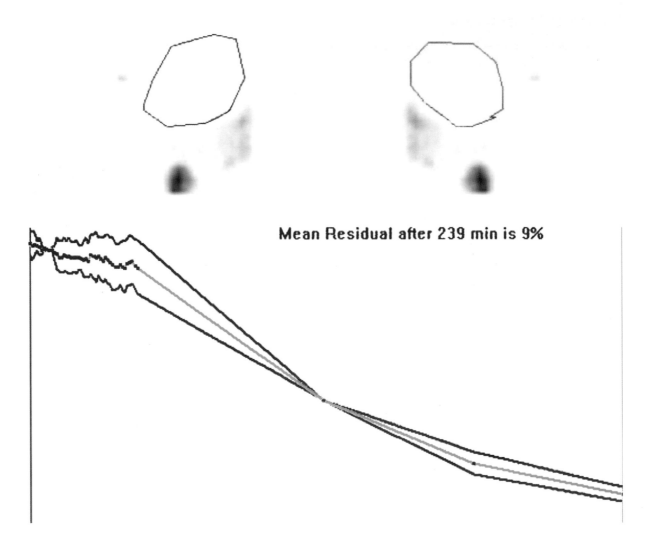

Fig. 141.2 0–239 minutes continuous acquisition.

Technique

Standard Meal:

- 120 ml egg whites labeled with 0.5 mCi ^{99m}Tc-sulfur colloid
- 120 ml water
- 2 slices white bread (or toast)
- 30 gm strawberry jam

Mix the sulfur colloid with the egg white and cook or microwave until done. Consume with bread, jelly and water. The meal should not take longer than 10 minutes to consume.

The patient is placed supine between the heads of a dual-headed gamma camera.

Anterior and posterior data is collected continuously for 45 minutes and divided into one-minute frames (**Fig. 141.1**).

Static images are obtained for one minute in anterior and posterior projections at 2 hours, 3 hours, and 4 hours after meal ingestion (as needed).

Anterior, posterior, and geometric mean time-activity curves (decay corrected) are generated from the region of interest (ROI) drawn around the stomach at each data point (**Fig. 141.2**).

Image Interpretation

The anterior/posterior cine images show emptying into the small bowel over the first 45 minutes of the study (not shown). A region-of-interest (ROI) is drawn around the anterior and posterior images and a time-activity emptying curve is generated for the initial dynamic curve (**Fig. 141.1**), as well as the hourly time points (**Fig. 141.2**). In the blue (anterior) curve, activity initially increases while the activity declines in the red (posterior) curve. This is due to movement of the stomach contents from the relatively posterior fundus to the more anterior antrum. As the contents approach the anterior detector, the counts increase. This is an artifact of the effect of soft tissue attenuation. The middle curve is the geometric mean (GM) correction (square root of the product of the anterior and posterior counts). This geometric mean curve helps to cancel out the effects of attenuation and therefore more accurately represent the true emptying from the gastric ROI. Over the course of the entire study, the geometric mean curve shows a relative plateau initially before emptying accelerates in a linear manner, until towards the end of emptying when the curve levels off. The final point at 4 hours shows less than 10% of the meal remains within the gastric ROI.

Differential Diagnosis

The residual activity in the stomach at 4 hours (less than 10%) is consistent with a normal study.

Diagnosis and Clinical Follow-Up

The patient was a normal student volunteer who enjoyed a free meal.

The Society of Nuclear Medicine (SNM) and the American Neurogastroenterological and Motility Society (ANMS) recently collaborated on a paper that addressed some of the prior weaknesses in the nuclear gastric motility study (see references below).

One of the major factors determining how rapidly the stomach empties is the meal content. Solid food (meat) empties more slowly than semisolids (eggs) or liquids. The more fat, protein and calories in the meal, the slower the emptying. Until recently, the meals used across the country could be substantially different from one another, with many facilities not properly establishing normal emptying values for their particular meal.

The paper written by the SNM and ANMS was written based on a multi-institutional study establishing normal values for the meal described above. At the present time this study represents the best demonstration of normal values and therefore has provided an opportunity for clinics around the world to develop a standardized protocol using readily available ingredients.

The standard protocol does not require continuous acquisition for the first portion of the study as is done here; however, continuous acquisition, as seen in this example, permits careful analysis of the movement of the ingested meal within the stomach, a factor that is important to some gastroenterologists.

PEARLS/PITFALLS

- The radionuclide gastric emptying study is the gold standard for diagnosis of gastroparesis.
- Recent standardization of the radiolabeled meal and imaging protocol has provided a more reliable normal value, and allows inter-institutional comparison of patient data.

- If the entire standardized meal is not ingested or if there are any other variations from the standardized protocol, they should be recorded in the study report.
- It is often helpful to interview the patient at the end of the study to determine if they had their usual symptoms during the study.

Suggested Reading

Tougas G, Chen Y, Coates G, Paterson W, Dallaire C, Pare P, Boivin M, Watier A, Daniels S, Diamant N. Standardization of a simplified scintigraphic methodology for the assessment of gastric emptying in a multicenter setting. American Journal of Gastroenterology 2000;95(1):78–86

Abell TL, Camilleri M, Donohoe K, Hasler WL, Lin HC, Maurer AH, McCallum RW, Nowak T, Nusynowitz ML, Parkman HP, Shreve P, Szarka LA, Snape WJ, Jr., Ziessman HA. Consensus recommendations for gastric emptying scintigraphy: a joint report of the American Neurogastroenterology and Motility Society and the Society of Nuclear Medicine. J Nucl Med Technol 2008;36(1):44–54

Waseem S, Moshiree B, Draganov PV. Gastroparesis: Current diagnostic challenges and management considerations. World J Gastroenterol 2009;15(1):25–37

CASE 142

Clinical Presentation

43-year-old insulin-dependent diabetic presenting with symptoms of post-prandial nausea, abdominal discomfort, and early satiety.

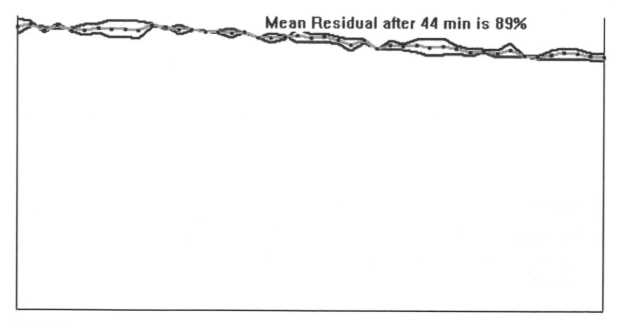

Fig. 142.1

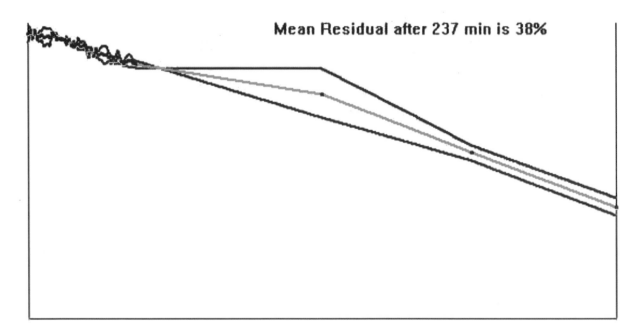

Fig. 142.2

Technique

Standard Meal:

- 120 ml egg whites labeled with 0.5 mCi ^{99m}Tc-sulfur colloid
- 120 ml water
- 2 slices white bread (or toast)
- 30 gm strawberry jam

Mix the sulfur colloid with the egg white and cook or microwave until done. Consume with bread, jelly and water. The meal should not take longer than 10 minutes to consume.

The patient is placed supine between the heads of a dual-headed gamma camera.

Anterior and posterior data is collected continuously for 45 minutes and divided into one-minute frames (**Fig. 142.1**).

Static images are obtained for one minute in anterior and posterior projections at 2 hours, 3 hours, and 4 hours after meal ingestion (as needed).

Anterior, posterior, and geometric mean time-activity curves (decay corrected) are generated from the region of interest (ROI) drawn around the stomach at each data point (**Fig. 142.2**).

Image Interpretation

Sequential one minute images (**Fig. 142.1**) show slow emptying of the radiolabeled meal from the stomach into the small bowel during the first 45 minutes of the study. The gastric emptying curves over 4 hours (**Fig. 142.2**) confirm delayed emptying. At 4 hours

Differential Diagnosis

- Diabetic gastroparesis
- Non-ulcer dyspepsia
- Gastric outlet obstruction
- Hypomotility secondary to medication or previous surgery
- Hypothyroidism
- Muscular dystrophy
- False positive secondary to overlapping small bowel

Diagnosis and Clinical Follow-Up

The study findings are consistent with diabetic gastroparesis as the cause of the symptoms. The patient was successfully treated with prokinetic drugs.

Discussion

Diabetic gastroenteropathy occurs in patients with long-standing insulin-dependent diabetes. The pathophysiology is related to vagal nerve damage as part of a generalized autonomic neuropathy. Symptoms are nonspecific and similar complaints may be due to various other causes in patients with diabetes mellitus. Gastroparesis can exacerbate the problem of diabetic glucose control.

An increasingly common clinical diagnosis is non-ulcer dyspepsia. It is characterized by various upper abdominal symptoms, ulcer-like in some, but dyspeptic in others. Approximately 40% of these patients have delayed gastric emptying. A variety of chronic systemic diseases have been associated with delayed gastric emptying, including Parkinson's disease, amyloidosis, myotonic dystrophy, and HIV infection.

Gastroparesis has also been associated with gastric operations, e.g., vagotomy with or without pyloroplasty, gastric bypass surgery, and fundoplication.

PEARLS/PITFALLS

- Gastric emptying studies must be corrected for radioactive decay or emptying will be overestimated and incorrect (Tc-99m has a half-life of 6 hours).
- Hyperglycemia may of itself be the cause of delayed gastric emptying. In diabetic patients a fasting serum glucose should be obtained at the time of the exam.

- Acute illnesses and metabolic disorders have been associated with gastroparesis including hypokalemia, hypercalcemia, physical and mental stress, and inner-ear disorders.
- Various drugs can cause delayed gastric emptying. These include beta adrenergic agonists, nifedipine, isoproterenol, theophylline, anticholinergics, narcotics and diazepam.
- Small bowel loops overlapping the gastric ROI may result in a false positive study. Review of images (particularly cine images) is helpful to determine the location of the bowel in relation to the gastric ROI.

Suggested Reading

Parkman H, Hasler W, Fisher R. American Gastroenterological Association medial Position Statement: Diagnosis and treatment of gastroparesis. *Gastroenterology* 127:1589–1591, 2004

Koch KL. Diabetic gastropathy: gastric neuromuscular dysfunction in diabetes mellitus: a review of symptoms, pathophysiology, and treatment. *Dig Dis Sci* 44:1061–1075, 1999

Samsom M, Smout AJ. Abnormal gastric and small intestinal motor function in diabetes mellitus. *Dig Dis Sci* 15: 263–274, 1997

CASE 143

Clinical Presentation

18-year-old obese male presenting with epigastric pain following meals.

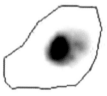
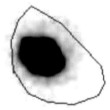

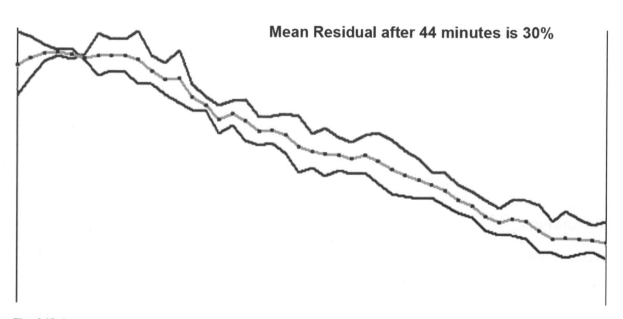

Mean Residual after 44 minutes is 30%

Fig. 143.1

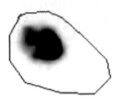

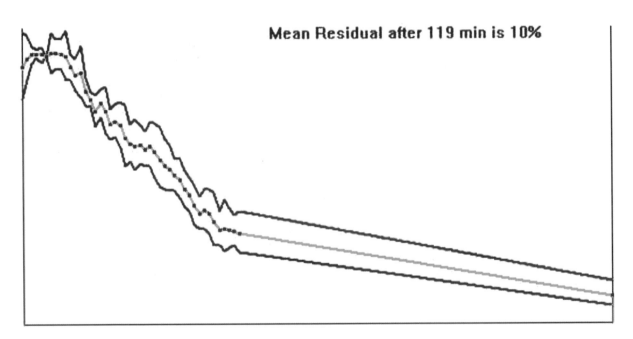

Fig. 143.2

Technique

Standard Meal:

- 120 ml egg whites labeled with 0.5 mCi ^{99m}Tc-sulfur colloid
- 120 ml water
- 2 slices white bread (or toast)
- 30 gm strawberry jam

Mix the sulfur colloid with the egg white and cook or microwave until done. Consume with bread, jelly and water. The meal should not take longer than 10 minutes to consume.

The patient is placed supine between the heads of a dual-headed gamma camera.

Anterior and posterior data is collected continuously for 45 minutes and divided into one-minute frames (**Fig. 143.1**).

Static images are obtained for one minute in anterior and posterior projections at 2 hours, 3 hours, and 4 hours after meal ingestion (as needed).

Anterior, posterior, and geometric mean time-activity curves (decay corrected) are generated from the region of interest (ROI) drawn around the stomach at each data point (**Fig. 143.2**).

Image Interpretation

Curves demonstrate rapid emptying of tracer from the stomach ROI.

Differential Diagnosis

- Diabetic gastroenteropathy with rapid emptying
- Dumping syndrome
- Hyperthyroidism
- Zollinger-Ellison syndrome
- Patient movement during the exam, with subsequent movement of the stomach out from under the ROI.

Diagnosis and Clinical Follow-Up

Gastroenteropathy with rapid emptying. The patient was treated successfully with anticholinergics.

Discussion

The symptoms associated with rapid gastric emptying demonstrate substantial overlap with those of gastroparesis. Some patients have more classical dumping syndrome symptoms such as weakness, sweating and dizziness, but even these symptoms may be seen with gastroparesis. Accelerated emptying occurs in some patients after partial gastrectomy, vagotomy, or pyloroplasty, and has also been reported in patients with duodenal ulcers.

PEARLS/PITFALLS _____

- The symptoms of rapid gastric emptying in diabetics can be identical to those with gastroparesis.
- The patient should ingest the meal in the imaging room with the gamma camera set up and ready for imaging. The patient can then be put into position quickly, before appreciable emptying has occurred.
- If the initial image shows substantial emptying into the small bowel, the ROI at time 0 should include all activity in the GI tract since it represents the meal ingested at time zero.
- Review of the cine images or with images showing the location of the ROI in relation to the stomach are helpful to rule out patient movement during the study.

Suggested Reading

Singh A, Gull H, Sing RJ. Clinical significance of rapid (accelerated) gastric emptying. Clin Nucl Med 28:658–662, 2003

Lipp RW, Schnedl WJ, Hammer HF, et al. Evidence of accelerated gastric emptying in longstanding diabetic patients after ingestion of a semisolid meal. J Nucl Med. 38:814–818, 1997

Nowak TV, Johnson CP, Kalbfleisch JH, et al. Highly variable gastric emptying in patients with insulin dependent diabetes mellitus. Gut. 37:23–29, 1995

Ziessman HA, Fahey FH, Collen MJ. Biphasic solid and liquid gastric emptying in normal controls and diabetics using continuous acquisition in LAO view. Dig Dis Sci 37:744–75, 1992

CASE 144

Clinical Presentation

A 43-year-old woman with abdominal pain, nausea, and vomiting cannot keep solid food down but can drink liquids. She is hospitalized because of dehydration and general deterioration.

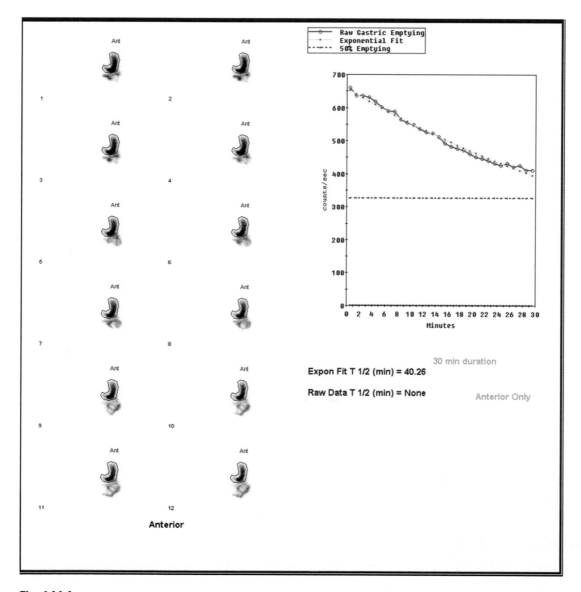

Fig. 144.1

Technique

- ⁹⁹ᵐTc-sulfur colloid (0.5 mCi) is mixed with 500 mL of water.
- The gamma camera is placed anteriorly.
- One-minute frames are acquired continuously for 30 minutes.

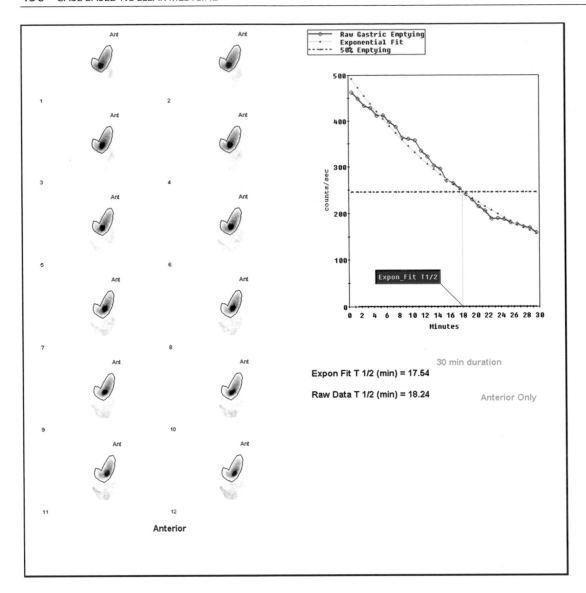

Fig. 144.2

- A region-of-interest is drawn around the stomach.
- A time–activity curve is generated.
- The half-time ($t_{1/2}$) of emptying is determined.

Image Interpretation

The clear liquid meal is emptying in a single exponential pattern (**Fig. 144.1**), although slowly, with a $t_{1/2}$ exponential fit of 40 minutes. The second study (**Fig. 144.2**), for comparison, is from a patient with a normal $t_{1/2}$ of emptying of 18 minutes (normal, 10–20 minutes).

Differential Diagnosis

- Gastric outlet obstruction
- Gastroparesis associated with non-ulcer dyspepsia syndrome
- Hypomotility secondary to medications that delay gastric emptying

- Gastroparesis secondary to metabolic causes, such as hypothyroidism, hypercalcemia, hypokalemia, and hyperglycemia

Diagnosis and Clinical Follow-Up

An upper gastrointestinal series was not remarkable. Once the patient's metabolic and fluid status had been reestablished, the vomiting resolved. The study was not repeated.

Discussion

Delayed liquid gastric emptying is often associated with delayed solid emptying. However, a liquid study can be abnormal when a solid study is normal. One publication has shown that this occurs in up to 32% of patients referred for gastric emptying evaluation. Unlike solids, liquids have no lag phase and empty in a single exponential pattern. The tonic contraction of the gastric fundus is responsible for liquid emptying.

Dual-isotope solid and liquid gastric-emptying studies can be done; however, they are usually reserved for investigative research. Dual-phase solid and liquid gastric-emptying studies are performed with two different isotopes that have different photopeaks (eg, ^{99m}Tc-sulfur colloid for the solid phase and ^{111}In-DTPA for the liquid phase). The pattern of liquid emptying will be similar to that of liquid-only studies, but the rate of emptying will be slower than that of liquid-only meals because of the higher caloric content.

PEARLS AND PITFALLS

- Liquids typically empty more rapidly than solids.
- The normal half-time of emptying of clear liquids is 10 to 20 minutes. Whereas there is a delay before solid emptying begins, there is no delay before liquid emptying begins, and emptying follows a single exponential pattern.

Suggested Reading

Chaudhuri TK. Use of 99mTc-DTPA for measuring gastric emptying time. J Nucl Med 1974;15(6): 391–395

Ziessman HA, Fahey FH, Collen MJ. Biphasic solid and liquid gastric emptying in normal controls and diabetics using continuous acquisition in LAO view. Dig Dis Sci 1992;37(5):744–750

Ziessman HA, Chander A, Clarke JO, Ramos O, Wahl RL. The added diagnostic value of liquid gastric emptying compared with solid emptying alone. J Nucl Med 2009;50:726–731

CASE 145

Clinical Presentation

A 44-year-old woman presents with a history of chronic constipation that has become difficult to treat. The patient had an episode of diarrhea 24 hours following the initial set of images, and therefore the study was rescheduled and repeated several weeks later.

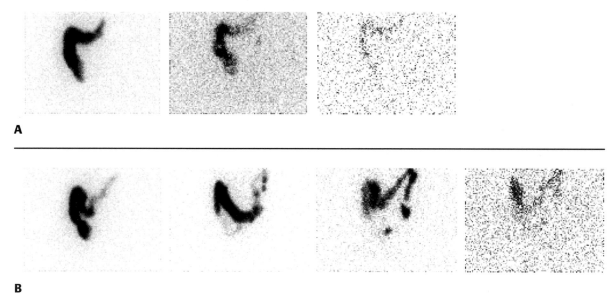

Fig. 145.1 **(A)** Initial study. **(B)** Second study.

Technique

- A 1 mCi dose of ^{111}In-DTPA is ingested in 500 mL of water.
- Anterior and posterior images of the abdomen are acquired at 6, 24, 48, and 72 hours after ingestion of the radiolabeled water.
- Regions-of-interest are defined for the cecum, ascending colon, transverse colon, descending colon, and rectum, and for excreted stool.
- The geometric mean of the anterior and posterior images is obtained for each imaging time point for each region.
- All counts are corrected for decay.
- The geometric center of activity (weighted average of the counts in each region) is determined at each imaging time for each region of the colon.

Image Interpretation

The initial set of images (**Fig. 145.1A**) demonstrates accumulation of tracer in the ascending and transverse colon. After an episode of diarrhea, the diminished tracer can still be seen collecting just behind the mid–transverse colon. A second study (**Fig. 145.1B**), done several days later, again shows prominent accumulation of radiotracer in the transverse colon on 24-hour images. At 48 hours, some tracer is seen to move beyond the transverse colon to the left side of the colon. At 72 hours, much of the activity has been evacuated.

Differential Diagnosis

- Anatomic obstruction
- Functional obstruction, including the following:
  - Chronic idiopathic constipation
  - Chronic idiopathic intestinal pseudo-obstruction
  - Hirschsprung disease (usually diagnosed in infancy)
  - Chagas disease (damage to myenteric plexus)
  - Anticholinergic drugs
  - Parasympathetic injury
  - Multiple sclerosis

Diagnosis and Clinical Follow-Up

After considering a partial bowel resection of the midcolon, the patient elected to pursue nonsurgical therapy. She continues to have problems with constipation, but medical therapy has reduced her symptoms.

Discussion

The optimal therapy for chronic constipation depends on whether there is diffuse slow colonic transit, regional dysfunction, pelvic floor dysfunction, or irritable bowel syndrome. Radiographs with opaque markers have been used to estimate the transit time; however, this method is not physiologic and not quantitative, and intracolonic localization can be difficult with limited anatomic landmarks. The radionuclide study can be quantified by dividing the colon into multiple segments and calculating a geometric center of activity to estimate the progression of colonic activity. The geometric center is a weighted average of the counts for various regions of the colon. Normal values have been published by Mayo Clinic and Temple University investigational groups.

Most anatomic causes of bowel obstruction should be ruled out with barium enema and/or colonoscopy studies before a scintigraphy study of colonic transit is ordered. Colonic transit scintigraphy can help distinguish between generalized slow-transit constipation, a regional problem, and normal transit.

Whole-gut transit studies may be done by combining a gastric-emptying study and an intestinal transit study. Different methodologies have been proposed. The simpler method uses eggs labeled with ^{99m}Tc for gastric emptying and ^{111}In-DTPA for small- and large-bowel transit.

PEARLS AND PITFALLS

- An important advantage of the ^{111}In-DTPA intestinal transit study is its ability to provide quantitative information.
- ^{111}In, which has a 2.8-day (67-hour) half-life, is often used because colonic transit analysis requires 72 hours of imaging. Thus, correction for decay is mandatory.
- The geometric mean (square root of the product of the anterior and posterior counts) is used to correct for variable soft tissue attenuation.

Suggested Reading

Charles F, Camilleri M, Phillips SF, Thomforde GM, Forstrom LA. Scintigraphy of the whole gut: clinical evaluation of transit disorders. Mayo Clin Proc 1995;70(2):113–118

Maurer AH, Krevsky B. Whole-gut transit scintigraphy in the evaluation of small-bowel and colon transit disorders. Semin Nucl Med 1995;25(4):326–338

Maurer AH, Parkman HP. Update on gastrointestinal scintigraphy. Semin Nucl Med 2006;36(2): 110–118

Roberts JP, Newell MS, Deeks JJ, Waldron DW, Garvie NW, Williams NS. Oral [111In]DTPA scintigraphic assessment of colonic transit in constipated subjects. Dig Dis Sci 1993;38(6):1032–1039

CASE 146

Clinical Presentation

A 3-year-old child is admitted to the hospital with rectal bleeding.

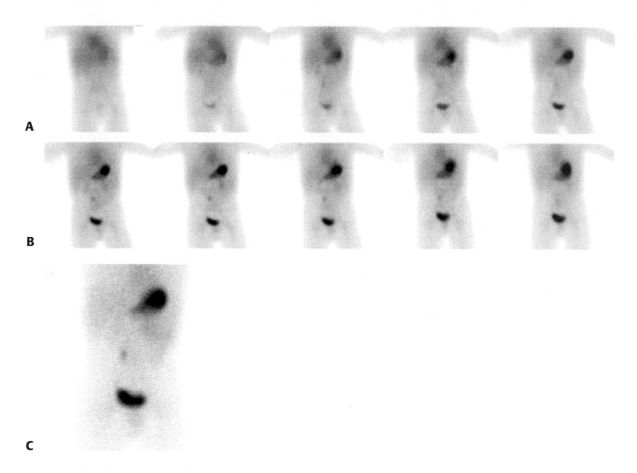

Fig. 146.1 Ten minute images.

Technique

- Cimetidine (20 mg/kg) is administered orally for 24 to 48 hours before the study.
- The patient is fasting for 4 hours before the radiopharmaceutical is injected.
- The patient should void before the study. Catheterization may be required.
- 99mTc-pertechnetate (0.1 mCi/kg) is administered intravenously.
- Sequential 5-minute images are acquired for 1 hour.
- Upright and oblique static images can be obtained as necessary to confirm localization or differentiate gastrointestinal activity from urinary tract activity.

Image Interpretation

Serial 5-minute anterior images over the abdomen (**Fig. 146.1A,B**) show a progressive focal increase in tracer accumulation in the right lower quadrant, although it appears decreased and blurred in the last few frames. A single anterior 10-minute image (**Fig. 146.1C**) acquired immediately after the initial 60-minute acquisition shows definite accumulation in the same region.

Differential Diagnosis

- Meckel diverticulum
- Intestinal duplication
- Ureterocele

Diagnosis and Clinical Follow-Up

Scintigraphy was diagnostic of a Meckel diverticulum. The patient was taken to surgery, and a Meckel diverticulum was resected.

Discussion

Meckel diverticulum is the most common congenital anomaly of the gastrointestinal tract. It results from failure of closure of the omphalomesenteric duct in the embryo. This true diverticulum arises on the antimesenteric side of the small bowel, usually 80 to 90 cm proximal to the ileocecal valve.

^{99m}Tc-pertechnetate is taken up by gastric mucosa and therefore within a Meckel diverticulum that possesses gastric mucosa. Uptake in the diverticulum generally occurs at the same rate as uptake in the stomach. The overall accuracy is reported to be high, with a sensitivity of 85% and a specificity of more than 90%.

Pre-treatment with cimetidine is recommended. Reports suggest that cimetidine increases the sensitivity of the study, and side effects are uncommon with a short, 2-day course. This histamine H$_2$-receptor antagonist increases sensitivity by inhibiting the release of ^{99m}Tc-pertechnetate from the gastric mucosa.

PEARLS AND PITFALLS

- Ectopic gastric mucosa is present in 10 to 30% of patients with a Meckel diverticulum, in 60% of patients with a symptomatic Meckel diverticulum, and in 98% of those with a bleeding Meckel diverticulum.
- ^{99m}Tc-pertechnetate is taken up by the mucinous cells, not the parietal cells, as is often assumed.
- The most common false-positive studies for Meckel diverticulum are in patients with a gastrointestinal duplication containing gastric mucosa or with accumulation in the genitourinary tract (eg, renal pelvis, ureterocele).
- False-negative results may be caused by small size (< 2 cm²), lack of sufficient gastric mucosa, or an impaired blood supply.

Suggested Reading

Emamian SA, Shalaby-Rana E, Majd M. The spectrum of heterotopic gastric mucosa in children detected by Tc-99m pertechnetate scintigraphy. Clin Nucl Med 2001;26(6):529–535

Kumar R, Tripathi M, Chandrashekar N, et al. Diagnosis of ectopic gastric mucosa using 99Tcm-pertechnetate: spectrum of scintigraphic findings. Br J Radiol 2005;78(932):714–720

Sfakianakis GN, Haase GM. Abdominal scintigraphy for ectopic gastric mucosa: a retrospective analysis of 143 studies. AJR Am J Roentgenol 1982;138(1):7–12

CASE 147

Clinical Presentation

A 65-year-old man presents with melena and acute gastrointestinal bleeding.

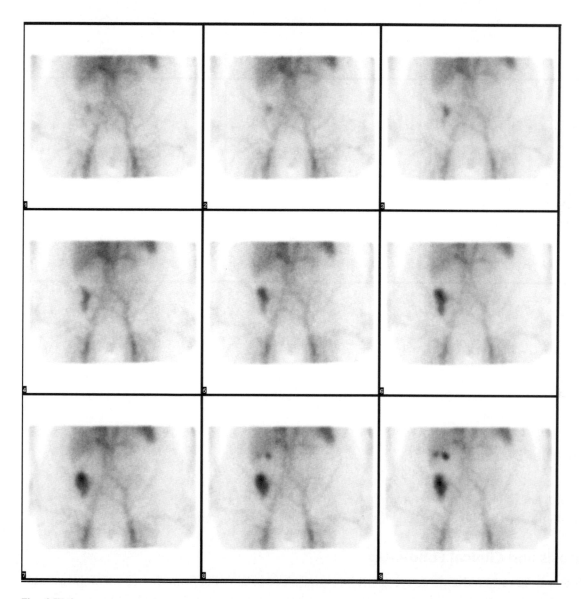

Fig. 147.1

Technique

- The in vitro or modified in vivo methodology is used to label autologous red blood cells with 25 mCi of ^{99m}Tc-pertechnetate.
- The patient is placed in a supine position beneath a gamma camera with a large field of view.
- Initial flow images are acquired at 1 to 3 seconds per frame for 1 minute (not shown).
- Dynamic images are acquired at 1 minute per frame for 89 minutes.

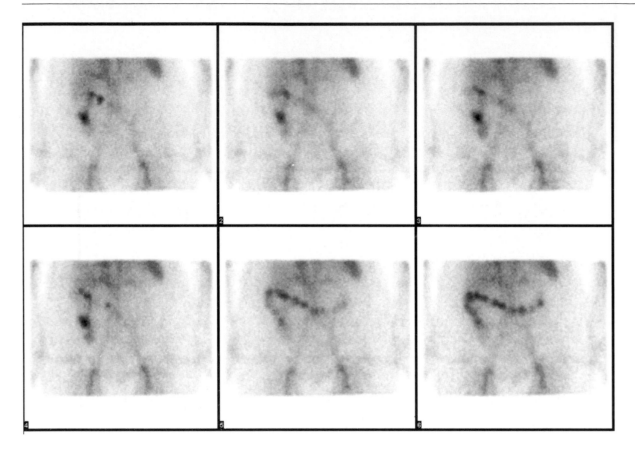

Fig. 147.2

Image Interpretation

Serial anterior images of the abdomen (**Fig. 147.1**) demonstrate progressively increasing focal activity in the right lower quadrant. On continued imaging (**Fig. 147.2**), the activity can be seen to be transiting to the transverse colon.

Differential Diagnosis

- Gastrointestinal bleeding in the region of the cecum
- Atypical site of bleeding in the small bowel
- Extraluminal site of bleeding, collecting in the left side of the abdomen

Diagnosis and Clinical Follow-Up

The study was interpreted as an active gastrointestinal bleed originating from the cecum of the ascending colon. Colonoscopy revealed a cecal mass. The pathology was carcinoma of the colon.

Discussion

Gastrointestinal scintigraphy can determine whether active bleeding is present and can localize the approximate site of origin of the bleeding. This information is valuable to angiographers. Bleeding is often intermittent. If no active bleeding is seen on the radionuclide study, contrast angiography is likely to be futile and is best postponed. Locating the bleeding vessel (superior mesenteric, inferior mesenteric, or celiac) with the radionuclide study saves time and contrast for the angiographer and the patient.

Localization of a site of bleeding should meet certain criteria. A focus of activity is seen where none was initially, the activity should increase in intensity over time, and the radiotracer should transit in a pattern conforming to the intestinal anatomy. The movement may be antegrade and/or retrograde.

Flow images (2–3 seconds per frame for 60 minutes) may on occasion detect a vascular blush, even if the subsequent dynamic 90-minute images show no active bleeding. This is seen most commonly with angiodysplasia or tumor.

An image of the head and neck region can determine the presence of free ^{99m}Tc-pertechnetate, demonstrated by salivary gland and thyroid uptake. If delayed images are indicated because of recurrent bleeding, dynamic imaging should be repeated in a manner similar to that used for the initial image acquisition (1-minute dynamic imaging for 30 minutes), and the same criteria should be used to diagnose the site of the bleeding. Static delayed images will not be able to reliably localize a site of bleeding, even if radiolabeled blood is noted in the bowel.

PEARLS AND PITFALLS

- Reviewing the study in cinematic format is helpful for detection and localization.
- When active bleeding is detected, imaging should be continued until the anatomic origin of the bleeding can be ascertained by the pattern of transit.
- In labeling red blood cells, stannous ion (tin) as stannous pyrophosphate is necessary for the ^{99m}Tc to bind to the β-chain of the hemoglobin.
- Poor labeling of the red blood cells can result in gastric secretion of free ^{99m}Tc-pertechnetate that can be mistaken for gastric bleeding.
- Genital blood pool activity can either mimic or hide rectal bleeding. A lateral view of the pelvis can help distinguish anterior genital and bladder activity from rectal blood.

Suggested Reading

Howarth DM. The role of nuclear medicine in the detection of acute gastrointestinal bleeding. Semin Nucl Med 2006;36(2):133–146

Maurer AH, Rodman MS, Vitti RA, Revez G, Krevsky B. Gastrointestinal bleeding: improved localization with cine scintigraphy. Radiology 1992;185(1):187–192

Zuckier LS. Acute gastrointestinal bleeding. Semin Nucl Med 2003;33(4):297–311

CASE 148

Clinical Presentation

A 75-year-old man on warfarin sodium (Coumadin) for atrial fibrillation presents with melena and anemia.

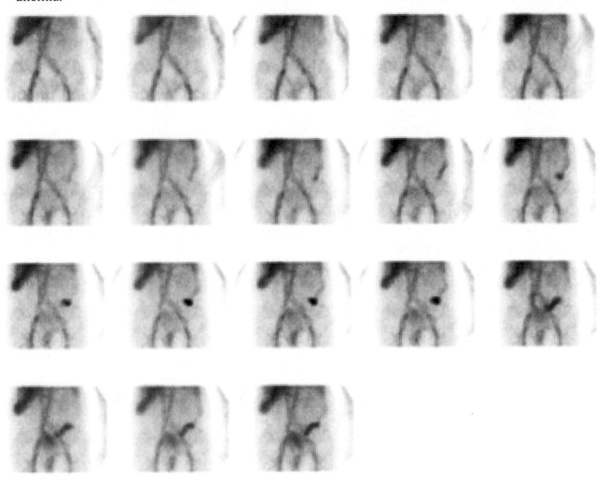

Fig. 148.1

Technique

- The in vitro or modified in vivo method is used to label autologous blood with 25 to 30 mCi of ^{99m}Tc-pertechnetate.
- The patient is placed in a supine position and imaged anteriorly with a gamma camera that has a large field of view.
- Initial flow images are acquired at 1 to 3 seconds per frame for 1 minute (not shown).
- Anterior abdominal 1-minute images are acquired continuously for 60 to 90 minutes.

Image Interpretation

Serial anterior images of the abdomen (**Fig. 148.1**) initially demonstrate no abnormality; then, slowly increasing focal activity is seen in the left lower quadrant that subsequently transits inferiorly and medially, consistent with a sigmoid colon pattern.

Differential Diagnosis

- Distal descending colon bleed
- Atypical site of bleeding in the small bowel
- Free ^{99m}Tc-pertechnetate
- Extraluminal site of bleeding, collecting in the left side of the abdomen

Diagnosis and Clinical Follow-Up

The study was interpreted as active gastrointestinal bleeding originating in the region of the distal descending colon at the junction with the sigmoid colon. Contrast angiography revealed a bleeding colonic diverticulum. The feeding vessel was occluded. Colonoscopy revealed diverticula throughout the colon.

Discussion

Gastrointestinal scintigraphy is a valuable test for the diagnosis of gastrointestinal bleeding. Bleeding at a rate of as little as 0.1 mL/min can be detected. A volume of blood as small as 2 to 3 mL can be detected.

Because gastrointestinal bleeding is often intermittent, the radionuclide study is best performed soon after arrival in the emergency department or admission to the hospital. Delaying the study until after colonoscopy or radiographic studies may result in a negative study. The bleeding study is most likely to be positive during the initial 90 minutes; however, delayed dynamic imaging can occasionally be valuable when initial imaging is negative.

The radionuclide study is used to document the presence of active bleeding and to localize the approximate site of bleeding. Contrast angiography is much more likely to be diagnostic if active bleeding is seen on the radionuclide study.

PEARLS AND PITFALLS

- Free ^{99m}Tc-pertechnetate is secreted in the stomach and will transit the bowel, which can result in an erroneous diagnosis of gastric or intestinal bleed.
- Routine anterior views of the neck can show evidence of free ^{99m}Tc-pertechnetate in the salivary glands and thyroid.
- Renal excretion of free ^{99m}Tc-pertechnetate in the urinary collecting system can mimic hemorrhage, particularly if hydronephrosis or hydroureter is present.
- Retrograde movement of tracer can falsely suggest a more proximal site of bleeding if continuous acquisition and cinematic display are not performed.

Suggested Reading

Emslie JT, Zarnegar K, Siegel ME, Beart RW Jr. Technetium-99m-labeled red blood cell scans in the investigation of gastrointestinal bleeding. Dis Colon Rectum 1996;39(7):750–754

Ng DA, Opelka FG, Beck DE, et al. Predictive value of technetium Tc 99m-labeled red blood cell scintigraphy for positive angiogram in massive lower gastrointestinal hemorrhage. Dis Colon Rectum 1997;40(4):471–477

Suzman MS, Talmor M, Jennis R, Binkert B, Barie PS. Accurate localization and surgical management of active lower gastrointestinal hemorrhage with technetium-labeled erythrocyte scintigraphy. Ann Surg 1996;224(1):29–36

CASE 149

Clinical Presentation

A 68-year-old man presents with intermittent melena and a recently falling hematocrit.

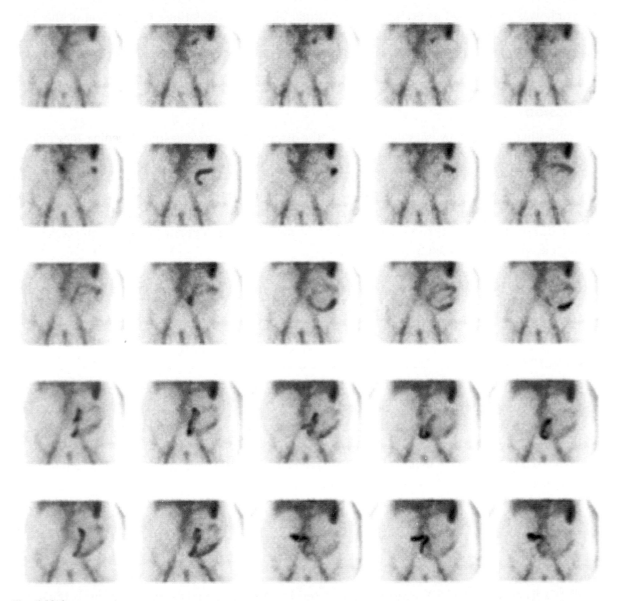

Fig. 149.1

Technique

- Three milliliters of autologous red blood cells are labeled with ^{99m}Tc-pertechnetate (25 mCi) and injected intravenously.
- The patient is placed in a supine position beneath a gamma camera with a large field of view.
- Flow images are acquired at 1 to 3 seconds per frame for 60 seconds (not shown).

- Anterior abdominal image data are acquired continuously (1 minute per frame for 90 minutes).
- Delayed dynamic images (1 minute per frame for 30 minutes) are acquired as needed.

Image Interpretation

Serial 1-minute anterior images over the abdomen (**Fig. 149.1**) show a collection of tracer at the upper edge of the field of view that moves inferiorly and outlines the duodenal C-loop before it crosses the midline to the left upper quadrant. The tracer then moves in a serpiginous pattern on the left side of the abdomen before crossing over to the right side of the abdomen. Later images, taken after repositioning of the camera (not shown), demonstrated the accumulation of tracer to be just distal to the stomach.

Differential Diagnosis

- Bleeding in the upper small bowel
- Biliary tract hemorrhage
- Intraperitoneal bleeding (the pattern of tracer movement in this study is very unlikely to be consistent with bleeding into any structure other than the bowel lumen)

Diagnosis and Clinical Follow-Up

Endoscopy demonstrated a bleeding duodenal ulcer.

Discussion

A radionuclide study is not usually indicated for upper gastrointestinal bleeding, although it can sometimes be diagnosed incidentally. In cases of lower gastrointestinal bleeding, colonoscopy and barium contrast studies are not possible during active bleeding.

Tracer movement in small-bowel bleeding will follow a serpentine pattern, much different from that seen with large-bowel bleeding. If bleeding is intermittent, however, and bowel motility is diminished, a focal accumulation of tracer that does not move can be difficult to localize. Continued acquisition of images is needed in these patients because delayed static images will identify the site of tracer accumulation only at the time the image is acquired. This may have little to do with the site of origin.

Because the tracer collection began at the edge of the field of view in this case, it was not clear whether the bleeding was coming from the duodenum or from above the duodenum. It is not uncommon that the gamma camera needs to be repositioned to better observe a site of bleeding. Careful review of the study during acquisition will indicate how to reposition the gamma camera to best visualize the source of hemorrhage.

PEARLS AND PITFALLS

- The in vitro method of radiolabeling has a higher percentage of labeling efficiency (> 97%) than that of the modified in vivo method (85%) or in vivo method (75%).
- Extreme care must be taken in handling and labeling blood, and in reinfusing blood, to avoid the potential problem of transferring bloodborne disease.
- A fixed region of uptake is not diagnostic of bleeding and may be caused by hemangioma, aneurysm, varices, accessory spleen, pelvic kidney, or renal transplant.

Suggested Reading

Dusold R, Burke K, Carpentier W, Dyck WP. The accuracy of technetium-99m-labeled red cell scintigraphy in localizing gastrointestinal bleeding. Am J Gastroenterol 1994;89(3):345–348

Lau WY, Yuen WK, Chu KW, Poon GP, Li AK. Obscure bleeding in the gastrointestinal tract originating in the small intestine. Surg Gynecol Obstet 1992;174(2):119–124

Section XIII

Vascular Scintigraphy

Steven C. Burrell and Annick D. Van den Abbeele

CASE 150

Clinical Presentation

A 51-year-old woman with breast cancer undergoes abdominal ultrasonography to assess (arrow) for possible liver metastases. This reveals a 2.5-cm echogenic focus in the right lobe of the liver (**Fig. 150.1**). Although the sonographic appearance is suggestive of a hemangioma, it is not specific. Given the history of cancer, a tagged red blood cell (RBC) blood pool study is requested for confirmation (**Figs. 150.2** and **150.3A**).

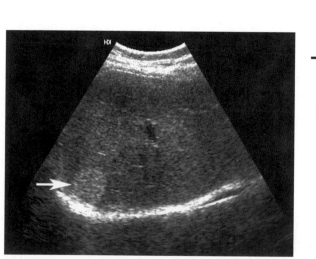

Fig. 150.1

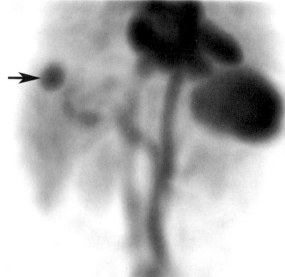

Fig. 150.2

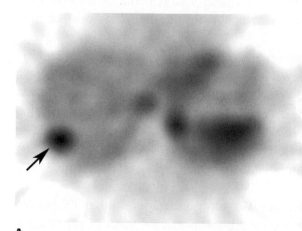

A

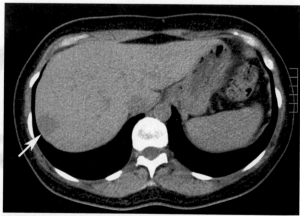

B

Fig. 150.3

Technique

- Three milliliters of autologous red blood cells are labeled with ⁹⁹ᵐTc-pertechnetate (25 mCi) and injected intravenously.
- The patient is placed in a supine position beneath a gamma camera with a large field of view.
- Flow images are acquired at 1 to 3 seconds per frame for 60 seconds (not shown).
- Anterior abdominal image data are acquired continuously (1 minute per frame for 90 minutes).
- Delayed dynamic images (1 minute per frame for 30 minutes) are acquired as needed.

Image Interpretation

Anterior maximum-intensity projection (MIP) image (**Fig. 150.2**) demonstrates an intense focus of RBC accumulation near the dome of the liver (arrow). Normal intense RBC activity is also seen in the heart, vasculature, and spleen. An axial slice from the SPECT scan (**Fig. 150.3A**) shows the location of the RBC accumulation to be in the liver (arrow), corresponding with a low-density lesion on a subsequent CT scan (**Fig. 150.3B** [*arrow*]) and with the original ultrasound. Note also the normal intense uptake in the spleen and vasculature, including the aorta and inferior vena cava.

Differential Diagnosis

- Cavernous hemangioma
- Angiosarcoma (rare)
- Hepatocellular carcinoma (rare to have this appearance)
- Vascular neuroendocrine tumor (rare to have this appearance)

Final Diagnosis

A cavernous hemangioma was diagnosed.

Discussion

Cavernous hemangiomas are the most common benign masses of the liver, occurring in 0.4 to 7% of the population; metastases are the most common liver masses overall. Cavernous hemangiomas are formed from large vascular channels, with capillary-like lumina between the channels. The vast majority of hemangiomas are asymptomatic and incidentally detected by other abdominal imaging modalities. Occasionally, hemangiomas can present with pain if they hemorrhage, or large hemangiomas can have a mass effect. The clinical significance of an incidentally discovered hemangioma is that it can be mistaken for a malignancy.

The premise of the tagged RBC study is that the large vascular capacitance of a hemangioma results in a marked accumulation of RBCs in the lesion on delayed imaging. Despite the large volume of blood, the rate of blood flow to the lesion is actually decreased relative to that in the surrounding liver parenchyma. Thus, hemangiomas characteristically show decreased activity on early flow phase imaging and increased activity on delayed imaging ("perfusion–blood pool mismatch"). Flow imaging should be performed in the projection that best demonstrates the lesion, based on correlation with other imaging modalities. Delayed imaging is performed at 2 hours or later, to allow blood pool equilibration. SPECT imaging is highly recommended.

Many cavernous hemangiomas have a typical appearance with ultrasonography, MRI, or CT, but the findings are not specific. The tagged RBC study has the highest positive predictive value of any imaging modality.

- As with other labeled blood cell studies, procedures to prevent injection into the wrong patient must be in place and strictly adhered to.
- Some, although not all, researchers strongly advocate an early flow phase. This should be performed in the projection that best demonstrates the suspected hemangioma based on knowledge acquired from other imaging. Most hemangiomas will demonstrate normal or decreased flow.
- The hallmark of the tagged RBC scan is increased uptake on delayed views, similar to that in the blood vessels. The SPECT images should be carefully followed to ensure that what is thought to be a hemangioma is not a blood vessel.
- SPECT imaging identifies smaller and deeper hemangiomas than planar imaging is generally considered essential.

Suggested Reading

Davis LP, McCarroll K. Correlative imaging of the liver and hepatobiliary system. Semin Nucl Med 1994;24(3):208–218

Front D, Israel O, Groshar D, Weininger J. Technetium-99m-labeled red blood cell imaging. Semin Nucl Med 1984;14(3):226–250

Ziessman H. Progress and direction of gastrointestinal nuclear medicine. Eur J Nucl Med 1994;21(11): 1263–1268

CASE 151

Clinical Presentation

A 44-year-old woman undergoes abdominal ultrasonography, which reveals multiple echogenic lesions within the liver. This leads to a nuclear medicine tagged red blood cell (RBC) study (**Figs. 151.1, 151.2,** and **151.3**).

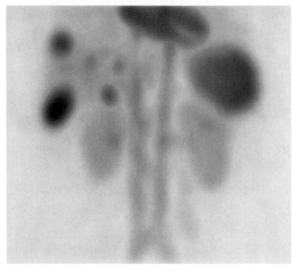

Fig. 151.1

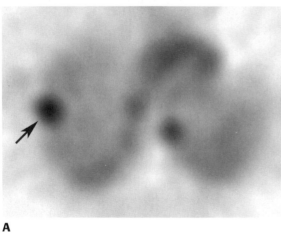

A   B

Fig. 151.2

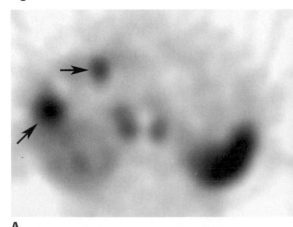

A   B

Fig. 151.3

Technique

- The in vitro or modified in vivo method is used to label autologous blood with 25 to 30 mCi of ^{99m}Tc-pertechnetate.
- The patient is placed in a supine position and imaged anteriorly with a gamma camera that has a large field of view. The gamma camera is placed over the abdomen.
- Initial flow images are acquired at 1 to 3 seconds per frame for 1 minute (not shown).
- Anterior abdominal 1-minute images are acquired continuously for 60 to 90 minutes.

Image Interpretation

Anterior maximum-intensity projection (MIP) view from the SPECT acquisition (**Fig. 151.1**) demonstrates multiple foci of intense uptake in the liver, correlating with the sonographic abnormalities (not shown). Axial SPECT slices (**Figs. 151.2A** and **151.3A**) confirm the location of several of these foci, which correlate with high-T2-signal lesions on subsequent MRI (**Figs. 151.2B** and **151.3B** [*arrows*]). Note also the normal intense uptake in the spleen, aorta, and inferior vena cava.

Differential Diagnosis

- Multiple hemangiomas
- Metastases from a vascular neuroendocrine tumor or a hepatocellular carcinoma (rare)
- Multiple angiosarcomas (rare)

Final Diagnosis

The diagnosis was multiple hemangiomas.

Discussion

The tagged RBC study is very specific (95–100%) for hemangiomas. Very rare false-positive studies have occurred with angiosarcomas, hepatocellular carcinomas, and vascular neuroendocrine metastases. Because hepatocellular carcinomas are hypervascular, the initial flow phase can help distinguish hepatocellular carcinomas from hemangiomas, and some consider this phase to be essential. However, not all researchers advocate including a flow phase because the vast majority of hepatocellular carcinomas do not mimic hemangiomas on delayed views, and the typical perfusion–blood pool mismatch is not entirely sensitive (some hemangiomas may not demonstrate decreased early flow) or specific (angiosarcomas and carcinoids have shown perfusion–blood pool mismatch).

The sensitivity of the tagged RBC study depends on the lesion size. Sensitivities as high as 100% have been reported for hemangiomas larger than 1.4 cm when three-headed SPECT was used. Although the sensitivity drops off for smaller lesions, hemangiomas as small as 0.5 cm have been detected. Detection also decreases close to vessels and in organs accumulating RBCs, such as the heart and spleen.

PEARLS AND PITFALLS

- The tagged RBC study is sensitive and very specific for cavernous hemangiomas.
- Causes of (rare) false-positive studies include angiosarcomas, hepatocellular carcinomas, and neuroendocrine tumor metastases.
- Causes of false-negative studies include small size of lesions, proximity to blood vessels or vascular organs, and hemangiomas with fibrosis or thrombosis.

Suggested Reading

Farlow DC, Little JM, Gruenewald SM, Antico VF, O'Neill P. A case of metastatic malignancy masquerading as a hepatic hemangioma on labeled red blood cell scintigraphy. J Nucl Med 1993;34(7):1172–1174

Front D, Israel O, Groshar D, Weininger J. Technetium-99m-labeled red blood cell imaging. Semin Nucl Med 1984;14(3):226–250

Ginsberg F, Slavin JD Jr, Spencer RP. Hepatic angiosarcoma: mimicking of angioma on three-phase technetium-99m red blood cell scintigraphy. J Nucl Med 1986;27(12):1861–1863

Rabinowitz SA, McKusick KA, Strauss HW. 99mTc red blood cell scintigraphy in evaluating focal liver lesions. AJR Am J Roentgenol 1984;143(1):63–68

Ziessman H. Progress and direction of gastrointestinal nuclear medicine. Eur J Nucl Med 1994;21(11): 1263–1268

Ziessman HA, Silverman PM, Patterson J, et al. Improved detection of small cavernous hemangiomas of the liver with high-resolution three-headed SPECT. J Nucl Med 1991;32(11):2086–2091

CASE 152

Clinical Presentation

A 78-year-old woman undergoes chest radiography because of a cough. A potential lung nodule is identified, and a CT scan of the thorax is obtained. Images through the upper abdomen reveal two masses adjacent to the spleen. This leads to the study summarized below (**Figs. 152.1, 152.2,** and **152.3**).

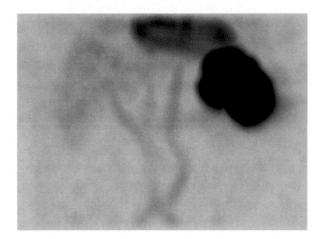

Fig. 152.1

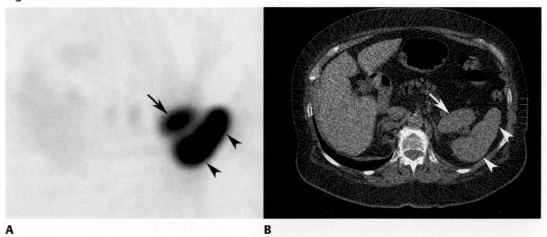

A   B

Fig. 152.2

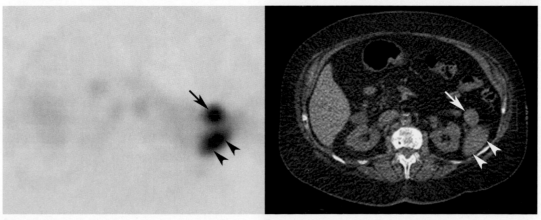

A   B

Fig. 152.3

Technique

- Heat-damaged red blood cells (RBCs) labeled with 1 to 3 mCi of technetium ^{99m}Tc
  - Autologous RBCs labeled in vitro
  - Heated at 49°C for 15 to 20 minutes
  - Cooled at room temperature for 15 minutes
- Slow intravenous injection over 1 minute
- Planar and SPECT images of the abdomen beginning 30 to 120 minutes after injection

Image Interpretation

Anterior maximum-intensity projection (MIP) view from the SPECT study (**Fig. 152.1**) reveals intense uptake in the left upper quadrant. There is mild uptake in the cardiac blood pool and faint uptake in the liver. An axial view from the SPECT study (**Fig. 152.2A**) reveals intense uptake in the spleen (arrowheads), as well as in a mass (arrow) immediately anterior to the spleen, correlating with one of the separate masses on the CT scan (**Fig. 152.2B**). Likewise, an axial image more inferiorly (**Fig. 152.3A**) demonstrates intense activity in the spleen and in the second mass (arrow) identified on the CT scan (**Fig. 152.3B**).

Differential Diagnosis

- Spleniculi

Final Diagnosis

The diagnosis was spleniculi.

Discussion

Accessory spleens (spleniculi, or splenules) are common, occurring in one-fifth to one-third of post-mortem studies. They are histologically and functionally identical to normal splenic tissue, reacting to the same stimuli. They are generally found in the gastrosplenic ligament or in the region of the tail of the pancreas, although sometimes in the omentum or mesenteries. Following splenic rupture, they may be found scattered throughout the peritoneal cavity, arising from transplants of splenic tissue. Spleniculi are clinically relevant because of their potential to be mistaken for disease on anatomic imaging, and because of their deleterious effects following splenectomy for conditions such as idiopathic thrombocytopenic purpura (ITP), thrombotic thrombocytopenic purpura (TTP), and hereditary spherocytosis.

Nuclear medicine imaging with heat-damaged (denatured) RBCs is a sensitive and specific method to assess for splenic tissue. Indications include the following:

1. Identify spleniculi after surgical splenectomy for thrombocytopenia.
2. Assess for spleniculi after trauma.
3. Assess whether a mass found on anatomic imaging is an accessory spleen.
4. Assess abnormalities of splenic number or position: asplenia, polysplenia, situs ambiguus, wandering spleen.

Splenic trauma results in a 50% incidence of splenosis, as cells from the splenic pulp seed the intraperiotoneal cavity and grow. Rarely, if the diaphragm has been violated, spleniculi may develop in the thoracic cavity. The heat-denatured RBC scan may be undertaken in the post-trauma setting to assess whether there is functioning splenic tissue or whether a mass in a patient with prior splenic trauma is simply a spleniculus.

The method involves removing a sample of the patient's blood and labeling RBCs in vitro with ^{99m}Tc-pertechnetate. The labeled RBCs are then heated at 49°C for 15 to 20 minutes. Normal RBCs are highly deformable and pass readily through the spleen. Heat-denatured RBCs, on the other hand, are stiff, having undergone fragmentation and spherocytosis. They pass slowly through the spleen and are irreversibly trapped. Thus, uptake is highly sensitive and specific for splenic tissue, although there will be some background blood pool activity and some excretion of ^{99m}Tc through the kidneys. Splenic tissue can also be identified with ^{99m}Tc-sulfur colloid, but uptake is less specific because colloid is also taken up by other components of the reticuloendothelial system—namely, liver and bone marrow.

PEARLS AND PITFALLS

- A heat-damaged RBC study is very specific for splenic tissue, more so than a ^{99m}Tc-sulfur colloid study.
- The study is useful in evaluating post-surgical or post-traumatic spleniculi, incidentally identified masses, and certain congenital anomalies.
- As with other labeled blood cell studies, procedures to prevent injection into the wrong patient must be in place and strictly adhered to.
- In vitro labeling is mandatory with heat-damaged RBC studies.

Suggested Reading

Armas RR. Clinical studies with spleen-specific radiolabeled agents. Semin Nucl Med 1985;15(3): 260–275

Kumar V, Abbas AK, Fausto N, eds. *Robbins and Cotran Pathologic Basis of Disease.* 7th ed. Philadelphia: Elsevier Saunders; 2005:702–705

Royal HD, Brown ML, Drum DE, et al. Society of Nuclear Medicine Procedure Guideline for Hepatic and Splenic Imaging 3.0, version 3.0, approved July 20, 2003. http://interactive.snm.org/docs/pg_ch10_0403.pdf. Accessed April 24, 2010

Srivastava SC, Chervu LR. Radionuclide-labeled red blood cells: current status and future prospects. Semin Nucl Med 1984;14(2):68–82

CASE 153

Clinical Presentation

A 43-year-old man presented 8 years previously with thrombocytopenia, and idiopathic thrombocytopenic purpura (ITP) was diagnosed. The disease initially responded to therapy with steroids but eventually became refractory, and the patient underwent splenectomy 5 years after diagnosis. At first, his platelet levels increased dramatically, but ultimately he relapsed, leading to the study presented below (**Figs. 153.1** and **153.2**).

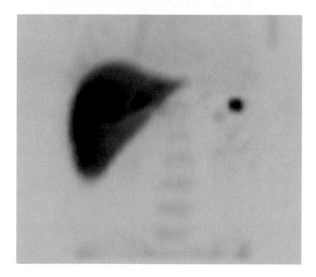

Fig. 153.1

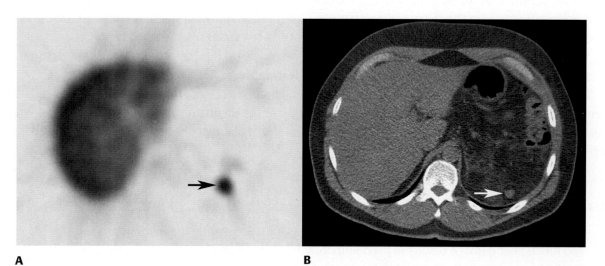

A   **B**

Fig. 153.2

Technique

- Heat-damaged red blood cells (RBCs) labeled with 1 to 3 mCi of technetium ^{99m}Tc
  - Autologous RBCs labeled in vitro
  - Heated at 49°C for 15 to 20 minutes
  - Cooled at room temperature for 15 minutes
- Planar and SPECT images of the abdomen beginning 30 to 120 minutes after injection

Image Interpretation

Anterior maximum-intensity projection (MIP) view from the SPECT study (**Fig. 153.1**) demonstrates a small focus of intense uptake of the heat-damaged RBCs in the left upper quadrant. There is normal moderate uptake in the liver. An axial slice from the SPECT study (**Fig. 153.2A**) confirms the abnormality to be in the splenic bed (arrow). A CT scan at the same level (**Fig. 153.2B**) reveals a tiny nodule in the splenic bed (arrow), correlating with the SPECT abnormality.

Differential Diagnosis

- Splenule

Final Diagnosis

The diagnosis was splenule.

Discussion

ITP is an autoimmune disorder in which thrombocytopenia arises from both decreased platelet production and increased platelet destruction in the spleen. Treatment is necessary for patients with severe and symptomatic thrombocytopenia. Therapy may include immunosuppressive agents, but splenectomy remains the most effective treatment for ITP. Following splenectomy, approximately 20% of patients may require further therapy. One option is to identify and remove any accessory residual splenic tissue not removed at the time of initial splenectomy. The heat-damaged RBC scan can be very helpful in this scenario because the sharp contrast between the intense uptake in splenic tissue and the uptake in the surrounding abdomen makes it possible to identify even small spleniculi.

The surgical removal of identified spleniculi can be aided by the intraoperative use of a gamma probe after the patient has been injected again with heat-damaged RBCs on the day of surgery.

Proper heat damaging of the RBCs is critically dependent on the temperature. A constant water bath temperature of 49 ± 0.5°C must be maintained throughout the incubation. Too little heat damage will result in little or no splenic uptake and a resultant high level of blood pool activity. Too much heat damage will result in predominantly liver uptake.

PEARLS AND PITFALLS

- It is critical to maintain a constant temperature of 49 ± 0.5°C during the heating process.
- Too much heat damage results in predominantly hepatic uptake.
- Too little uptake results in mainly blood pool activity.
- Other potential causes of a high level of blood pool activity include too little time between injection and imaging, splenic dysfunction, and poor labeling efficiency.

- During an assessment for ectopic splenic tissue, the entire abdomen and pelvis must be imaged. Furthermore, if prior trauma has possibly disrupted the diaphragm, the chest must be imaged as well.

Suggested Reading

Armas RR. Clinical studies with spleen-specific radiolabeled agents. Semin Nucl Med 1985;15(3): 260–275

George JN. Management of patients with refractory immune thrombocytopenic purpura. J Thromb Haemost 2006;4(8):1664–1672

Royal HD, Brown ML, Drum DE, et al. Society of Nuclear Medicine Procedure Guideline for Hepatic and Splenic Imaging 3.0, version 3.0, approved July 20, 2003. http://interactive.snm.org/docs/pg_ch10_0403.pdf. Accessed April 24, 2010

Srivastava SC, Chervu LR. Radionuclide-labeled red blood cells: current status and future prospects. Semin Nucl Med 1984;14(2):68–82

CASE 154

Clinical Presentation

A 5-year-old boy presents with blood in his stool, as well as abdominal pain and constipation. Results of endoscopy of the upper and lower gastrointestinal tract are normal. A Nuclear Medicine study was requested (**Figs. 154.1, 154.2,** and **154.3**).

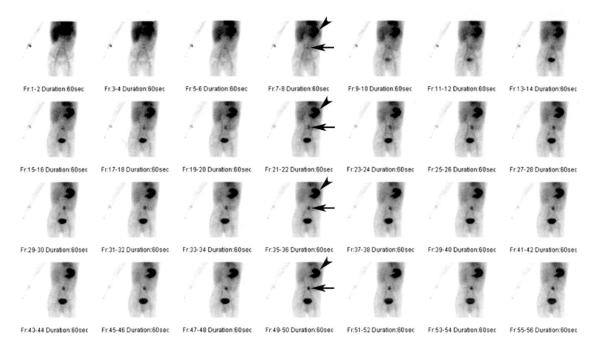

Fig. 154.1

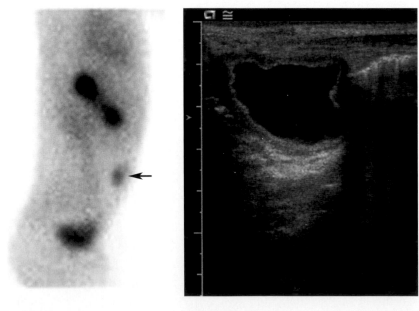

Fig. 154.2

Fig. 154.3

Technique

- ^{99m}Tc-pertechnetate
- Nothing by mouth for 4 to 12 hours.
- No barium or Gastrografin for 2 to 3 days before the study. If there is uncertainty as to whether residual oral contrast may interfere with the scan, obtain a radiograph of the abdomen.
- Pharmacologic intervention with pentagastrin, histamine H$_2$-receptor blockers, or glucagon has been advocated. These are further discussed in Case 156.
- 10 mCi
- Intravenous injection
- Low-energy, all-purpose collimator
- 140-keV photopeak, 20% window
- Dynamic imaging of the abdomen and pelvis
  - 1 frame per second for 60 seconds
  - 1 frame per minute for 30 minutes
- Post-void view

Image Interpretation

The flow images (not shown) were normal. The 1-minute images acquired over the ensuing 30 minutes (**Fig. 154.1**) demonstrate a focus of abnormal accumulation of ^{99m}Tc-pertechnetate in the lower abdomen, immediately to the left of midline (arrows). The intensity of uptake in this lesion increases over time in parallel with the normal accumulation within the stomach (arrowheads). There is normal physiologic excretion into the bladder. A single lateral view (**Fig. 154.2**) confirms the location of the abnormality just deep to the anterior abdominal wall (arrow). A subsequent ultrasound examination (**Fig. 154.3**) reveals a corresponding fluid-filled structure closely related to the umbilicus, with a "gut signature" wall (alternating hyperechoic and hypoechoic layers).

Differential Diagnosis

- Meckel diverticulum
- Enteric duplication or duplication cyst
- Vesicoureteral reflux
- Regional enteritis
- Vascular mass

Diagnosis and Clinical Follow-Up

Meckel diverticulum. The lesion was surgically removed and found to be a Meckel diverticulum measuring 4 × 3 × 3 cm and containing extensive gastric mucosa and a focal area of ulceration.

Discussion

Meckel diverticulum is a congenital anomaly arising from incomplete involution of the omphalomesenteric (vitelline) duct, a tubular structure connecting the fetal intestine at the future site of the ileum to the embryonic yolk sac. It is the most common congenital anomaly of the small intestine, occurring in 2% of the population. Meckel diverticula occur on the antimesenteric side of the bowel and contain all three layers of intestine. Most symptoms are caused by ectopic mucosa within the Meckel diverticulum, most commonly gastric mucosa but occasionally pancreatic, duodenal, or colonic mucosa. Such ectopic mucosa has been reported in 95% of Meckel diverticula resected because of gastrointestinal bleeding and in 30 to 65% of asymptomatic patients. Between 4 and 35% of Meckel diverticula become symptomatic, 50% of these before the age of 2 years. The most common complications are gastrointestinal bleeding and abdominal pain, which develop when hydrochloric acid and pepsin ulcerate adjacent mucosa. The bleeding tends to be painless, in distinction to the bleeding in pediatric patients resulting from intussusception. Meckel diverticula usually occur within 40 to 100 cm of the ileocecal valve and vary in length from 1 to 12 cm.

The premise of the Nuclear Medicine Meckel scan is that ^{99m}Tc-pertechnetate is avidly taken up in the mucous cells of gastric mucosa, both in the stomach and in ectopic locations. Thus, in the normal scan, visualization of the stomach increases in intensity over the first 10 to 20 minutes. Later in the study, some of this activity may leave the stomach and travel distally in the bowel, a potentially false-positive finding. Urinary activity is seen in the bladder and increases throughout the study. A positive Meckel scan is characterized by a small, focal accumulation of ^{99m}Tc-pertechnetate that occurs at approximately the same time as the stomach activity and increases in intensity in parallel with the stomach activity. Rarely, the activity may decrease later in the study because of downstream washout. The activity should remain in the same position relative to the bowel, whereas any physiologic ^{99m}Tc-pertechnetate in the bowel will move with peristalsis. On the other hand, activity in a Meckel diverticulum may move along with other mesenteric structures if the patient moves, unlike retroperitoneal renal activity.

As the uptake of ^{99m}Tc-pertechnetate is predicated on the presence of gastric mucosa, not all Meckel diverticula will be identified. However, the vast majority of symptomatic cases present with bleeding or ulcerative pain due to the presence of gastric mucosa, so the test is very useful in symptomatic patients, with a sensitivity of 85% and a specificity of 95%.

PEARLS AND PITFALLS

- Symptoms will develop in 4 to 35% of patients with a Meckel diverticulum at some point in their life, most commonly gastrointestinal bleeding or abdominal pain.
- Ectopic gastrointestinal mucosa, usually gastric, is contained in 30 to 65% of Meckel diverticula.
- The preoperative diagnosis of a Meckel diverticulum can be challenging. The ^{99m}Tc-pertechnetate scan is the most accurate method to identify a Meckel diverticulum preoperatively.
- The premise of the Meckel scan is the identification of ectopic gastric mucosa with ^{99m}Tc-pertechnetate.
- Although the Meckel scan will thus identify only those Meckel diverticula that contain ectopic gastric mucosa, the vast majority of symptoms are caused by ectopic gastric mucosa.
- A positive Meckel scan is characterized by a small, focal accumulation of ^{99m}Tc-pertechnetate that occurs at approximately the same time as the stomach activity and increases in intensity in parallel with the stomach activity.
- When both a Meckel scan and a labeled red blood cell (RBC) scan are planned for the assessment of gastrointestinal bleeding, the Meckel scan should be performed first because the stannous pyrophosphate used in RBC labeling may reduce the uptake of ^{99m}Tc-pertechnetate in gastric mucosa for several weeks.

Suggested Reading

Emamian SA, Shalaby-Rana E, Majd M. The spectrum of heterotopic gastric mucosa in children detected by Tc-99m pertechnetate scintigraphy. Clin Nucl Med 2001;26(6):529–535

Ford PV, Bartold SP, Fink-Bennett DM, et al.; Society of Nuclear Medicine. Procedure guideline for gastrointestinal bleeding and Meckel's diverticulum scintigraphy. J Nucl Med 1999;40(7):1226–1232

Gosche JR, Vick L, Boulanger SC, Islam S. Midgut abnormalities. Surg Clin North Am 2006;86(2):285–299, viii

Howarth DM. The role of nuclear medicine in the detection of acute gastrointestinal bleeding. Semin Nucl Med 2006;36(2):133–146

Levy AD, Hobbs CM. From the archives of the AFIP. Meckel diverticulum: radiologic features with pathologic correlation. Radiographics 2004;24(2):565–587

McCollough M, Sharieff GQ. Abdominal pain in children. Pediatr Clin North Am 2006;53(1):107–137, vi

Wilton G, Froelich JW. The "false-negative" Meckel's scan. Clin Nucl Med 1982;7(10):441–443

Yahchouchy EK, Marano AF, Etienne JC, Fingerhut AL. Meckel's diverticulum. J Am Coll Surg 2001;192(5):658–662

CASE 155

Clinical Presentation

A 7-year-old boy presents with two episodes of blood in his stool. A Nuclear Medicine study was requested (**Figs. 155.1** and **155.2**).

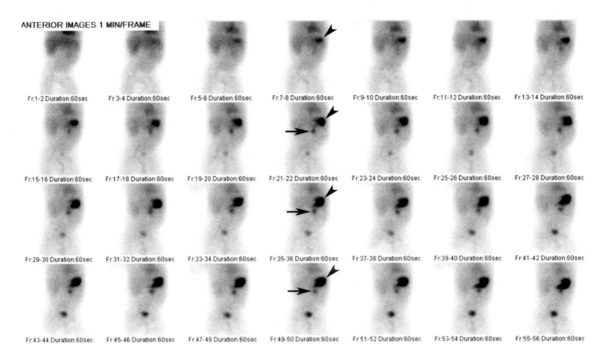

ANTERIOR IMAGES 1 MIN/FRAME

Fr:1-2 Duration:60sec Fr:3-4 Duration:60sec Fr:5-6 Duration:60sec Fr:7-8 Duration:60sec Fr:9-10 Duration:60sec Fr:11-12 Duration:60sec Fr:13-14 Duration:60sec

Fr:15-16 Duration:60sec Fr:17-18 Duration:60sec Fr:19-20 Duration:60sec Fr:21-22 Duration:60sec Fr:23-24 Duration:60sec Fr:25-26 Duration:60sec Fr:27-28 Duration:60sec

Fr:29-30 Duration:60sec Fr:31-32 Duration:60sec Fr:33-34 Duration:60sec Fr:35-36 Duration:60sec Fr:37-38 Duration:60sec Fr:39-40 Duration:60sec Fr:41-42 Duration:60sec

Fr:43-44 Duration:60sec Fr:45-46 Duration:60sec Fr:47-48 Duration:60sec Fr:49-50 Duration:60sec Fr:51-52 Duration:60sec Fr:53-54 Duration:60sec Fr:55-56 Duration:60sec

Fig. 155.1

Technique

- ^{99m}Tc-pertechnetate
- Nothing by mouth for 4 to 12 hours.
- No barium or Gastrografin for 2 to 3 days before the study. If there is uncertainty as to whether residual oral contrast may interfere with the scan, obtain a radiograph of the abdomen.
- Pharmacologic intervention with pentagastrin, histamine H_2-receptor blockers, or glucagon has been advocated (see below).
- 10 mCi
- Intravenous injection
- Low energy, all purpose collimator
- 140-keV photopeak, 20% window
- Dynamic imaging of the abdomen and pelvis
  - 1 frame per second for 60 seconds
  - 1 frame per minute for 30 minutes
- Post-void view, as a Meckel diverticulum may be located adjacent to the bladder

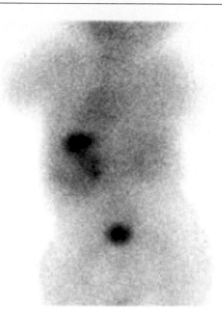

Fig. 155.2

Image Interpretation

The flow study (not shown) was normal. The ensuing 30-minute study (**Fig. 155.1**) demonstrates normal accumulation within the stomach (arrowheads) and excretion into the bladder. There is also accumulation throughout the study within a structure in the upper abdomen to the left of midline (arrows). A posterior image (**Fig. 155.2**) reveals this activity to be within the left renal collecting system.

Differential Diagnosis

- Meckel diverticulum
- Enteric duplication or duplication cyst
- Hydronephrosis
- Regional enteritis
- Vascular mass

Diagnosis and Clinical Follow-Up

Hydronephrosis. No Meckel diverticulum. The accumulation of ^{99m}Tc-pertechnetate in the upper abdomen was within the renal collecting system.

Discussion

In a normal Meckel scan, visualization of the stomach increases in intensity over the first 10 to 20 minutes. Later in the study, some of this activity may leave the stomach and travel distally in the bowel, potentially causing a false-positive study. Renal activity is seen early and is another possible cause of a false-positive study. Urinary activity is seen in the bladder, increasing throughout the study, and occasionally focal urinary activity is seen in a ureter as it passes over the pelvic brim. Other potential causes of false-positive scans include entities other than gastric mucosa, such as Barrett esophagus and enteric duplication cysts, and abnormalities associated with hyperemia, such as appendicitis, regional enteritis, and vascular masses. A positive Meckel scan is characterized by a small, focal accumulation of ^{99m}Tc-pertechnetate occurring at approximately the same time as the stomach activity and increasing in intensity in parallel with the stomach activity. Rarely, the activity may decrease later in the study because of downstream washout. The activity should remain in the same position relative to the bowel, whereas any physiologic ^{99m}Tc-pertechnetate in the bowel will move with peristalsis. On the other hand, activity in a Meckel diverticulum may move along with other mesenteric structures if the patient moves, unlike retroperitoneal urinary activity.

A variety of pharmacologic interventions have been advocated to further increase the sensitivity of the scan, although the benefits have not been universally accepted:

- Pentagastrin
  - A dose of 6 μg/kg is administered subcutaneously 15 to 20 minutes before imaging.
  - Pentagastrin increases the uptake of ^{99m}Tc-pertechnetate in the mucous cells.
- Cimetedine or ranitidine
  - Cimetidine: a dose of 300 mg is given orally four times daily for 2 days before the scan.
  - Ranitidine: a dose of 1 mg/kg (maximum of 50 mg) is infused intravenously over 20 minutes 1 hour before the scan.
  - These agents block the washout of ^{99m}Tc-pertechnetate from gastric glands in the stomach and ectopic tissue.
- Glucagon
  - A dose of 50 μg/kg is administered intravenously 10 minutes after the ^{99m}Tc-pertechnetate injection.
  - Glucagon promotes the retention of activity at the Meckel diverticulum by reducing downstream transit.

PEARLS AND PITFALLS

- Causes of false-positive Meckel scans include the following:
  - Other entities containing gastric mucosa
    - Enteric duplication or duplication cyst
    - Barrett esophagus
    - Occasionally an area of small intestine without any morphologic abnormality
  - Urinary activity, particularly with associated abnormalities
    - Hydronephrosis
    - Ectopic or horseshoe kidney
    - Vesico-ureteral reflux
    - Bladder diverticulum
  - Abnormalities causing hyperemia of the bowel
    - Appendicitis
    - Regional enteritis
  - Vascular masses
- Causes of false-negative Meckel scans include the following:
  - Meckel diverticulum containing no gastric mucosa or only a small amount
  - Small size of diverticulum
  - Obscuration by other structures containing ^{99m}Tc-pertechnetate
  - Downstream transit of ^{99m}Tc-pertechnetate from the Meckel diverticulum
- The sensitivity of the Meckel scan can be increased through the use of pharmacologic interventions, including the following:
  - Cimetidine or ranitidine
  - Pentagastrin
  - Glucagon

Suggested Reading

Emamian SA, Shalaby-Rana E, Majd M. The spectrum of heterotopic gastric mucosa in children detected by Tc-99m pertechnetate scintigraphy. Clin Nucl Med 2001;26(6):529–535

Ford PV, Bartold SP, Fink-Bennett DM, et al. Society of Nuclear Medicine. Procedure guideline for gastrointestinal bleeding and Meckel's diverticulum scintigraphy. J Nucl Med 1999;40(7):1226–1232

Gosche JR, Vick L, Boulanger SC, Islam S. Midgut abnormalities. Surg Clin North Am 2006;86(2): 285–299, viii

Howarth DM. The role of nuclear medicine in the detection of acute gastrointestinal bleeding. Semin Nucl Med 2006;36(2):133–146

Levy AD, Hobbs CM. From the archives of the AFIP. Meckel diverticulum: radiologic features with pathologic correlation. Radiographics 2004;24(2):565–587

McCollough M, Sharieff GQ. Abdominal pain in children. Pediatr Clin North Am 2006;53(1):107–137, vi

Wilton G, Froelich JW. The "false-negative" Meckel's scan. Clin Nucl Med 1982;7(10):441–443

Yahchouchy EK, Marano AF, Etienne JC, Fingerhut AL. Meckel's diverticulum. J Am Coll Surg 2001; 192(5):658–662

CASE 156

Clinical Presentation

A 68-year-old woman presents with breast cancer and an indwelling left-sided central line (single-lumen Port-A-Cath; Smiths Medical, Dublin, OH). Blood return from the central line is poor. The study is performed to rule out obstruction or thrombus (**Figs. 156.1, 156.2,** and **156.3**).

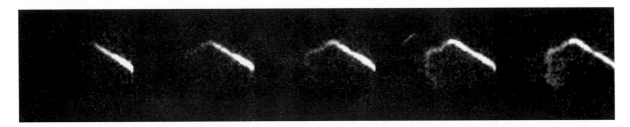

Fig. 156.1

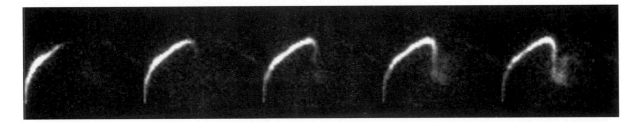

Fig. 156.2

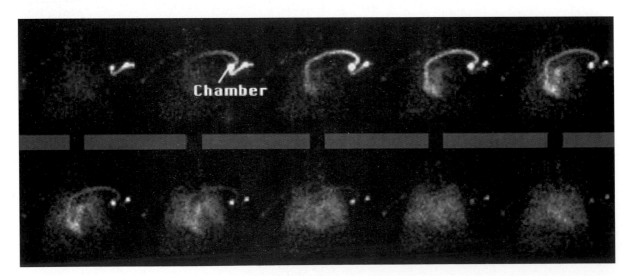

Fig. 156.3

Technique

- To block thyroid uptake, potassium perchlorate (400 mg) is administered by mouth 15 minutes before ^{99m}Tc-pertechnetate.
- Indwelling catheters with subcutaneous chambers (such as those of the Port-A-Cath) need to be accessed with sterile technique.
- With the patient lying supine, butterfly needles are attached to a three-way stopcock connected to the accessed central line ports and also placed into a vein in each upper extremity.
- Connected to the stopcocks are 1-mL syringes containing approximately 5 mCi of ^{99m}Tc-pertechnetate in a volume of 0.1 to 0.3 mL and 10-mL syringes containing 10 mL of normal saline.
- Gamma camera with a large field of view
- Low-energy, parallel-hole, high-resolution collimator
- Energy window 20% centered at 140 keV
- The camera is positioned over the anterior chest and shoulders with the heart in the center of the field of view.
- The tracer is administered as a bolus injection, followed by the infusion of 10-mL flushes of normal saline in rapid sequence: first into the upper extremity ipsilateral to the central line, then the contralateral arm, and finally the central line.
- Digital dynamic images are obtained in a 64 × 64 matrix at 1 frame per second for 120 seconds. At the completion of the study, the central line is flushed with 5 mL of heparin lock flush solution.
- Data are reviewed in a cine format as well as 1 second per frame digital images.

Image Interpretation

The injection into the left arm (**Fig. 156.1**) shows normal transit of tracer through the left axillary, subclavian, and brachiocephalic veins into the superior vena cava and cardiac chambers.

The flow study obtained following injection of the tracer into the right upper extremity (**Fig. 156.2**) demonstrates normal flow of tracer through the right axillary, subclavian, and brachiocephalic veins into the superior vena cava and cardiac chambers.

The injection through the port of the left-sided central line (**Fig. 156.3**) shows activity flowing from the subcutaneous chamber through the central line into the superior vena cava and right cardiac chambers, followed by activity into the lungs and return to the left side of the heart.

Diagnosis and Clinical Follow-Up

The diagnosis was normal venous flow in the upper extremity and normal flow through the central line. The central line and venous system of the upper extremity were patent.

Discussion

Radionuclide venography provides a quick answer to any clinical question regarding the patency of a vessel and that of the central line within it. It is faster than conventional venography, is less expensive, and results in less exposure to radiation and lower procedural risks (eg, reaction to iodinated contrast).

It is important to keep in mind the normal, relatively oblique route of the left brachiocephalic vein compared with the more vertical route of the right subclavian vein. Activity seen transiting from the left subclavian vein in a horizontal fashion to the right side of the neck, followed by filling of right-sided vessels, may be due to total obstruction of the left brachiocephalic vein and transit to the right-sided vessels via collaterals such as the jugular arch.

Note that after injection of the left-sided central line, the activity clears from the chamber, the line, and the vessels. The focus to the left of the chamber represents residual activity within tubing that lies on the patient's chest.

PEARLS AND PITFALLS

- If the patient is scheduled for another nuclear medicine study, the radiopharmaceutical for that study may be used for the flow study instead of ^{99m}Tc-pertechnetate. Also, because of the short acquisition time and high count rate, these studies can be performed even if the patient has recently undergone another nuclear medicine study.
- It is important to inject not only the line but also the ipsilateral arm vein. The arm injection will allow the detection of thrombus around the line that may be occluding the vessel lumen while the central line remains patent. If injections of the line and ipsilateral arm vein fail to demonstrate the superior vena cava, the contralateral arm vein should be injected to confirm patency of the superior vena cava.
- Note the relatively oblique route of the left brachiocephalic vein compared with the more vertical route of the right brachiocephalic vein.
- If activity does not clear from the chamber or increases over time, infiltration into the chest wall should be considered. This is why the injection into the line should always be the last one; residual activity in the chest wall will prevent the visualization of venous structures, given the short acquisition time.
- If the patient experiences pain during the injection, the tracer may have infiltrated the chest wall, or the tip of the catheter may have moved out of the superior vena cava (eg, cephalad into the jugular vein, which may result in pain or an unusual sensation in the neck upon injection).
- If there is significant resistance to an injection, the injection should be stopped. A forced injection into an obstructed system may result in disconnection of the syringe, with the risk for contamination. It may also cause dislodgment of a downstream thrombus, resulting in pulmonary embolism or even rupture of the line.
- Radionuclide venography should not be performed to differentiate extrinsic from intrinsic obstruction. Morphologic modalities such as CT and MRI should be used for that purpose.

Suggested Reading

Chasen MH, Charnsangavej C. Venous chest anatomy: clinical implications. Categorical course in chest radiology. Oak Brook, IL: Radiological Society of North America; 1992:121–134

Horattas MC, Wright DJ, Fenton AH, et al. Changing concepts of deep venous thrombosis of the upper extremity—report of a series and review of the literature. Surgery 1988;104(3):561–567

Maxfield WS, Meckstroth GR. Technetium-99m superior vena cavography. Radiology 1969;92(4):913–917

Miyamae T. Interpretation of 99m Tc superior vena cavograms and results of studies in 92 patients. Radiology 1973;108(2):339–352

Muramatsu T, Miyamae T, Dohi Y. Collateral pathways observed by radionuclide superior cavography in 70 patients with superior vena caval obstruction. Clin Nucl Med 1991;16(5):332–336

Savolaine ER, Schlembach PJ. Scintigraphy compared to other imaging modalities in benign superior vena caval obstruction accompanying fibrosing mediastinitis. Clin Imaging 1989;13(3):234–238

CASE 157

Clinical Presentation

A 44-year-old patient with colon cancer has been receiving chemotherapy through an indwelling central line. There is no problem with injecting, but there is difficulty in withdrawing blood from the central line. A flow study is requested to assess the patency of the central line (**Fig. 157.1**).

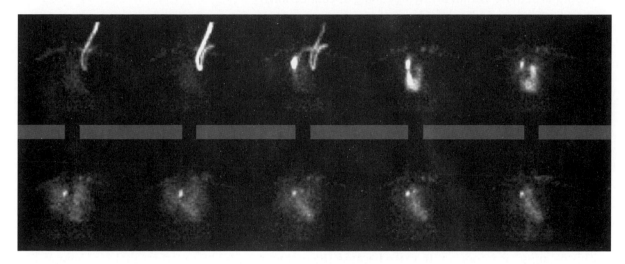

Fig. 157.1

Technique

- To block thyroid uptake, potassium perchlorate (400 mg) is administered by mouth 15 minutes before ^{99m}Tc-pertechnetate.
- Indwelling catheters with subcutaneous chambers (such as those of the Port-A-Cath) need to be accessed with sterile technique.
- With the patient lying supine, butterfly needles attached to a three-way stopcock are connected to the accessed central line ports and also placed into a vein in each upper extremity.
- Connected to the stopcocks are 1-mL syringes containing approximately 5 mCi of ^{99m}Tc-pertechnetate in a volume of 0.1 to 0.3 mL and 10-mL syringes containing 10 mL of normal saline.
- Gamma camera with a large field of view
- Low-energy, parallel-hole, high-resolution collimator
- Energy window 20% centered at 140 keV
- The camera is positioned over the anterior chest and shoulders with the heart in the center of the field of view.
- The tracer is administered as a bolus injection, followed by the infusion of 10-mL flushes of normal saline in rapid sequence: first into the upper extremity ipsilateral to the central line, then the contralateral arm, and finally the central line.
- Digital dynamic images are obtained in a 64 × 64 matrix at 1 frame per second for 120 seconds. At the completion of the study, the central line is flushed with 5 mL of heparin lock flush solution.
- Data are reviewed in a cine format as well as 1 second per frame digital images.

Image Interpretation

Serial dynamic images **(Fig. 157.1)** demonstrate normal transit of the tracer through the central line into the superior vena cava and cardiac chambers. Following the clearance of activity from the vessels and the cardiac chambers, there is persistent tracer uptake in the region of the tip of the line despite continuous flushing. The venous blood flow through both upper extremities was normal (images not shown).

Differential Diagnosis

- Retention at the tip of the catheter lumen
- Residual activity within overlying tubing or connections
- Residual activity in the vessel
- Residual activity within a collateral vessel

Diagnosis and Clinical Follow-Up

The findings are suggestive of a "fibrin sheath" deposit at the tip of the catheter. The patient received urokinase, and blood return improved following urokinase therapy.

Discussion

Fibrin deposits are found around almost all indwelling catheters after 1 week. When the fibrin sheath extends over the tip of the line, it may cause difficulties in withdrawing blood because it can be pulled against or into the tip of the catheter during the drawing process. Injecting into the lines is less of a problem because the fibrin deposits form a loose mesh through which fluid can flow.

This diagnosis is important to make because the patient requires "local" thrombolytic therapy, like urokinase, rather than systemic anticoagulant therapy with heparin.

PEARLS AND PITFALLS_____

- Avoid placing connective tubing over the regions-of-interest so as not to confuse retention at the tip of the catheter with residual activity in connecting lines or hubs lying on the chest surface.
- The diagnosis should be made after thorough flushing of the line and clearance of activity from the vessels and right cardiac chambers. It is normal to see a blush of activity at the tip of the line as the tracer exits the line and enters the vessel. In normal circumstances, this blush of activity clears after continuous flushing of the line with normal saline.
- Fibrin sheaths may be considered a risk factor for thrombus formation, and the treatment of fibrin sheaths that do not significantly obstruct the line tip remains controversial. However, not being able to draw blood from a central line may be a serious inconvenience to patients, who then require peripheral venous punctures. Diagnosing this problem and then administering local thrombolytic therapy with urokinase may improve the functionality of the lines, on which patients depend.

Suggested Reading

Chasen MH, Charnsangavej C. Venous chest anatomy: clinical implications. Categorical course in chest radiology. Oak Brook, IL: Radiological Society of North America; 1992:121–134

Horattas MC, Wright DJ, Fenton AH, et al. Changing concepts of deep venous thrombosis of the upper extremity—report of a series and review of the literature. Surgery 1988;104(3):561–567

Maxfield WS, Meckstroth GR. Technetium-99m superior vena cavography. Radiology 1969;92(4): 913–917

Miyamae T. Interpretation of 99m Tc superior vena cavograms and results of studies in 92 patients. Radiology 1973;108(2):339–352

Muramatsu T, Miyamae T, Dohi Y. Collateral pathways observed by radionuclide superior cavography in 70 patients with superior vena caval obstruction. Clin Nucl Med 1991;16(5):332–336

Savolaine ER, Schlembach PJ. Scintigraphy compared to other imaging modalities in benign superior vena caval obstruction accompanying fibrosing mediastinitis. Clin Imaging 1989;13(3):234–238

CASE 158

Clinical Presentation

A 44-year-old woman with breast cancer who has been receiving chemotherapy through an indwelling right-sided central line has recently had swelling of the right upper extremity (**Figs. 158.1, 158.2,** and **158.3**).

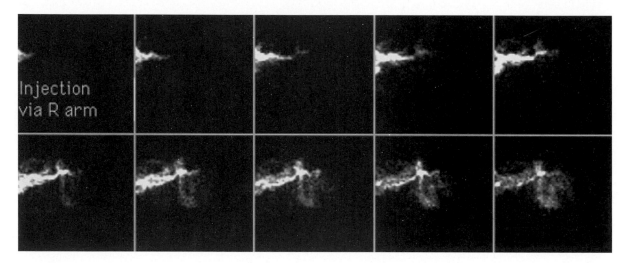

Fig. 158.1

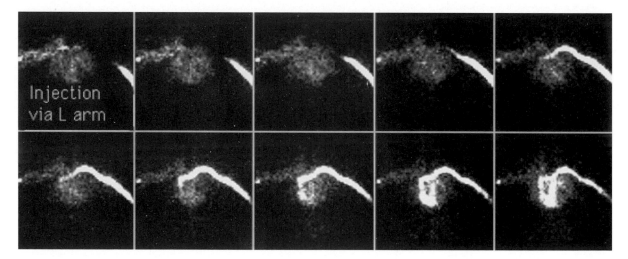

Fig. 158.2

Technique

- To block thyroid uptake, potassium perchlorate (400 mg) is administered by mouth 15 minutes before technetium ^{99m}Tc-pertechnetate.
- Indwelling catheters with subcutaneous chambers (such as those of the Port-A-Cath) need to be accessed with sterile technique.

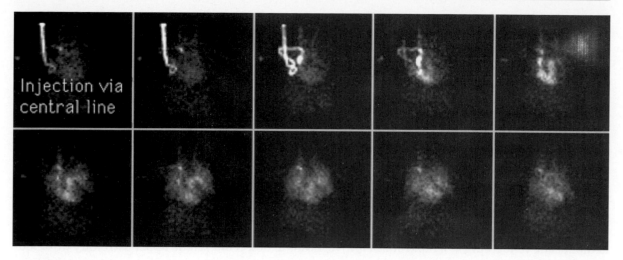

Fig. 158.3

- With the patient lying supine, butterfly needles attached to a three-way stopcock are connected to the accessed central line ports and also placed into a vein in each upper extremity.
- Connected to the stopcocks are 1-mL syringes containing approximately 5 mCi of ^{99m}Tc-pertechnetate in a volume of 0.1 to 0.3 mL and 10-mL syringes containing 10 mL of normal saline.
- Gamma camera with a large field of view
- Low-energy, parallel-hole, high-resolution collimator
- Energy window 20% centered at 140 keV
- The camera is positioned over the anterior chest and shoulders with the heart in the center of the field of view.
- The tracer is administered as a bolus injection followed by the infusion of 10-mL flushes of normal saline in rapid sequence: first into the upper extremity ipsilateral to the central line, then the contralateral arm, and finally the central line.
- Digital dynamic images are obtained in a 64 × 64 matrix at 1 frame per second for 120 seconds. At the completion of the study, the central line is flushed with 5 mL of heparin lock flush solution.
- Data are reviewed in a cine format as well as 1 second per frame digital images.

Image Interpretation

Injection into the right upper extremity (**Fig. 158.1**) demonstrates filling of collateral vessels extending from the level of the right axillary vein along the right brachiocephalic vein up to the right jugular vein. The right brachiocephalic vein and superior vena cava are not visualized. The activity progresses across the neck into another collateral (the jugular arch), and the cardiac chambers are filling via the collaterals.

Injection into the left arm (**Fig. 158.2**) shows normal progression of tracer through the left axillary, subclavian, and brachiocephalic veins into the superior vena cava, confirming patency of the superior vena cava.

The last injection, into the central line (**Fig. 158.3**), shows normal progression of tracer through the line, superior vena cava, and cardiac chambers.

Differential Diagnosis

- Intrinsic causes: thrombi, emboli, tumors, webs, foreign bodies
- Extrinsic causes: impression from masses or musculoskeletal structures; cicatrizing processes (eg, mediastinal fibrosis)

Diagnosis and Clinical Follow-Up

The findings are consistent with a high-grade obstruction of the right subclavian vein, possibly extending into the right axilla. Based on the clinical and scintigraphic findings, a thrombus of the upper extremity was diagnosed, and the patient was placed on heparin.

Discussion

Radionuclide venography is a rapid and sensitive means to detect or exclude upper extremity thrombosis. It is also a useful means to assess the patency of central lines and an early way to detect the formation of fibrin mesh at the tip of an indwelling line.

At our institution, the majority of patients who undergo this test have indwelling central lines and frequently an underlying malignancy. These factors predispose to thrombus formation.

The study in this patient demonstrated that a patent central line does not exclude venous thrombus. Second, the contralateral arm injection was helpful in defining patency of the superior vena cava when a high-grade obstruction in the ipsilateral venous system prevented definite visualization of the superior vena cava via the right upper extremity injection because of collateral formation.

Although this patient's central line was patent, the vein in which it lay was totally obstructed, based on the significant collateral formation demonstrated by the ipsilateral arm injection. The right subclavian and brachiocephalic veins, as well as the superior vena cava, could not be explicitly assessed in this study because tracer was shunted to collateral vessels around the venous obstruction. The right brachiocephalic vein and the superior vena cava could be involved with thrombus, or they could conceivably be patent. From the left-sided injection, we knew that the superior vena cava in this patient was patent.

PEARLS AND PITFALLS

- Radionuclide venography may be performed in conjunction with other nuclear medicine studies.
- Careful attention should always be paid to the region at the tip of a central line. A persistent focus of tracer activity at this location suggests the presence of a fibrin mesh at the line tip. This can be the cause of a central line that flushes well but from which it is difficult to withdraw blood.
- Both upper extremities should always be imaged. If an abnormality is detected on one side, the contralateral study provides an assessment of the superior vena cava.
- The central line should be injected last, after the arm veins. This is done in case extravasation from the line into the soft tissues of the thorax obscures subsequent imaging.
- A patent central line does not exclude thrombus. Thrombus may form concentrically around a catheter without obstructing the lumen. The ipsilateral injection is essential to evaluate the patency of a central line.
- Radionuclide venography is not an effective means by which to distinguish intrinsic from extrinsic causes of venous stenosis or obstruction. If there is reason to suspect a cause of obstruction other than thrombus, anatomic imaging, such as CT of the chest, may be useful.

Suggested Reading

Fielding JR, Nagel JS, Pomeroy O. Upper extremity DVT. Correlation of MR and nuclear medicine flow imaging. Clin Imaging 1997;21(4):260–263

Kida T. Demonstration of collateral pathways in superior vena cava syndrome by means of radionuclide venography. Clin Nucl Med 1985;10(3):195–196

Podoloff DA, Kim EE. Evaluation of sensitivity and specificity of upper extremity radionuclide venography in cancer patients with indwelling central venous catheters. Clin Nucl Med 1992;17(6):457–462

Van Houtte P, Frühling J. Radionuclide venography in the evaluation of superior vena cava syndrome. Clin Nucl Med 1981;6(4):177–183

Section XIV

Pediatric Scintigraphy

Laura A. Drubach, Leonard P. Connolly, and S. Ted Treves

CASE 159

Clinical Presentation

A 7-year-old girl presents with a 2-day history of abdominal pain, dysuria, and fever of 102° to 103°F. Physical examination shows right costovertebral angle tenderness. Initial laboratory evaluation includes a complete blood cell count (white blood cells, 13,200/mm³), urinalysis (white blood cells, 20–40 per high-power field; red blood cells, 10–20 per high-power field), blood culture, and urine culture. A ^{99m}Tc-DMSA study and a radionuclide cystography are requested for the evaluation of renal involvement and for the detection of vesicoureteral reflux. The patient was started on intravenous antibiotics for suspected pyelonephritis.

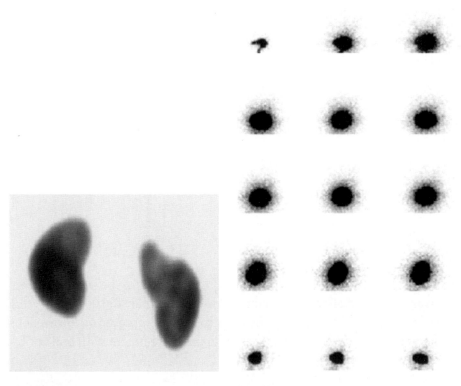

Fig. 159.1   **Fig. 159.2**

Technique

^{99m}Tc-DMSA Study

- ^{99m}Tc-DMSA (0.5 mCi/kg) is given intravenously; the minimum dose is 0.2 mCi and the maximum dose is 3.0 mCi.
- Use a high-resolution or ultra-high-resolution, low-energy, parallel-hole collimator for SPECT acquisition; perform planar imaging with a pinhole collimator for young infants.
- Energy window is 20% centered at 140 keV.
- Imaging is done 4 hours after radiotracer injection. SPECT acquisition is performed with 40 stops per detector or 120 stops with a three-detector imaging system.

Radionuclide Cystography

- ^{99m}Tc-pertechnetate (2 mCi) is given. The patient is asked to urinate before the examination. A catheter is placed into the bladder under sterile technique. A 500-mL bag of saline is connected to the catheter. The radiotracer is injected as a bolus into the catheter. The bladder is filled with saline at a pressure of 70 to 90 cm H_2O.
- A high-resolution, low-energy, parallel-hole collimator is used.
- Energy window is 20% centered at 140 keV.
- Dynamic images are acquired of the filling and voiding. Once the voiding is complete, the computer recording is terminated and the catheter is removed.

Image Interpretation

A reprojected image of the kidneys (**Fig. 159.1**) shows a cortical defect in the upper pole of the right kidney. The left kidney is normal. The differential cortical uptake is 52% for the left kidney and 48% for the right kidney.

A radionuclide cystogram (**Fig. 159.2**) shows no evidence of vesicoureteral reflux.

A normal ^{99m}Tc-DMSA scan (**Fig. 159.3**) from a different patient is shown for comparison. There is symmetric uptake by the two kidneys. The contour of both kidneys is smooth, with no cortical defect. There is relatively lower tracer uptake in the medulla and collecting systems than in the renal cortex. The differential cortical uptake is 50% for each kidney.

Differential Diagnosis

- Pyelonephritis
- Scarring
- Renal infarction
- Renal trauma
- Vesicoureteral reflux

Diagnosis and Clinical Follow-Up

Urinary tract infection (UTI) was confirmed after a urine culture grew more than 100,000 *Escherichia coli* organisms. The patient was treated for acute pyelonephritis, her condition improved on intravenous antibiotics, and she was discharged after 6 days of hospitalization to finish treatment with oral antibiotics as an outpatient.

Discussion

In the pre-antibiotic era, UTI was a serious disease with significant mortality, but antibiotic therapy and aggressive diagnostic approaches have reduced the mortality to zero. Even in the modern era, however, UTI still carries the potential for long-term consequences. Of children entering dialysis, 10 to 20% have a history of UTI or reflux, or both.

There are several approaches to the diagnostic imaging evaluation of UTI. It is now universally accepted that all children presenting with an initial episode of UTI should be evaluated for predisposing factors. The risk factors for the development of scarring related to UTI include: (1) obstruction, (2) reflux, (3) young age, (4) delay in treatment, (5) high number of pyelonephritic attacks, and (6) unusual causative bacteria. Imaging with ^{99m}Tc-DMSA is superior to sonography and to intravenous pyelography for the detection of both acute pyelonephritis and scarring. The number of defects detected by ^{99m}Tc-DMSA scintigraphy in patients with repeated episodes of pyelonephritis may increase over time as scarring replaces the renal parenchyma. Abnormalities noted on ^{99m}Tc-DMSA scintigraphy usually manifest one of two recognizable patterns of uptake: (1) generalized decreased uptake, or (2) focally decreased uptake with or without loss of volume. It has been reported that ^{99m}Tc-DMSA imaging has a sensitivity of 96% and a specificity of 98% for the detection of changes induced by pyelonephritis.

Vesicoureteral reflux is the most significant host risk factor for the development of UTI and renal scarring, but renal scarring can occur in the absence of demonstrable vesico-ureteral reflux in a large percentage of children. Radionuclide cystography is indicated in children in whom UTI is diagnosed for the evaluation of genitourinary reflux. Three degrees of reflux can be recognized with radionuclide cystography. Grade 1 (**Fig. 159.4A**) corresponds to reflux into the ureter; grade 2 (**Fig. 159.4B**) corresponds to reflux into the ureter reaching the renal pelvis, which does not appear dilated; grade 3 (**Fig. 159.4C**) corresponds to reflux reaching a dilated renal pelvis, with or without a dilated, tortuous ureter.

There is a correlation between the grade of reflux and the severity of scarring detected by ^{99m}Tc-DMSA imaging. Higher grades of reflux lead to more severe abnormalities on ^{99m}Tc-DMSA scintigraphy.

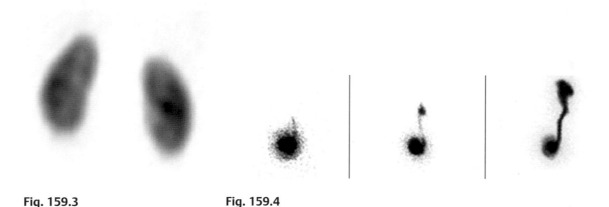

Fig. 159.3   **Fig. 159.4**

Suggested Reading

Björgvinsson E, Majd M, Eggli KD. Diagnosis of acute pyelonephritis in children: comparison of sonography and 99mTc-DMSA scintigraphy. AJR Am J Roentgenol 1991;157(3):539–543

Conway JJ. The role of scintigraphy in urinary tract infection. Semin Nucl Med 1988;18(4):308–319

Kass EJ, Fink-Bennett D, Cacciarelli AA, Balon H, Pavlock S. The sensitivity of renal scintigraphy and sonography in detecting nonobstructive acute pyelonephritis. J Urol 1992;148(2 Pt 2):606–608

Sty JR, Wells RG, Schroeder BA, Starshak RJ. Diagnostic imaging in pediatric renal inflammatory disease. JAMA 1986;256(7):895–899

Treves ST, Majd M, Kuruc A, Packard AB, Harmon W. Kidneys. In: Treves ST, ed. *Pediatric Nuclear Medicine*. 2nd ed. New York: Springer-Verlag; 1995:339–399

Treves ST, Gelfand M, Willi UV. Vesicoureteric reflux and radionuclide cystography. In: Treves ST, ed. *Pediatric Nuclear Medicine*. 2nd ed. New York: Springer-Verlag; 1995:411–429

CASE 160

Clinical Presentation

A 15-month-old child presents with the passage of bright red blood per rectum for 1 day and no abdominal pain or vomiting. Physical examination shows a pale infant with otherwise normal examination findings. Laboratory evaluation shows a hemoglobin level of 8 mg/dL. A bleeding Meckel diverticulum is considered as a possible diagnosis, and a Meckel scan is ordered.

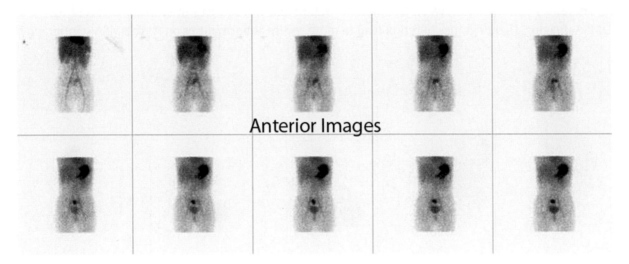

Anterior Images

Fig. 160.1

Technique

Meckel Scan

- ^{99m}Tc-pertechnetate, 100 µCi (3.7 MBq) per kilogram. The maximum dose is 10 mCi (370 MBq), and the minimum dose is 200 µCi (7.5 MBq).
- Ultra-high-resolution collimator, matrix 128 × 128. The acquisition of 1 frame per second for 60 seconds is followed by the acquisition of 1 frame per minute for 30 minutes. Static image matrix 256 × 256 for 60 seconds.
- Nothing by mouth for 4 hours before the study. Images are taken anteriorly and posteriorly.

Image Interpretation

The Meckel scan shows an abnormal focus of uptake in the lower midabdomen, just above the urinary bladder (**Fig. 160.1**). There is normal uptake in the stomach and normal excretion of tracer in the urinary bladder.

Differential Diagnosis

- Enteric duplication cysts
- Vascular malformations

544

- Intussusception
- Gastrogenic cyst
- Inflammatory bowel disease

Diagnosis and Clinical Follow-Up

The Meckel scan identified a diverticulum in the lower abdomen. The patient underwent exploratory laparotomy with resection. Pathologic evaluation of the resected specimen revealed a diverticulum containing ulcerated gastric mucosa. The patient recovered postoperatively without complications and was discharged home.

Discussion

Meckel diverticulum is a remnant of the vitelline duct that connects the yolk sac to the gut in the fetus. The failure of the vitelline duct to involute gives rise to the diverticulum. It contains all layers of the intestinal wall. Ectopic tissue is present in approximately 50% of cases, most commonly gastric tissue and less commonly pancreatic tissue.

A Meckel diverticulum is present in 2% of the population. It is usually localized within 2 ft of the ileocecal junction, with a length of 2 in. and a diameter of 2 cm. It is usually symptomatic before the age of 2 years, and female-to-male ratio is 2:1.

Ulceration of the diverticulum gives rise to gastrointestinal bleeding. Painless bleeding is the most common presentation of Meckel diverticulum. The Meckel scan is the procedure of choice for the diagnosis of Meckel diverticula. ^{99m}Tc-pertechnetate is taken up by the mucus-producing cells of the ectopic gastric mucosa. The sensitivity of this test is 90% for the detection of ectopic gastric mucosa. The uptake by the gastric cells increases over time and parallels the uptake in the stomach (**Fig. 160.1**). After the intravenous injection of ^{99m}Tc-pertechnetate, images of the abdomen and pelvis are obtained over 60 minutes. The tracer is excreted in the urinary system. Visualization of the renal pelves is common and may be a source of error in interpretation, as this can be confused with abnormal uptake in the diverticulum. Another source of interpretive error is the proximity of a Meckel diverticulum to the urinary bladder. Post-void images or SPECT images may help in difficult cases.

Several pharmacologic interventions have been advocated in the past to help the detection of abnormal uptake. Histamine H_2-receptor antagonists impair the secretion of pertechnetate by the gastric mucous cells, allowing better visualization of localization in abnormal gastric tissue. In children, the recommended dose of cimetidine is 20 mg/kg per day for 1 to 2 days before the test.

Glucagon has been recommended to decrease peristalsis in the intestine and therefore the rate of clearance of ^{99m}Tc-pertechnetate from the stomach. An unwanted effect of glucagon is a decrease in the uptake of ^{99m}Tc-pertechnetate, making visualization of the ectopic gastric mucosa more difficult.

PEARLS AND PITFALLS

- Care should be taken not to confuse excretion in the renal pelvis with abnormal uptake in a Meckel diverticulum.
- Obtain a post-void image so as not to miss abnormal uptake in close proximity to the urinary bladder.
- Not all Meckel diverticula will take up ^{99m}Tc-pertechnetate, only those containing gastric mucosa.
- Do not give Lugol solution to the patient before the study. It will interfere with uptake by the gastric mucosa.

Suggested Reading

Rudolph AM, et al. Rudolph's Pediatrics. Rudolph CD, ed. New York: McGraw-Hill, 2003. http://online.statref.com/document.aspx?fxid=13&docid=942

Saremi F, Jadvar H, Siegel ME. Pharmacologic interventions in nuclear radiology: indications, imaging protocols, and clinical results. Radiographics 2002;22(3):477–490

Sfakianakis GN, Haase GM. Abdominal scintigraphy for ectopic gastric mucosa: a retrospective analysis of 143 studies. AJR Am J Roentgenol 1982;138(1):7–12

Bar-Sever Z. Gastrointestinal bleeding. In: Treves ST, ed. *Pediatric Nuclear Medicine*. 2nd ed. New York: Springer-Verlag; 1995:453–462

CASE 161

Clinical Presentation

A hepatobiliary scan is requested to help differentiate between biliary atresia and neonatal hepatitis in a 2-week-old infant with extreme lethargy, poor feeding, and a high direct bilirubin level. Sepsis and metabolic disorders have been ruled out.

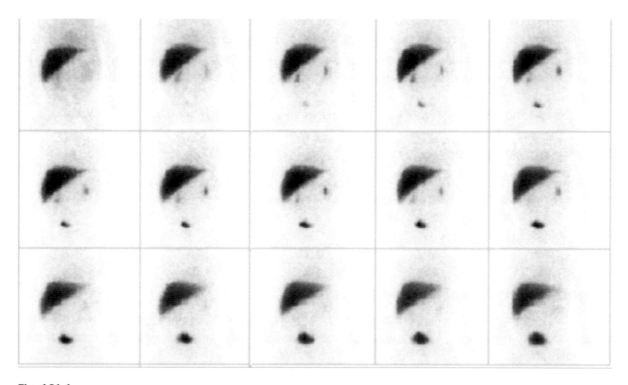

Fig. 161.1

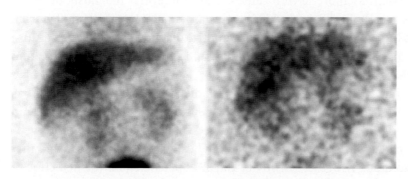

Fig. 161.2

547

Technique

- ^{99m}Tc-disofenin is administered intravenously at a dose of 0.05 mCi/kg at the beginning of the acquisition. The minimum dose is 0.25 mCi, and the maximum dose is 3.0 mCi.
- Use a high-resolution or ultra-high-resolution, low-energy, parallel-hole collimator.
- Energy window is 20% centered at 140 keV.
- Imaging time for the initial series is 0.5 minute per frame for 60 minutes. Additional images are obtained at 4 and 24 hours.
- Pre-treatment with phenobarbital is administered at 2.5 mg/kg twice a day for 3 to 5 days before hepatobiliary scintigraphy.

Image Interpretation

Images displayed as 5-minute frames after the injection of ^{99m}Tc-disofenin (**Fig. 161.1**) demonstrate prompt hepatic uptake of tracer. The high early liver-to-background ratio and the clear definition of the liver boundaries indicate that there is good hepatic extraction of ^{99m}Tc-disofenin, although the prominent renal excretion suggests a mild degree of hepatic dysfunction. Tracer is not identified in the small intestine.

Images at 4 and 24 hours (**Fig. 161.2**) show no evidence of tracer in the bowel.

Differential Diagnosis

- Biliary atresia
- Severe hepatocellular disease
- Complete common duct obstruction
- Intrahepatic cholestasis
- Ascending cholangitis

Diagnosis and Clinical Follow-Up

Hepatoportoenterostomy was performed after an intraoperative cholangiogram confirmed the diagnosis of biliary atresia. The patient improved clinically after surgery, and the direct bilirubin level normalized.

Discussion

Hyperbilirubinemia in the neonate is very common. In the majority of cases, neonatal hyperbilirubinemia reflects increased indirect bilirubin. This is usually physiologic and benign. Direct hyperbilirubinemia, which is less common, has more severe causes. The differential diagnosis of direct hyperbilirubinemia includes sepsis, metabolic disorders, biliary atresia, neonatal hepatitis, choledochal cyst, α_1-antitrypsin deficiency, and Alagille syndrome. The differential diagnosis is difficult because these disorders share many clinical features. Hepatobiliary scintigraphy helps in the differentiation between neonatal hepatitis and biliary atresia.

Biliary atresia has been detected in 1 per 10,000 live births, and idiopathic neonatal hepatitis has been found in 1 per 5,000. With either condition, jaundice usually develops at 3 to 6 weeks of age in an otherwise well-appearing, thriving infant, and the stools become acholic. Early surgical intervention is essential in biliary atresia; neonatal hepatitis is managed medically. It has been reported that hepatobiliary scintigraphy is 91% accurate, with 97% sensitivity and 82% specificity, for the detection of biliary atresia. Phenobarbital improves the accuracy of hepatobiliary scintigraphy by inducing hepatic enzymes and acting as a choleretic. Tracer uptake is thereby enhanced and its excretion promoted.

The recommended dose is 2.5 mg/kg twice a day for 3 to 5 days before scintigraphy. Biliary atresia is excluded when hepatobiliary scintigraphy demonstrates tracer excretion into the small intestine. Nonvisualization of tracer within the bowel in the presence of efficient hepatic extraction is presumptive evidence of biliary atresia. To make this determination, imaging beyond the first hour is required. We obtain an image at 4 hours. If the bowel is not visualized on that image, we obtain an image at 24 hours. Frequently, only the 24-hour image shows tracer in the bowel. Occasionally, because of rapid bowel transit, tracer in the small intestine will be evident on the 4-hour image but will not be present at 24 hours.

Other causes of the pattern of preserved hepatic tracer uptake with nonvisualization of the bowel include bile plug syndrome in patients with cystic fibrosis, severe dehydration, sepsis, prolonged parenteral nutrition, and Alagille syndrome. When the hepatic extraction of tracer is poor, a diagnosis of neonatal hepatitis is more likely. Failure to identify tracer excretion in the small intestine, however, prevents the exclusion of biliary atresia in cases with both decreased liver extraction and nonvisualization of the small intestine.

PEARLS AND PITFALLS

- Pre-treatment with phenobarbital increases hepatic uptake and excretion of the radiotracer, improving accuracy in the diagnosis of biliary atresia.
- In infants with neonatal hepatitis, excretion of radiotracer into the bowel may not be visualized within the first 60 minutes of serial imaging. Imaging at 4 and 24 hours is required in many cases.
- Portoenterostomy (Kasai procedure) is performed in infants in whom biliary atresia is diagnosed. The usefulness of this procedure is controversial in infants who are older than 3 months and who have advanced fibrosis of the liver. The 5-year survival rate for these children is 10%, compared with 70 to 90% if surgery is performed before 3 months of age.

Suggested Reading

Gerhold JP, Klingensmith WC III, Kuni CC, Lilly SR, Silverman A, Fritzberg AR, Nixt TL. Diagnosis of biliary atresia with radionuclide hepatobiliary imaging. Radiology 1983;146(2):499–504

Hirsig J, Rickham PP. Early differential diagnosis between neonatal hepatitis and biliary atresia. J Pediatr Surg 1980;15(1):13–15

Majd M, Reba RC, Altman RP. Effect of phenobarbital on 99mTc-IDA scintigraphy in the evaluation of neonatal jaundice. Semin Nucl Med 1981;11(3):194–204

Majd M, Reba RC, Altman RP. Hepatobiliary scintigraphy with 99mTc-PIPIDA in the evaluation of neonatal jaundice. Pediatrics 1981;67(1):140–145

Treves ST, Jones AG, Markisz J. Liver and spleen. In: Treves ST, ed. *Pediatric Nuclear Medicine.* 2nd ed. New York: Springer-Verlag; 1995:466–495

CASE 162

Clinical Presentation

A 6-year-old girl with a 4-year history of partial complex seizures that proved refractory to medical treatment is being considered for surgical cortical resection of an epileptogenic focus pending its localization. Results of CT and MRI of the brain are within normal limits. Electroencephalography is nonlocalizing. A SPECT study with 99mTc-bicisate is obtained.

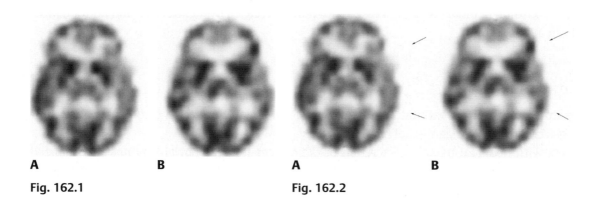

A   **B**   **A**   **B**

Fig. 162.1   **Fig. 162.2**

Technique

- 99mTc-bicisate is administered at a dose of 0.3 mCi/kg of body weight. The minimum dose is 5 mCi; the maximum dose is 20 mCi.
- Use an ultra-high-resolution collimator.
- Energy window is 20% centered at 140 keV.
- SPECT acquisition on a 128 × 128 matrix with a triple-detector system takes approximately 20 minutes. A usual technique includes 40 stops over 360 degrees per detector, 20 to 30 seconds per stop.
- The ictal study is performed in an inpatient setting, preferably in an epilepsy monitoring unit. Continuous electroencephalography (EEG) and video telemetry are essential to ensure ictal injection of tracer. Venous access is established before any seizure activity so that radiotracer can be quickly injected at the onset of a seizure.

Image Interpretation

Interictal perfusion brain SPECT (**Fig. 162.1A**) demonstrates relatively low regional blood flow to the left temporal and posterior frontal regions. Ictal brain SPECT (**Fig. 162.1B**) reveals a well-defined increase in blood flow to the left temporal and posterior frontal regions. These correspond to the areas of decreased perfusion on the interictal study. *Arrows* indicate the location of the finding on the interictal (**Fig. 162.2A**) and ictal (**Fig. 162.2B**) images.

Differential Diagnosis

- Epilepsy
- Encephalitis

- Tumor
- Luxury perfusion
- Environmental or motor stimulation of cortical activity

Diagnosis and Clinical Follow-Up

Subdural grid placement demonstrated abnormal EEG activity in the posterior frontal and temporal regions, confirming the ^{99m}Tc-bicisate SPECT findings. Left temporal and partial frontal lobectomy was performed. The patient has been seizure-free postoperatively.

Discussion

Epilepsy is a recurrent convulsive or nonconvulsive disorder caused by partial or generalized epileptogenic discharge in the cerebrum. It is estimated that seizures become refractory to medical treatment in 10 to 20% of patients with epilepsy. Some patients with medically refractory epilepsy benefit from surgery, with limited cortical resection providing the best results. Identifying the ictal focus and delineating its relationship to the language and motor centers are essential in directing cortical resection. This is accomplished with a multimodality approach that includes clinical evaluation, EEG, and imaging. Clinical evaluation alone is extremely inaccurate, and scalp EEG has a 10 to 15% rate of false lateralization.

Perfusion brain SPECT has emerged as an important tool in the detection of the seizure focus. Tracers such as ^{99m}Tc-bicisate and ^{99m}Tc-exametazime, which are distributed in the brain in proportion to regional cerebral blood flow, have been used. Interictally, the level of perfusion in the region of the epileptogenic focus is often low in relation to perfusion in the normal brain. During ictus, perfusion to the epileptogenic focus is greater than it is to the normal brain. Its location is more easily identified on ictal than on interictal studies. The sensitivity for the detection of an ictal focus has been found to be 97% when tracer is administered ictally. The sensitivity decreases to approximately 50 to 70% if tracer is injected interictally.

PET has also been used in the workup of patients with intractable seizures. Oxygen use, glucose metabolism, blood flow, and receptor distribution can be mapped and quantified with PET. PET with 2-deoxy-2-^{18}F-FDG is usually done interictally and shows a relatively low rate of metabolism in the region of the epileptogenic focus. Ictal ^{18}F-FDG-PET shows a high metabolic rate in the ictal focus.

PEARLS AND PITFALLS

- Ictal ^{99m}Tc-bicisate SPECT and ^{18}F-FDG-PET have a higher sensitivity for the detection of seizure foci than that of interictal studies.
- MRI is valuable for the detection of structural abnormalities, but findings are often normal in patients with intractable seizures. Brain SPECT is valuable for the localization of epileptogenic foci in this circumstance.
- SPECT with ^{99m}Tc-bicisate has been found to have a higher sensitivity in the detection of ictal foci located in the temporal region than of those in the frontal cortex.
- Sedatives are often required to obtain technically satisfactory examinations and do not have any effect on tracer distribution if given after the radiotracer injection.
- Proper timing of the injection for an ictal ^{99m}Tc-bicisate SPECT study is essential. The radiotracer should be injected as soon as the seizure is detected. If tracer is injected postictally, the localization of an ictal focus is much less reliable because of extended brain activation.

- EEG monitoring with surgically implanted subdural electrode grids is highly accurate in the detection and localization of epileptogenic foci. However, this procedure is associated with a high risk for infection, cerebral edema, and hemorrhage.

Suggested Reading

Harvey AS, Bowe JM, Hopkins IJ, Shield LK, Cook DJ, Berkovic SF. Ictal 99mTc-HMPAO single photon emission computed tomography in children with temporal lobe epilepsy. Epilepsia 1993;34(5):869–877

Ives JR. Video recording during long-term EEG monitoring of epileptic patients. Adv Neurol 1987;46: 1–11

Krausz Y, Cohen D, Konstantini S, Meiner Z, Yaffe S, Atlan H. Brain SPECT imaging in temporal lobe epilepsy. Neuroradiology 1991;33(3):274–276

Packard AB, Roach PJ, Davis RT, Carmant L, Davis R, Riviello J, Holmes G, Barnes PD, O'Tuama LA, Bjornson B, Treves ST. Ictal and interictal technetium-99m-bicisate brain SPECT in children with refractory epilepsy. J Nucl Med 1996;37(7):1101–1106

Ryvlin P, Philippon B, Cinotti L, Froment JC, Le Bars D, Mauguière F. Functional neuroimaging strategy in temporal lobe epilepsy: a comparative study of 18FDG-PET and 99mTc-HMPAO-SPECT. Ann Neurol 1992;31(6):650–656

CASE 163

Clinical Presentation

A 10-year-old boy presents with persistent vague abdominal pain, fever, decreased appetite, and diarrhea. Abdominal ultrasonography and CT reveal a left suprarenal mass.

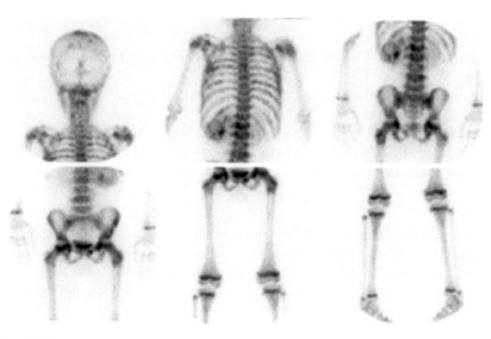

Fig. 163.1

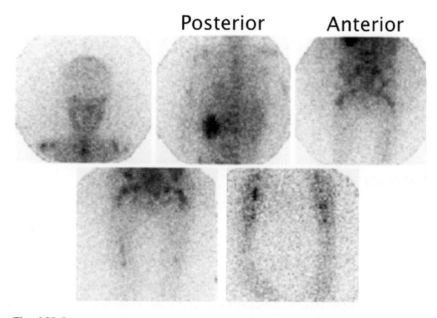

Posterior   Anterior

Fig. 163.2

Technique

99mTc-MDP Bone Scan

- 99mTc-MDP at 0.2 mCi/kg of body weight is given intravenously. The minimum dose is 1 mCi; the maximum dose is 20 mCi.
- Use a high- or ultra-high-resolution, low-energy, parallel-hole collimator. Supplemental pinhole magnification images may be obtained for improved detail. SPECT is performed for better three-dimensional localization.
- Planar whole-body or spot views of the entire skeleton are obtained 4 hours after tracer injection.

123I-MIBG Scintigraphy

- 123I-MIBG at a dose of 0.2 mCi/kg is given intravenously. The minimum dose is 1 mCi, and the maximum dose is 10 mCi.
- Use a high- or ultra-high-resolution, low-energy, parallel-hole collimator.
- Energy window is 20% centered at 159 keV.
- Whole-body images and SPECT are obtained as needed 24 hours after injection.
- Thyroid uptake can be blocked by the administration of saturated solution of potassium iodide, one drop three times a day, beginning 1 day before imaging and continuing for 3 days.

Image Interpretation

The workup for metastatic disease includes 99mTc-MDP bone scan (**Fig. 163.1**) and 123I-MIBG scintigraphy (**Fig. 163.2**). Scintigraphy with 99mTc-MDP shows areas of abnormal tracer uptake in the calvarium, spine, pelvis, ribs, femora, and tibiae. In addition, tracer is concentrated in the left adrenal mass. Scintigraphy with 123I-MIBG demonstrates an intense focus of radiotracer uptake in the left upper abdomen and diffuse involvement of the skeleton.

Differential Diagnosis

(MIBG uptake)

- Neuroblastoma
- Pheochromocytoma
- Paraganglioma
- Gastrinoma
- Insulinoma
- Medullary thyroid carcinoma
- Infantile myofibromatosis

Diagnosis and Clinical Follow-Up

The presumptive diagnosis was neuroblastoma. Laparotomy with resection of the mass confirmed the diagnosis. Chemotherapy was begun postoperatively.

Discussion

Neuroblastoma, the most common extracranial solid malignancy of childhood, arises from the embryonal neural crest anywhere along the sympathetic nervous system. The most common primary site is the adrenal gland, where 40 to 50% of neuroblastomas originate. Other sites of origin include the paravertebral and presacral sympathetic chains, the organs of Zuckerkandl, the posterior mediastinal sympathetic ganglia, and the cervical sympathetic plexuses. Disseminated disease is present in up to 70% of cases at diagnosis. This most commonly involves cortical bone and bone marrow but also liver, skin, and occasionally lung. The most characteristic sites of cortical involvement are the calvarium, periorbital facial bones, and long bones, where a metaphyseal location is typical.

Scintigraphy with MIBG has a sensitivity of more than 85% for detecting neuroblastoma. At the doses used for imaging, the cellular uptake of MIBG in neuroblastoma is through a neuronal sodium- and energy-dependent transport mechanism. MIBG can be labeled with either ^{131}I or [123]I. Currently, only ^{131}I-MIBG is available commercially in the United States; ^{123}I-MIBG is available for investigational use in some pediatric centers. Normal tracer distribution is to the heart, liver, thyroid gland, salivary and lacrimal glands, kidneys, urine, adrenal glands, bowel, and muscle. There is no uptake by normal marrow or bone.

In comparison with MIBG, ^{99m}Tc-MDP has equal sensitivity for detecting metastatic disease on a per-patient basis but tends to depict the overall extent of disease less accurately. The accurate identification of metastases with skeletal scintigraphy, but not MIBG imaging, frequently requires experience in interpreting pediatric studies. Metaphyseal metastases, which are often symmetric, may be particularly difficult for less experienced observers to detect.

PEARLS AND PITFALLS

- Because of the different mechanisms by which MIBG and MDP localize in neuroblastoma, the two agents complement each other, resulting in a high sensitivity for the detection of metastases.
- The pre-treatment and post-treatment administration of saturated solution of potassium iodide decreases the thyroidal radiation dose from MIBG.
- MIBG should be administered slowly over 20 to 30 seconds to reduce the possibility of a hypertensive crisis resulting from the competitive displacement of norepinephrine from storage granules.
- Numerous medications may interfere with the uptake of MIBG in neuroblastoma. Although few children with neuroblastoma are on these medications, some are receiving nonprescription medications for upper respiratory or ear infections that contain ephedrine, phenylephrine, or other potentially interfering agents. A careful medication history is therefore essential.
- The uptake of ^{99m}Tc-MDP may be increased at bone marrow biopsy sites, and this should not be mistaken for metastatic disease.

Suggested Reading

Brodeur GM, Pritchard J, Berthold F, Carlsen NL, Castel V, Castleberry RP, DeBernardi B, Evans AE, Favrot M, Hedborg F, et al. Revisions of the international criteria for neuroblastoma diagnosis, staging, and response to treatment. J Clin Oncol 1993;11(8):1466–1477

Bousvaros A, Kirks DR, Grossman H. Imaging of neuroblastoma: an overview. Pediatr Radiol 1986;16(2):89–106

Connolly LP, Treves ST. *Pediatric Skeletal Scintigraphy with Multimodality Imaging Correlation.* New York: Springer-Verlag; 1997

Connolly LP, Treves ST, Conway JJ. Pediatric skeletal scintigraphy. In: Henkin RE, Boles MA, Dillehay GL, Halama J, Karesh S, Wagner R, Zimmer M. eds. Nuclear Medicine. St. Louis, MO: Mosby Year Book; 1996:1690–1724

Farahati J, Mueller SP, Coennen HH, Reiners C. Scintigraphy of neuroblastoma with radioiodinated m-iodobenzylguanidine. In: Treves ST, ed. *Pediatric Nuclear Medicine*. 2nd ed. New York: Springer-Verlag; 1995:528–545

Gelfand MJ, Elgazzar AH, Kriss VM, Masters PR, Golsch GJ. Iodine-123-MIBG SPECT versus planar imaging in children with neural crest tumors. J Nucl Med 1994;35(11):1753–1757

Krenning EP, Kwekkeboom DJ, Bakker WH, Breeman WA, Kooij PP, Oei HY, van Hagen M, Postema PT, de Jong M, Reubi JC, et al. Somatostatin receptor scintigraphy with [111In-DTPA-D-Phe1]- and [123I-Tyr3]-octreotide: the Rotterdam experience with more than 1000 patients. Eur J Nucl Med 1993;20(8):716–731

Rufini V, Fisher GA, Shulkin BL, Sisson JC, Shapiro B. Iodine-123-MIBG imaging of neuroblastoma: utility of SPECT and delayed imaging. J Nucl Med 1996;37(9):1464–1468

Treves ST, Connolly LP, Kirkpatrick JA, Packard AB, Roach P, Jaramillo D. Bone. In: Treves ST, ed. *Pediatric Nuclear Medicine*. 2nd ed. New York: Springer-Verlag; 1995:233–301

CASE 164

Clinical Presentation

A 4-year-old boy presents with swelling and pain in his left leg for 2 days and fever and a limp for 1 day. There is no history of trauma. Radiographic evaluation of the left leg is within normal limits. Laboratory workup demonstrates a white blood cell count of 13,200/mm³ and a sedimentation rate of 48 mm/h. Blood cultures are obtained.

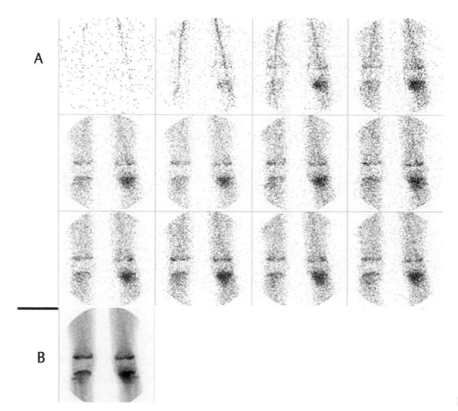

Fig. 164.1

Technique

- ⁹⁹ᵐTc-MDP at 0.2 mCi/kg of body weight is given intravenously. The minimum dose is 1 mCi; the maximum dose is 20 mCi.
- Use a high- or ultra-high-resolution, low-energy, parallel-hole collimator. Supplemental pinhole magnification images are obtained for improved detail. SPECT is performed for better three-dimensional localization.
- The imaging time for an initial radionuclide angiogram is 3-second frames for 1 minute. A static blood pool image should be obtained within 5 to 10 minutes of tracer injection. A planar static view of the region-of-interest should be obtained 4 hours after injection. There should be whole-body or spot views of the entire skeleton.

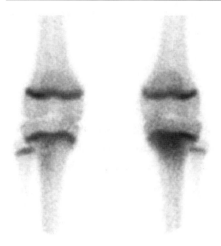

Fig. 164.2

Image Interpretation

An anterior radionuclide angiogram shows increased blood flow to the proximal left tibia (**Fig. 164.1A**). The distribution of increased tracer concentration depicted in the tissue phase imaging corresponds to the area with increased flow demonstrated on the radionuclide angiogram (**Fig. 164.1B**). Anterior views of the tibiae (**Fig. 164.2**) in the skeletal phase reveal abnormal uptake in the proximal left tibial metaphysis.

Differential Diagnosis

- Osteomyelitis
- Soft tissue infection/inflammation
- Acute trauma
- Malignancy
- Sarcoidosis

Diagnosis and Clinical Follow-Up

Following skeletal scintigraphy, bone biopsy was performed. Cultures grew *Staphylococcus aureus* (*S. aureus*). Intravenous antibiotic treatment was initiated based on a presumptive diagnosis of acute osteomyelitis. The patient's condition improved on antibiotic treatment, and he was discharged in good condition after 1 week of hospitalization. He completed the course of antibiotic treatment as an outpatient.

Discussion

Acute osteomyelitis is a common pediatric problem. It usually results from the hematogenous spread of infection related to transient and often asymptomatic bacteremia. *S. aureus* is the most frequent infective organism.

Approximately 75% of cases involve the long bones, with a metaphyseal location typical. The metaphyseal predominance reflects the regional vascularity and the slow blood flow in looping metaphyseal arterial and venous sinusoidal vessels. The most rapidly growing and larger metaphyses are more commonly involved. Transphyseal vessels allow infection to spread from metaphysis to epiphysis in infants and children younger than 18 months of age. After these vessels are obliterated, the relatively avascular physis serves as a natural barrier to the spread of infection. Epiphyseal involvement is, therefore, uncommon between 18 months of age and the time of physeal closure. The flat and irregular bones, such as the pelvis, are involved in approximately 25% of cases. Acute osteomyelitis of the flat and irregular bones characteristically develops in bone adjacent to cartilage.

The early diagnosis of acute osteomyelitis is necessary to prevent significant complications, such as sepsis, chronic infection, arrested growth, and bone deformity. Unfortunately, the clinical diagnosis of acute osteomyelitis is difficult in young children, who frequently present only with limping or refusal to bear weight. Pain is often not well localized, and swelling and tenderness are often absent. Fever may be the only sign or may be absent in children of all age groups with acute osteomyelitis.

The imaging evaluation usually begins within radiography. A radiographic diagnosis in the early stages of acute osteomyelitis is difficult, however, because the early radiographic manifestations are neither consistently observed nor specific. In contrast, skeletal scintigraphy, which is typically abnormal with 24 to 48 hours of symptom onset, has proved invaluable in providing a prompt, early diagnosis of acute osteomyelitis, allowing timely treatment.

As in the adult, scintigraphic evaluation is accomplished with multiphase imaging to help distinguish acute osteomyelitis from cellulitis. The clinically apparent site of infection is imaged with blood flow and blood pool phases of the three-phase bone scan, followed by delayed images of the entire skeleton. The whole-body evaluation is important because of the significant incidence of multifocal involvement, particularly in neonates (22% incidence of multifocality), and the frequent absence of localizing signs in young children. Whole-body imaging is also valuable in cases in which diseases such as metastatic neuroblastoma and leukemia clinically mimic acute osteomyelitis.

Regionally increased blood flow and localization to the infected bone and adjacent soft tissues are typically revealed on angiographic and tissue phase images. Skeletal phase images usually demonstrate focally increased tracer uptake in an infected bone. Rarely, there is focally decreased to absent uptake that likely reflects regional ischemia caused by vascular tamponade resulting from inflammation and edema.

PEARLS AND PITFALLS_____

- Skeletal scintigraphy in children is best performed with high- or ultra-high-resolution collimation.
- Pinhole imaging is useful for demonstrating more convincingly or delineating more accurately an abnormality that is identified on standard images. When images of a clinically suspected area initially appear normal, pinhole images help to confirm the absence of focal abnormalities adjacent to the intensely tracer-avid physis.
- SPECT is often valuable for the evaluation of the pelvis.
- Skeletal scintigraphy is the most effective means of screening children with suspected osteomyelitis and a normal radiographic evaluation.
- Skeletal phase imaging must encompass the whole body in children with suspected acute osteomyelitis.
- Failure to position the extremities symmetrically and the physes perpendicular to the face of the camera may result in findings that mimic or obscure metaphyseal pathology.
- During image processing, care must be taken not to overexpose the epiphyseal-metaphyseal complex. Resultant "blooming" of the image may mimic or obscure metaphyseal pathology.
- An extended pattern of increased localization involving the adjacent physis and bones distal or proximal to an involved metaphysis may be observed. This reflects reactive hyperemia and should not be viewed as evidence of either physeal involvement or multifocal osteomyelitis. The role of MRI relative to that of scintigraphy in evaluating suspected acute osteomyelitis has been debated.

Although these modalities appear equally sensitive when symptoms are well localized, poor symptom localization in young children and the high incidence of multifocal involvement favor the use of scintigraphy.

Suggested Reading

Applegate KA, Connolly LP, Treves ST. Neuroblastoma presenting clinically as hip osteomyelitis: a "signature" diagnosis on skeletal scintigraphy. Pediatr Radiol 1995;25(Suppl 1):S93–S96

Asmar BI. Osteomyelitis in the neonate. Infect Dis Clin North Am 1992;6(1):117–132

Bressler EL, Conway JJ, Weiss SC. Neonatal osteomyelitis examined by bone scintigraphy. Radiology 1984;152(3):685–688

Connolly LP, Treves ST. *Pediatric Skeletal Scintigraphy with Multimodality Imaging Correlation.* New York: Springer-Verlag; 1997

Connolly LP, Treves ST, Conway JJ. Pediatric skeletal scintigraphy. In: Henkin RE, Boles MA, Dillehay GL, et al., eds. Nuclear Medicine. St. Louis, MO: MosbyYear Book; 1996:1690–1724

Faden H, Grossi M. Acute osteomyelitis in children: reassessment of etiologic agents and their clinical characteristics. Am J Dis Child 1991;145(1):65–69

Jones DC, Cady RB. "Cold" bone scans in acute osteomyelitis. J Bone Joint Surg Br 1981;63-B(3): 376–378

Mok PM, Reilly BJ, Ash JM. Osteomyelitis in the neonate: clinical aspects and the role of radiography and scintigraphy in diagnosis and management. Radiology 1982;145(3):677–682

Treves ST, Connolly LP, Kirkpatrick JA, Packard AB, Roach P, Jaramillo D. Bone. In: Treves ST, ed. *Pediatric Nuclear Medicine.* 2nd ed. New York: Springer-Verlag; 1995:233–301

Treves S, Khettry J, Broker FH, Wilkinson RH, Watts H. Osteomyelitis: early scintigraphic detection in children. Pediatrics 1976;57(2):173–186

CASE 165

Clinical Presentation

A 10-year-old boy presents with a 6-week history of right leg pain after falling while playing football. Radiographs are suggestive of osteosarcoma.

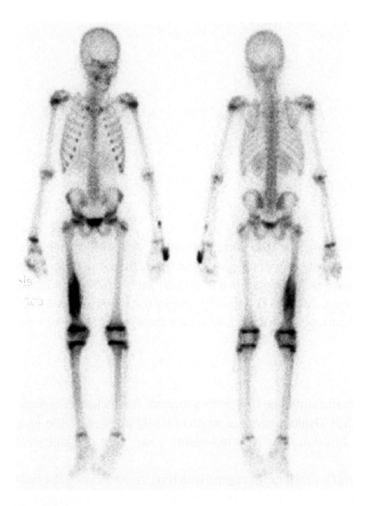

Fig. 165.1

Technique

- 99mTc-MDP at 0.2 mCi/kg of body weight is given intravenously. The minimum dose is 1 mCi; the maximum dose is 20 mCi.
- Use a high- or ultra-high-resolution, low-energy, parallel-hole collimator. Supplemental pinhole magnification images are obtained in addition to the planar images for improved detail. SPECT is performed for better three-dimensional localization.
- The imaging time for an initial radionuclide angiogram is 3-second frames for 1 minute. A static blood pool image should be obtained within 5 to 10 minutes following tracer injection. Whole-body or spot views of the entire bony skeleton should be obtained 4 hours after tracer injection. Spot planar or SPECT views of the region-of-interest should be obtained as needed.

Image Interpretation

Whole-body ⁹⁹ᵐTc-MDP images (**Fig. 165.1**) demonstrate a focal area of intense increased uptake in the distal diaphyseal region of the right femur. This corresponds to the area of abnormality seen on radiography. No metastatic disease is visualized. Retained tracer is present in the intravenous line of the left hand and wrist.

Differential Diagnosis

(Solitary site of focal bony tracer uptake)

- Benign primary tumor
- Trauma
  - Accidental
  - Post-surgical
- Primary bone malignancy
- Bony metastasis
- Osteomyelitis
- Bony infarct
- Skin contamination overlying bone structure

Diagnosis and Clinical Follow-Up

Biopsy of the primary site proved it to be osteosarcoma. The initial metastatic workup was negative. Chemotherapy was initiated, and wide tumor excision with allograft reconstruction was performed. Follow-up skeletal scintigraphy and CT of the chest were obtained at regular intervals for metastatic evaluation. In the fourth year of clinical follow-up, skeletal scintigraphy demonstrated widespread skeletal metastatic disease with soft tissue localization of tracer in pulmonary metastases that was confirmed by CT (**Fig. 165.2**).

Discussion

Osteosarcoma is the most common primary malignant bone tumor of childhood. The incidence is highest in persons between 10 and 25 years of age. Osteosarcoma is predominantly a lesion of the long bones, where it is typically metaphyseal in location. This case represents a rare case of diaphyseal involvement by the tumor.

The treatment of choice is wide resection and limb-sparing surgery, which is performed in 80% of patients. This treatment approach requires an accurate delineation of the tumor extent and an assessment of the response to preoperative chemotherapy at the primary site as well as the identification of metastatic foci, which most commonly involve lung and bone. Survival rates are highest in patients without metastatic disease at presentation whose tumor shows more than 90 to 95% necrosis before resection. Skeletal scintigraphy typically reveals marked tracer uptake in osteosarcomas, although it is not unusual for regions of decreased uptake to be present as well. Increased tracer uptake in the lesion often extends beyond the pathologic margins of the tumor secondary to hyperemia or reactive bone. The assessment of local extent is best based on MRI and ²⁰¹Tl imaging, which is especially valuable for estimating tumor viability. Skeletal scintigraphy is the primary means by which skeletal metastases are detected at diagnosis and during follow-up. Skeletal metastases, which appear as areas of increased radionuclide uptake, are often radiographically occult or asymptomatic, or both, at the time of scintigraphic detection. Occasionally, pulmonary metastases accumulate ⁹⁹ᵐTc-MDP because of osteoid production by the

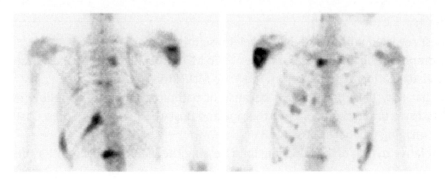

Fig. 165.2

metastatic deposits. There are also rare reports of metastases to other sites, including the liver, kidneys, and lymph nodes, that have been identified with skeletal scintigraphy.

Tumor viability is accurately assessed with ^{201}Tl scintigraphy. The intense uptake of this tracer in untreated osteosarcoma reflects cellular viability and a high rate of metabolic activity. Imaging with ^{201}Tl is valuable when used in combination with MRI in assessing the local extent of disease at diagnosis and following chemotherapy, and in evaluating the response to chemotherapy before limb salvage surgery is performed. The uptake of ^{201}Tl in osteosarcoma markedly decreases with a favorable pathologic response, which is defined histologically as more than 90 to 95% necrosis. This can be assessed visually by comparing tumor and cardiac or background ^{201}Tl uptake, or it can be assessed quantitatively. Various quantitative methods have been proposed, with the optimal method yet to be defined. In another case (**Fig. 165.3**), the absence of ^{201}Tl uptake after therapy reflects a good response to treatment. The upper images in **Fig. 165.3** show ^{99m}Tc-MDP (left) and ^{201}Tl (right) uptake in the bone and tumor, respectively, before therapy. The lower left image in **Fig. 165.3** shows post-therapeutic irregular residual ^{99m}Tc-MDP tracer uptake, consistent with expected bony repair, and the lower right image shows no evidence of abnormal ^{201}Tl uptake, suggesting the absence of residual viable tumor.

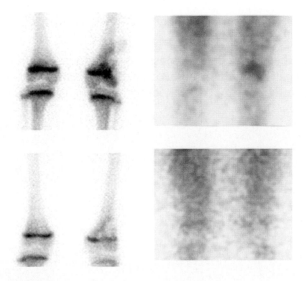

Fig. 165.3

- Skeletal metastases are best revealed with whole-body skeletal scintigraphy.
- The results of ^{201}Tl scintigraphy performed 24 hours after ^{99m}Tc-MDP imaging may be inaccurate because of the persistent visualization of activity from the ^{99m}Tc-MDP study.
- Attenuation from a cast that may have been placed because of pathologic fracture or following biopsy can limit the ability to accurately compare pre-therapy and post-therapy ^{201}Tl studies. Casts should be removed before imaging whenever possible.
- The role of dynamic MRI relative to that of ^{201}Tl imaging for assessing the viability of tumor has not been established.
- The ability to distinguish malignant from benign bone lesions on the basis of ^{201}Tl uptake (or lack of uptake) is uncertain.

Suggested Reading

Chew FS, Hudson TM. Radionuclide bone scanning of osteosarcoma: falsely extended uptake patterns. AJR Am J Roentgenol 1982;139(1):49–54

Connolly LP, Treves ST. *Pediatric Skeletal Scintigraphy with Multimodality Imaging Correlation*. New York: Springer-Verlag; 1997

Connolly LP, Treves ST, Conway JJ. Pediatric skeletal scintigraphy. In: Henkin RE, Boles MA, Dillehay GL, et al., eds. *Nuclear Medicine*. St. Louis, MO: Mosby Year Book; 1996:1690–1724

Hoefnagel CA, Bruning PF, Cohen P, Marcuse HR, van der Schoot JB. Detection of lung metastases from osteosarcoma by scintigraphy using 99mTc-methylene diphosphonate. Diagn Imaging 1981;50(5): 277–284

Kirks DR, McCook TA, Merten DF, Sullivan DC. The value of radionuclide bone imaging in selected patients with osteogenic sarcoma metastatic to lung. Pediatr Radiol 1980;9(3):139–143

Rees CR, Siddiqui AR, duCret R. The role of bone scintigraphy in osteogenic sarcoma. Skeletal Radiol 1986;15(5):365–367

Sehweil AM, McKillop JH, Milroy R, Wilson R, Abdel-Dayem HM, Omar YT. Mechanism of 201Tl uptake in tumours. Eur J Nucl Med 1989;15(7):376–379

Thrall JH, Geslien GE, Corcoron RJ, Johnson MC. Abnormal radionuclide deposition patterns adjacent to focal skeletal lesions. Radiology 1975;115(3):659–663

Treves ST, Connolly LP, Kirkpatrick JA, Packard AB, Roach P, Jaramillo D. Bone. In: Treves ST, ed. *Pediatric Nuclear Medicine*. 2nd ed. New York: Springer-Verlag; 1995:233–301

Vanel D, Henry-Amar M, Lumbroso J, Lemalet E, Couanet D, Piekarski JD, Masselot J, Boddaert A, Kalifa C, Le Chevalier T, Lemoine G. Pulmonary evaluation of patients with osteosarcoma: roles of standard radiography, tomography, CT, scintigraphy, and tomoscintigraphy. AJR Am J Roentgenol 1984;143(3):519–523

CASE 166

Clinical Presentation

A 7-week-old infant boy presents with severe right hydronephrosis detected by prenatal ultrasonography. Postnatal ultrasonography also demonstrates severe pelvicaliectasis of the right collecting system, consistent with right ureteropelvic junction obstruction. Voiding cystourethrography shows no reflux. A ^{99m}Tc-MAG-3 study is obtained to evaluate for the presence and severity of obstruction.

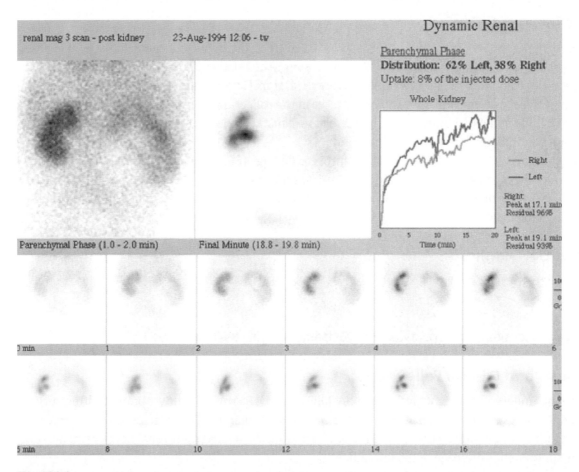

Fig. 166.1

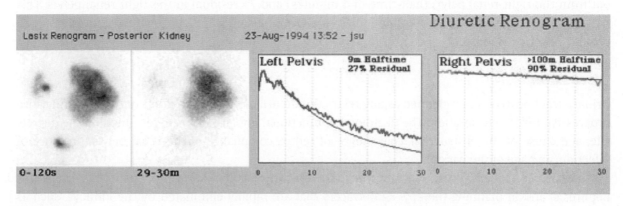

Fig. 166.2

Technique

- ^{99m}Tc-MAG-3 is administered at a dose of 0.2 mCi/kg. The minimum dose is 2 mCi; the maximum dose is 10 mCi.
- Use a high- or ultra-high-resolution, low-energy, parallel-hole collimator.
- Energy window is 20% centered at 140 keV.
- Dynamic images are acquired for a minimum of 20 minutes (or until tracer is seen in the collecting system). For the diuretic phase, after the administration of furosemide (dose, 1 mg/kg; maximum dose, 40 mg), dynamic images are acquired for 30 minutes.
- Bladder catheterization and intravenous access are established before the injection of radiotracer.

Image Interpretation

The parenchymal phase (**Fig. 166.1**) shows an enlarged right kidney with a central area of decreased tracer uptake representing the dilated collecting system. The relative uptake of radiotracer is 38% by the right kidney and 62% by the left kidney. The cortical transit time, defined as the time between the injection of tracer and the first appearance of tracer in the collecting system, is longer than 20 minutes for the right side and 4 to 5 minutes for the left. There is marked retention of tracer in the right collecting system before administration of the diuretic.

Thirty minutes after the administration of furosemide (**Fig. 166.2**), there is 91% residual radiotracer in the right pelvis, and a half-time of longer than 100 minutes is noted. These findings indicate a right ureteropelvic junction obstruction. Tracer washout from the left kidney is augmented by furosemide, indicating no obstruction.

Differential Diagnosis

- Obstructed urinary collecting system
- Urinoma
- Ureterocele
- Surgical diversion of the urinary collecting system overlying the kidney

Diagnosis and Clinical Follow-Up

The patient underwent a right pyeloplasty. A follow-up ^{99m}Tc-MAG-3 study obtained after surgery (**Fig. 166.3**) shows a cortical transit time of 4 to 5 minutes bilaterally. The relative uptake of tracer by the right kidney is 49% and by the left is 51%. Drainage from the dilated right renal pelvis remains slow. There is spontaneous drainage of the left kidney.

Following the administration of furosemide (**Fig. 166.4**), there is prompt and nearly complete washout from the right renal pelvis (half-time of 4 minutes) and 7% residual in the right renal pelvis. This nonobstructive response to furosemide indicates a favorable surgical result. The left kidney shows a normal diuretic response.

Discussion

Urinary tract obstruction is defined as any restriction to urinary flow that, if left untreated, will cause progressive renal deterioration. The likelihood of functional impairment is determined by the degree, site, and cause of the obstruction, coexistence of reflux, compliance of the renal pelvis, presence of infection, and age of the patient.

Nuclear medicine plays an important role in the evaluation and monitoring of patients with hydronephrosis, and in planning therapy. Radiotracers that are rapidly eliminated by the kidneys, such as ^{99m}Tc-MAG-3, ^{99m}Tc-DTPA, and ^{99m}Tc-glucoheptonate, may be used for the evaluation of obstruction. We

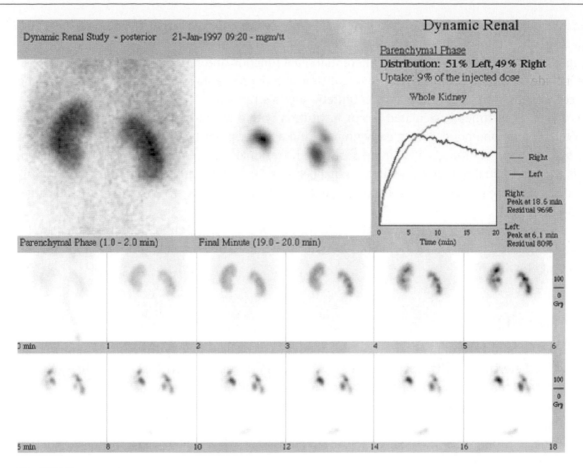

Fig. 166.3

favor ^{99m}Tc-MAG-3 because of its higher kidney-to-background ratio and rapid excretion, which provide good temporal resolution.

Studies performed to assess suspected renal obstruction most often consist of standard parenchymal imaging from 1 to 2 minutes after the injection of tracer, drainage phase imaging through 20 minutes after injection, and, when spontaneous drainage is not observed, dynamic imaging after furosemide. An alternative method entails administering furosemide 15 minutes before tracer administration.

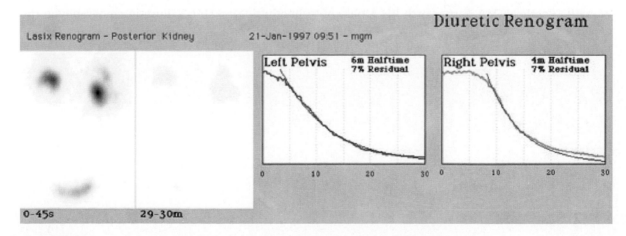

Fig. 166.4

The interpretation of a dynamic renal scan includes evaluation of the parenchymal phase, cortical transit time, and drainage phase. In children with suspected obstruction, the parenchymal phase provides important information regarding differential renal function and renal morphology. The diuretic phase includes a calculation of the washout half-time and the percentage of initial activity remaining in the collecting system at 30 minutes after diuretic administration.

The diuretic half-time is calculated in our institution with a mono-exponential interpolation between two points: one point during early diuresis and another point before the curve changes from monotonic decay. In addition, a 30-minute post-diuretic residual is calculated. In cases of obstruction, there is a large residual of radiotracer in the renal pelvis at 30 minutes after the administration of furosemide. In the case presented, a half-time longer than 100 minutes and a 90% residual are indicative of obstruction.

In a newborn infant, renal uptake of the radiotracer, cortical transit time, and excretion may be physiologically delayed. However, ^{99m}Tc-MAG-3 has been found to be reliable in this age group for the detection of obstruction.

PEARLS AND PITFALLS

- It is important to ensure that radiotracer has filled the renal pelvis before diuretic is administered.
- Vesical catheterization with open drainage of the bladder during the entire examination should be used to avoid the false-positive results that occur when a full bladder delays drainage.
- Careful attention should be paid to the selection of regions-of-interest and background.
- Be aware of the presence of reflux.
- The value of the diuretic half-time has been overemphasized. It should be one of several parameters considered during diuretic renography.

Suggested Reading

Koff SA, Thrall JH, Keyes JW Jr. Assessment of hydroureteronephrosis in children using diuretic radionuclide urography. J Urol 1980;123(4):531–534

Thrall JH, Koff SA, Keyes JW Jr. Diuretic radionuclide renography and scintigraphy in the differential diagnosis of hydroureteronephrosis. Semin Nucl Med 1981;11(2):89–104

Treves ST. The ongoing challenge of diagnosis and treatment of urinary tract infection, vesicoureteral reflux and renal damage in children. J Nucl Med 1994;35(10):1608–1611

Wong JC, Rossleigh MA, Farnsworth RH. Utility of technetium-99m-MAG3 diuretic renography in the neonatal period. J Nucl Med 1995;36(12):2214–2219

APPENDIX

Properties of Radioisotopes

Isotope	$T_{1/2}$	Energies (keV)*	Type of Decay	Uses
99mTc (Technetium)	6.0 h	140	IT	Wide variety of nuclear medicine studies
99Mo (Molybdenum)	66 h	181,740,780	β⁻	99mTc generator parent isotope
123I (Iodine)	13.2 h	159	EC	Thyroid uptake and scan
124I (Iodine)	4.2 d	Gamma: numerous β⁺ 511	EC Positron	PET imaging of thyroid cancer (nwu)
125I (Iodine)	60.2 d	35	EC	In-vitro radioimmunoassay
131I (Iodine)	8.1 d	Gamma: 364 β⁻: 606	EC β⁻	Thyroid uptake, thyroid therapy
111In (Indium)	2.8 d	172,247	EC	White blood cells, octreotide imaging, cisternograms
67Ga (Gallium)	78.2 h	93,185,300,394	EC	Infection, neoplastic disease (eg, lymphoma)
201Th (Thallium)	73 h	Gamma: 135,167 x-rays: 69-83	EC Hg x-rays	Myocardial perfusion, some neoplastic disease
57Co (Cobalt)	270 d	122,136	EC	Flood sources, string markers
81mKr (Krypton)	13 sec	191	IT	Lung ventilation studies (nwu)
127Xe (Xenon)	36.4 d	172,203,375	EC	Lung ventilation studies (nwu)
133Xe (Xenon)	5.3 d	Gamma: 81	β⁻	Lung ventilation studies when not using 99mTc aerosols
153Sm (Samarium)	46.3 h	Gamma:103 β⁻ 825	β⁻	Therapies (eg, bone pain from metastases)
89Sr (Strontium)	50.5 d	1463	β⁻	Therapies (eg, bone pain from metastases)
223Ra (Radium)	11.4 d	5650	Alpha	Therapies (eg, bone pain from metastases) (nwu)
90Y (Yttrium)	64 h	2280	β⁻	Therapies (eg, Radioimmunotherapy of Non-Hodgkin's Lymphoma, synovectomies)
32P (Phosphorus)	14.3 d	1710	β⁻	Therapies (eg, synovectomies)
186Re (Rhenium)	3.7 d	1069	β⁻	Therapies (eg, synovectomies) (nwu)
169Er (Erbium)	9.4 d	351	β⁻	Therapies (eg, synovectomies) (nwu)
177Lu (Lutetium)	6.7 d	498	β⁻	Therapies (eg, synovectomies) (nwu) Therapies (neuroendocrine tumors)
18F (Fluorine)	109 min	511	Positron	Most PET studies (eg, oncology, brain metabolism, myocardial viability)
11C (Carbon)	20.4 min	511	Positron	PET (eg, oncology, metabolism)
13N (Nitrogen)	10.0 min	511	Positron	PET (eg, myocardial perfusion)
15O (Oxygen)	2 min	511	Positron	PET (eg, flow studies, myocardial perfusion)
82Rb (Rubidium)	75 sec	Gamma: 777 β⁺ 511	EC Positron	PET (eg, myocardial perfusion)

*Unless otherwise specified, energies listed for IT and EC decay are for gamma photons. Energies listed for β⁻ decay are maximum β⁻ energies. Energies listed for Positron decay are energies of coincident photons.
IT – Isomeric transition
EC – Electron capture
nwu – not widely used

INDEX

Radiocolloid images, 367
Radioimmunotherapy, 329–331
Radioiodine
    scan, 327–328
    therapy, 197, 326
Radioisotope therapy, 305, 320, 331
Radionuclide lymphoscintigraphy, 438
Radionuclide renography, 392
Radionuclide salivagram, 475, 476
Radionuclide venography, 529–530, 536
Radiotherapy
    intensity-modulated (IMRT), 263
^{82}Rb, 81, 82
Recombinant TSH, 321
Rectal bleeding, 495
Rectilinear scanners, 57
Reflex sympathetic dystrophy, 40. *See also*
        Chronic Regional Pain Syndrome (CRPS 1)
Reflux
    of bile in the stomach, 421
    in infants, 475, 476
    vesicoureteral, 541
Renal artery stenosis, 407–409
Renal cell carcinoma, 53–54
    metastatic, 68
Renal disease, 379
Renal failure
    chronic, 400
    cause, 396
    patients at risk for, 400
    treatment, 396
Renal function
    diminished, 391
    measure of, 399–401
Renal pelves, abnormal amounts of tracer, 43
Renal scarring, 543
Renal stones, 197
Renal transplant, 379, 398
    complications, 381–382
    donor evaluation, 398–399
Retroperitoneum, 295
Revascularization, 113, 126, 130
Rheumatoid arthritis, 337–338
Ribs
    abnormalities, 63
    lesion, 75, 77
    removal of, 53, 54
Rim signs, 417
Rituximab, 330
^{82}Rb rest perfusion, 129

S
Sacral metastasis, 5
Sacral prominence, 5
Sacroiliac joint, 357
Sacroiliitis, 357
Sacrum, 85, 240
Salivary glands, 185, 256, 259
^{153}Sm, 47, 334–335

^{153}Sm-EDTMP
Sarcoidosis, 220, 221, 352–354
Sarcomas, 281
    detection of, 281
    metastatic spread, 281
    neoadjuvant chemotherapy response, 281
    PET, 281
    staging, 281
    Wilms, 305
Satiety, early, 481
Scan results, 113
Scars, severe, 113
Sclerotic lesion, 22
Scores, using global, 113
Seizures
    evaluation of, 455, 550–551
    intractable complex partial, 455
Septic arthritis, 7, 29, 31
Serial scanning, 231
Serotonin, 291
Sestamibi, 202, 203, 204
Sharpey fibers, 83
Shin
    pain, 38
    splint, 83
Shoulder pain, 9
Shunt, right-to-left, 164, 166, 167
Sickle cell disease
    correlative imaging with 67Ga-citrate or
        ^{111}In-WBC scintigraphy, 33
    osteomyelitis, concurrent, 33
^{99m}Tc-MDP
Sigmoid colon, 240, 500
Sigmoidoscopy, 240
SI joints, asymmetric tracer activity in, 28
Simvastatin, 100
Sincalide challenge, 432
Single-photon emission tomography (SPECT), 4,
        27, 43, 64, 88, 90, 93, 94, 103, 124, 205,
        508
    abnormal WBC accumulation, 372
    cardiac, 93
    and planar imaging, 205, 375, 509
    radionuclide brain perfusion, 451
Sinus, mass in piriform, 255
Skeletal scintigraphy
    agents, 20
    biodistribution patterns, 350
    metastatic disease, use in accessing, 13
    in primary malignant bone tumors, 13, 14
    three-phase, 31
Skip lesions, role of skeletal scintigraphy in, 13
^{153}Sm, 335
^{153}Sm-EDTMP, 333
Skull metastasis, 5
Soft tissue
    and bony structure, 64
    changes in, 110
    mass, 13

Your *Case-Based* book includes free bonus access to RadCases online!

RadCases is an extensive online database of key cases for your rounds, rotations and exams.

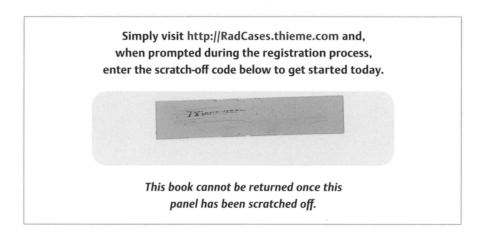

Simply visit http://RadCases.thieme.com and, when prompted during the registration process, enter the scratch-off code below to get started today.

This book cannot be returned once this panel has been scratched off.

Expand on your *Case-Based* book with access to 250 core cases online.

The scratch-off code above provides 12 months of access to an additional 250 nuclear medicine cases via **RadCases.thieme.com**, our searchable online database of must-know cases.

You can also purchase e-subscriptions to key cases in other subspecialties by visiting **RadCases.thieme.com**.

Features of RadCases online include:

- A **user-friendly layout** that is ideal for self-study or quick reference
- Stress-free way to **study and review the most common and most critical cases**
- **Clearly labeled, high-quality radiographs** allow you to absorb key findings at-a-glance
- A **flexible search function** that lets you locate specific cases by age, differential diagnosis, modality, and more
- The ability to **bookmark cases** you want to revisit or **'hide' cases** you've already learned

System requirements for optimal use of RadCases online

	WINDOWS	MAC
Recommended Browser(s) **	Microsoft Internet Explorer 7.0 or later, Firefox 2.x, Firefox 3.x	Firefox 2.x, Firefox 3.x, Safari 3.x, Safari 4.x
	** all browsers should have JavaScript enabled	
Flash Player Plug-in	Flash Player 8 or Higher*	
	* Mac users: ATI Rage 128 GPU does not support full-screen mode with hardware scaling	
Minimum Hardware Configurations	Intel® Pentium® II 450 MHz, AMD Athlon™ 600 MHz or faster processor (or equivalent)	PowerPC® G3 500 MHz or faster processor. Intel Core™ Duo 1.33 GHz or faster processor
	128 MB of RAM	128 MB of RAM
Recommended for optimal usage experience	Monitor resolutions: • Normal (4:3) 1024×768 or Higher • Widescreen (16:9) 1280×720 or Higher • Widescreen (16:10) 1440×900 or Higher. DSL/Cable internet connection at a minimum speed of 384.0 Kbps or faster	